Antithrombotic Therapy

Third Edition

Richard C. Becker, MD

Professor of Medicine
Duke University School of Medicine
Director, Cardiovascular Thrombosis Center
Duke University Medical Center

Dan J. Fintel, MD

Associate Professor of Medicine
Feinberg School of Medicine of Northwestern University
Director of Coronary Care Unit
Northwestern Memorial Hospital

David Green, MD, PhD

Professor of Medicine
Director of Atherosclerosis Program
Feinberg School of Medicine of Northwestern University
Northwestern Memorial Hospital

PROFESSIONAL
COMMUNICATIONS, INC.

Copyright 2004
Richard C. Becker, MD, Dan J. Fintel, MD,
and David Green, MD, PhD

Professional Communications, Inc.

A Medical Publishing Company

Marketing Office:
400 Center Bay Drive
West Islip, NY 11795
(t) 631/661-2852
(f) 631/661-2167

Editorial Office:
PO Box 10
Caddo, OK 74729-0010
(t) 580/367-9838
(f) 580/367-9989

ISBN: 1-884735-91-6

For orders, please call
1-800-337-9838
or visit our website
www.pcibooks.com

DISCLAIMER

The opinions expressed in this publication reflect those of the authors. However, the authors make no warranty regarding the contents of the publication. The protocols described herein are general and may not apply to a specific patient. Any product mentioned in this publication should be taken in accordance with the prescribing information provided by the manufacturer.

This text is printed on recycled paper.

DEDICATION

Dedicated to the investigation and optimal care of patients with atherothrombosis involving the cardiovascular, peripheral vascular, and cerebrovascular systems.

ACKNOWLEDGMENT

We graciously acknowledge the tireless and unconditional dedication of physicians, nurses, and support staff at Northwestern Memorial Hospital and Duke University Medical Center.

TABLE OF CONTENTS

Part 1 *Physiology of Thrombosis*	**Role of Clotting Factors and Fibrinolysis in Thrombus Formation**	1
	Role of the Platelet	2
Part 2 *Antithrombotic Agents*	**Heparins, Selective Factor Xa Inhibitors, Direct Thrombin Inhibitors, and Warfarin**	3
Part 3 *Plasminogen Activators*	**Fibrinolytic Agents**	4
Part 4 *Antiplatelet Agents*	**Aspirin**	5
	Ticlopidine	6
	Clopidogrel	7
	Platelet Glycoprotein IIb/IIIa Receptor Antagonists	8
Part 5 *Monitoring Therapy*	**Monitoring of Anticoagulants**	9
	Monitoring of Platelet Activity	10
Part 6 *Thrombotic Disorders*	**Inherited/Acquired Coagulation and Platelet Disorders (Thrombophilia)**	11
Part 7 *Clinical Syndromes: Arterial and Venous Diseases*	**Acute Coronary Syndromes**	12
	Acute Myocardial Infarction	13
	Noncardiac Arterial Disease: Peripheral Arterial Vascular Disease and Stroke	14
	Native and Prosthetic Valvular Heart Disease	15
	Atrial Fibrillation	16
	Venous Thromboembolic Disease and Pulmonary Embolism	17
Part 8 *Complications*	**Complications of Antithrombotic Therapy**	18
Index		19

TABLES

Table 1.1   Procoagulant and Anticoagulant Factors 16

Table 3.1   Currently Available LMWH Preparations and Synthetic Factor Xa Antagonists for Thromboprophylaxis 39

Table 3.2   Currently Available LMWH Preparations for Treatment of Venous and/or Arterial Thrombotic Disorders 40

Table 3.3   Properties of Heparins, Hirudin, and Bivalirudin 46

Table 3.4   Level-1 Evidence of Drug Interactions With Warfarin 51

Table 4.1   Clinical Features of Established Fibrinolytic Agents 63

Table 4.2   Clinical Features of Newly Developed Fibrinolytic Agents 68

Table 4.3   Contraindications and Cautions for Fibrinolytic Use in STEMI 74

Table 5.1   Recommendations for Aspirin Administration 83

Table 5.2   The Strengths and Weaknesses of Aspirin Therapy 94

Table 6.1   Randomized Clinical Trials of Ticlopidine in Patients With Vascular Disease 102

Table 6.2   Study End Points of Randomized Clinical Trials of Ticlopidine in Patients With Vascular Disease 104

Table 7.1   Clinical Outcomes in CAPRIE (Intention-to-Treat Analysis) 114

Table 8.1   Clinical Trials of Abciximab (ReoPro): Long-Term Follow-Up in the EPIC Study 132

Table 8.2   Clinical Trials of Tirofiban (Aggrastat): The PRISM and PRISM-Plus Studies 140

Table 8.3   Individual Characteristics of the GPIIb/IIIa Receptor Antagonists 145

Table 8.4   Intravenous GPIIb/IIIa Receptor Antagonists: Strategies for Clinical Practice 152

Table 9.1   Intensity of Oral Anticoagulant Therapy in Patients With Prosthetic Heart Valves (ACCP Recommendations) 159

Table 9.2   Regimens Using Unfractionated Heparin
             for the Treatment of Venous
             Thromboembolism 161

Table 9.3   Monitoring Direct Thrombin Inhibitors 163

Table 10.1   Hereditary Platelet Disorders 170

Table 10.2   Causes of Acquired Defects in Platelet
             Function 173

Table 10.3   Clinical Settings in Which Platelet
             Monitoring Might Be Useful 178

Table 11.1   Causes of Thrombophilia 183

Table 11.2   Causes of Hyperhomocysteinemia 186

Table 11.3   Acquired Causes of Antithrombin, Protein C,
             and Protein S Deficiency 190

Table 11.4   Diagnostic Approach to Thrombophilia 193

Table 12.1   Patient Characteristics and Electrocardiographic
             Features Useful in Determining the Probability
             of Myocardial Ischemia 204

Table 12.2   Early Evaluation Steps for Patients With
             Suspected Myocardial Ischemia 205

Table 12.3   High-Risk Features in Patients With
             Unstable Angina 210

Table 12.4   The TIMI Risk Score for UA/NSTEMI 211

Table 12.5   Medical Therapy for Acute Coronary
             Syndromes 213

Table 12.6   Summary of Antithrombotic Therapy
             in Acute Coronary Syndromes 214

Table 12.7   Patient-Specific Heparin-Dosing Nomogram ... 217

Table 12.8   Clinical Experience With LMWH
             Administered for PCI 220

Table 12.9   Enoxaparin Dosing Guidelines and Algorithm
             for NSTE-ACS Patients Undergoing PCI 222

Table 12.10 Revascularization in Acute Coronary
             Syndromes Without ST-Segment Elevation 229

Table 12.11 ACC/AHA Recommendations for Antiplatlet
             Therapy in ACS 230

Table 12.12 ACC/AHA Recommendations for
             Anticoagulant Therapy in ACS 232

Table 13.1   Mortality Outcome in Comparative
Trials of Fibrinolytic Therapy 242

Table 13.2   Diagnostic and Treatment Measures in Patients
With ST Elevation or Bundle Branch Block ... 246

Table 13.3   Factors That Increase the Risk of Systemic
Embolization Following Myocardial
Infarction 253

Table 13.4   Aspirin vs Warfarin Therapy After STEMI 256

Table 14.1   Randomized Trials in Patients With Either
Ischemic Stroke or Transient Ischemic Attacks
Receiving Platelet Antagonist Therapy 270

Table 14.2   The Pathogenesis of Acute Occlusion of
Peripheral Arteries 272

Table 14.3   Clinical Classification of Acute
Limb Ischemia 273

Table 14.4   Clinically Based Antithrombotic Therapy in
Peripheral Vascular Disease 278

Table 14.5   The Role of Specific Antithrombotic Agents in
Peripheral Vascular Disease 280

Table 15.1   Thromboembolic Risk Scale 292

Table 15.2   Hemorrhagic Risk Scale 293

Table 15.3   Antithrombotic Therapy for Patients
With Native Valvular Heart Disease 294

Table 15.4   Antithrombotic Therapy for Patients
With Bioprosthetic Heart Valves or
Valve Repair 296

Table 15.5   Summary of Recommendations for Patients
With Mechanical Heart Valves 297

Table 16.1   Stroke Predictors With Atrial Fibrillation:
Risk-Stratification Scheme 305

Table 16.2   Stroke Predictors With Atrial Fibrillation:
Echocardiographic Findings 306

Table 16.3   Stroke Reduction By Warfarin Therapy 306

Table 16.4   Number of Atrial Fibrillation Patients
Treated With Warfarin to Prevent a Stroke 308

Table 16.5   Risk of Bleeding: Annual Occurrence
of Major Bleeding Events 309

Table 16.6   Recommended Strategy for Managing
Patients With Atrial Fibrillation 312

Table 16.7 CHEST 2001 Summary of Recommendations 312

Table 16.8 Monitoring Anticoagulation Outcomes:
Anticoagulation Clinics vs Usual
Medical Care 317

Table 17.1 Low Molecular Weight Heparins Used for
the Treatment of Thromboembolism 334

Table 17.2 Regimens Approved by the Food and Drug
Administration for the Treatment of
Pulmonary Embolism 342

Table 18.1 Adverse Reactions Associated With
Antithrombotic Agents 350

Table 18.2 Factors Influencing the Risk of
Warfarin-Induced Bleeding 351

Table 18.3 Drug-Warfarin Interactions 353

Table 18.4 Guidelines for the Use of Anesthetics
and Anticoagulants in Patients
Undergoing Surgery 359

Table 18.5 Anticoagulant Therapy in Patients With
Heparin-Induced Thrombocytopenia 361

FIGURES

Figure 1.1 Activation of Blood Coagulation 17

Figure 1.2 Regulation of Thrombin Activity 18

Figure 1.3 Endogenous Fibrinolysis and Release
of D-Dimers 19

Figure 1.4 Components of the Fibrinolytic System 20

Figure 1.5 Hemostatic Effects of Statins 22

Figure 2.1 Chain of Events in Arterial Thrombosis 26

Figure 2.2 A Cell-Based Model of Coagulation 29

Figure 2.3 Multistep Adhesive and Signaling Interactions
of Leukocytes and Platelets With Vascular
Surfaces in Flow 30

Figure 2.4 Platelet-Binding Proteins Important
to Coagulation 32

Figure 3.1 Phase 3 Clinical Trials of Fondaparinux
(Synthetic Pentasaccharide) for Prevention of
Venous Thromboembolism 42

Figure 3.2 Reocclusion Rates in Patients With TIMI
            Grade 3 Flow or TIMI Grades 2 or 3 Flow
            at 90 Minutes 44

Figure 4.1 Pathways of Thrombolysis 60

Figure 4.2 Chemical Structure of Tissue Plasminogen
            Activator 61

Figure 4.3 Mechanism of Action of Tissue Plasminogen
            Activator 62

Figure 4.4 The Streptokinase-Plasminogen Activator
            Complex 64

Figure 4.5 Mechanism of Action of Anistreplase 67

Figure 4.6 Clinical Outcomes in the GUSTO V and
            ASSENT-3 Trials 70

Figure 5.1 Benefits of Aspirin Administration Based
            on Risk for Vascular Events 82

Figure 5.2 Absolute Effects of Antiplatelet Therapy on
            Vascular Events in Five Main High-Risk
            Categories 85

Figure 5.3 Association Between Prior Aspirin Use
            and Clinical Outcomes at 30 Days 86

Figure 5.4 Indirect Comparisons of Proportional
            Effects of Different Antipatelet Regimens
            on Vascular Events in High-Risk Patients
            (Excluding Those With Acute Stroke) 88

Figure 5.5 Mechanisms of Aspirin Resistance 93

Figure 6.1 Reduced Cardiac Events With Antiplatelet
            Therapy vs Anticoagulant Therapy Following
            Coronary Arterial Stenting 106

Figure 7.1 Inhibition of ADP-Mediated Platelet Aggregation
            With Clopidogrel vs Ticlopidine 112

Figure 7.2 Cumulative Risk of Ischemic Stroke,
            Myocardial Infarction, or Vascular Death 116

Figure 7.3 Kaplan-Meier Curves for Clopidogrel vs
            Aspirin 117

Figure 7.4 Kaplan-Meier Cumulative Hazard Rates for
            Primary Outcome of Cardiovascular Death,
            Myocardial Infarction, or Urgent Target-Vessel
            Revascularization at 30 Days After
            Percutaneous Coronary Intervention 119

Figure 7.5   Kaplan-Meier Cumulative Hazard Rates for
             Cardiovascular Death or Myocardial Infarction
             From Randomization to Follow-Up After
             Percutaneous Coronary Intervention 120

Figure 7.6   Cumulative Hazard Rates for the First Primary
             Outcome of Death From Cardiovascular Causes,
             Nonfatal Myocardial Infarction, or Stroke
             During the 12 Months of the CURE Trial 121

Figure 7.7   Rates and Relative Risks of the First Primary
             Outcome of Death From Cardiovascular Causes,
             Nonfatal Myocardial Infarction, or Stroke in
             Various Subgroups With Consistency of
             Benefit With Clopidogrel 122

Figure 7.8   Combined End-Point Results at 28 Days
             for Clopidogrel vs Placebo 125

Figure 7.9   Combined End-Point Results at 1 Year for
             Clopidogrel vs Placebo 126

Figure 8.1   Duration of GPIIb/IIIa Receptor Blockade
             and Inhibition of Platelet Aggregation With
             Abciximab 131

Figure 8.2   Death, Reinfarction, or Urgent Target-Vessel
             Revascularization at 30 Days Using Adjunctive
             Abciximab for Percutaneous Coronary
             Intervention in Acute Myocardial
             Infarction Trials 136

Figure 8.3   Impact of GPIIb/IIIa Receptor Inhibition
             on Fibrinolysis 137

Figure 8.4   Incidence of Death or Nonfatal
             Myocardial Infarction Illustrated
             by Kaplan-Meier Curves 143

Figure 8.5   Restoration of Platelet Aggregability
             Following Cessation of GPIIb/IIIa
             Receptor Antagonists 146

Figure 8.6   In Vitro GPIIb/IIIa Receptor-Directed
             Platelet Inhibition and Its Reversibility
             With Fibrinogen Supplementation 147

Figure 8.7   Major Clinical Outcomes in
             the TARGET Trial 148

Figure 8.8   Major Outcomes in Trials of Oral GPIIb/IIIa
             Receptor Antagonists 150

Figure 10.1 Pharmacologic Control of Thrombus
Formation 172

Figure 10.2 Correlation of Absolute Rate of Platelet
Aggregation With Percent Aggregation at
Various Time Points Following Start
of Abciximab Therapy 175

Figure 10.3 Association Between Early GPIIb/IIIa
Antagonist-Mediated Platelet Inhibition and
Clinical Events Following Percutaneous
Coronary Intervention 176

Figure 10.4 The Threshold Level of Platelet Inhibition
Required to Achieve Optimal Outcome With
GPIIb/IIIa Receptor Antagonists in
Percutaneous Coronary Intervention 177

Figure 10.5 Individual Variability in Platelet
Procoagulant Function 179

Figure 11.1 Prevalence of Thrombophilia 184

Figure 12.1 Distinct Pathobiologic Features of Stable
Angina and Acute Coronary Syndromes 202

Figure 12.2 ST/T-Wave Changes in Patient With
Myocardial Ischemia 206

Figure 12.3 Deep Symmetric T-Wave Inversions in
Patient With Myocardial Ischemia 207

Figure 12.4 12-Lead Electrocardiogram Used as a
Diagnostic and Management Tool 208

Figure 12.5 Rates of All-Cause Mortality, Myocardial
Infarction, and Severe Recurrent Ischemia
Leading to Urgent Revascularization 212

Figure 12.6 Narrow Therapeutic Index With
Unfractionated Heparin in Percutaneous
Coronary Intervention 218

Figure 12.7 Risk for Hemorrhage With Unfractionated
Heparin During Percutaneous
Coronary Intervention 219

Figure 12.8 Strategies for Mechanical and Pharmacologic
Intervention in Acute Coronary Syndrome
Patients 226

Figure 13.1 Mortality Outcomes From ISIS-2 238

Figure 13.2 30-Day and 1-Year Mortality Rates in
GUSTO I Trial 244

Figure 13.3 Thrombolytic Resistance Due to Activation
            of Thrombin and Platelets 249

Figure 13.4 Results From TIMI-14: Infarct Artery
            Patency Following Abciximab and Reduced-
            Dose tPA 250

Figure 13.5 30-Day Mortality in the GUSTO V and
            ASSENT-3 Trials 252

Figure 14.1 Thrombotic Processes Associated With
            Atherosclerosis Progression 268

Figure 14.2 Clinician's Approach to Antiplatelet
            Therapy in Patients With
            Atherosclerotic Vascular Disease 276

Figure 15.1 Characteristics of Blood Flow Across
            the Aortic Valve 288

Figure 15.2 Characteristics of Blood Flow Across
            the Mitral Valve 289

Figure 16.1 Stroke: Emboli of Cardiac Origin 303

Figure 16.2 Stroke Predictors With Atrial Fibrillation 304

Figure 16.3 Risks vs Benefits of Anticoagulation
            Therapy 310

Figure 16.4 Age-Related Effective Daily Warfarin Dose ... 313

Figure 16.5 Lowest Effective Intensity for Warfarin
            Therapy 314

Figure 16.6 Risk of Intracranial Hemorrhage
            (Outpatients) 315

Figure 16.7 Therapeutic Window 316

Figure 16.8 Warfarin Utilization 317

Figure 17.1 Gross Anatomy of the Systemic Venous
            System 322

Figure 17.2 Diagnostic Algorithm for Suspected
            Deep Vein Thrombosis 327

Figure 17.3 Diagnostic Algorithm for Suspected
            Nonmassive Pulmonary Embolism 330

1

Role of Clotting Factors and Fibrinolysis in Thrombus Formation

Introduction

The fluidity of the blood is maintained by a balance of procoagulants and anticoagulants. Activation of coagulation initially tips the balance in favor of the procoagulants, but as these proteins become activated they not only increase the clotting ability of the blood but also participate in the activation of the anticoagulant proteins, serving to restore the hemostatic balance. Thus coagulation is a dynamic process, with thrombin generation and inhibition, and fibrin formation and fibrin lysis, all occurring in varying degrees at any given moment.

Procoagulant and anticoagulant factors, their plasma concentrations, and half-lives are listed in **Table 1.1**.[1]

Initiation of Thrombosis

The initiating event in blood coagulation is injury to the vessel wall. Monocytes, neutrophils, and macrophages are attracted to the site of injury and elaborate tissue factor, an integral membrane glycolipoprotein of 50 kd.[2] To express its procoagulant activity, tissue factor must be anchored to a phospholipid membrane; it then forms a complex with factor VII and activated factor VII (VIIa), which constitutes about 1% of the circulating factor VII[3] (**Figure 1.1**). The binding of tissue factor to VIIa produces a powerful procoagulant complex, which cleaves its substrates, factor IX and factor X. With the cleavage of factor X to its active form, factor Xa, anticoagulant mechanisms are set into motion. Tissue factor pathway inhibitor (TFPI) is a 32-kd protein that is a potent protease inhibitor that binds to and inactivates Xa. Furthermore, the TFPI-Xa complex inhibits the tissue factor–VIIa complex.

TABLE 1.1 — PROCOAGULANT AND ANTICOAGULANT FACTORS

Protein	Concentration (nM)	$t^{\frac{1}{2}}$ (days)
Fibrinogen	7000	3 to 5
Prothrombin	1400	2.5
Factor V	20	0.5
Factor VII	10	0.25
Factor VIII	0.7	0.5
Factor IX	90	1
Factor X	170	1.25
Factor XI	30	3
Factor XIII	30	9
TFPI	2.5	*
Protein C	60	0.25
Protein S	300	1.75
Antithrombin	2400	3

Abbreviations: $t^{\frac{1}{2}}$, half-life; TFPI, tissue factor pathway inhibitor.

* 80 minutes in animals.

Mann KG, et al. In: *Hematology.* 5th ed. New York, NY: McGraw-Hill Inc; 1995:1206.

Factor IXa may be formed from factor IX by the contact activation system, which consists of factor XII, high molecular weight kininogen (HMWK), prekallikrein (PK), and factor XI.[4-6] Factor XI binds to activated platelets, where it is activated by thrombin to factor XIa and subsequently activates factor IX. Activated factor XI that escapes from the platelet surface is inactivated by protease nexin 2.

Thrombin is formed in trace amounts by the action of Xa on prothrombin (right half of **Figure 1.1**). Thrombin also activates factors V (Va) and VIII (VIIIa), which serve as cofactors for Xa and IXa, respectively. A complex forming on the surface of activated platelets consisting of IXa, VIIIa, and calcium ions activates factor X (Xa); it is termed the tenase complex. The Xa generated that escapes TFPI forms a complex on the platelet membrane with Va and calcium

FIGURE 1.1 — ACTIVATION OF BLOOD COAGULATION

Tissue factor (TF), presented by fibroblasts or monocytes, binds factor VIIa. While most of the TF-VIIa complex is inactivated by factor Xa-tissue factor pathway inhibitor (TFPI), TF-VIIa escaping inactivation converts factor X to factor Xa. Factor Xa along with factor Va activates prothrombin (II) to thrombin (IIa), which in turn activates platelets, converts factor V to Va, factor XI to XIa, and factor VIII to VIIIa after factor VIII dissociates from von Willebrand's factor (vWF). The TF-VIIa complex also activates factor IX to IXa, which, along with VIIIa on the activated platelet surface, converts X to Xa. Factor Xa with Va activates II to thrombin (IIa). XIa on the activated platelet surface also activates IX to IXa.

Roberts HR, et al. *Haemophilia.* 1998;4:331-334.

and cleaves prothrombin to thrombin; this complex is termed the prothrombinase complex.

As is apparent from the above description, platelets play a critical role in thrombus formation (see Chapter 2, *Role of the Platelet*). Platelets become adherent to collagen exposed at the site of injury and platelets are also trapped in the developing thrombus. Platelets in both of these locations become activated and release membrane vesicles known as microparticles, which are highly thrombogenic.[7]

Platelet glycoprotein Ib is the receptor for factor XI, and platelet glycoprotein IIb/IIIa is the receptor for prothrombin.[8] The soluble thrombin generated by platelets is a major contributor to clot formation and propagation.

Regulation of Thrombin Generation

Thrombin generation is limited by thrombomodulin (TM) (**Figure 1.2**).[9] TM binds thrombin, inhibiting its protease activity. The TM-thrombin complex then activates protein C (APC). APC inactivates VIIIa, and along with factor V and free protein S, inactivates Va. Protein S, a 64-kd glycoprotein, is present in free (40%) and bound (60%) forms; the binding protein (BP) of protein S is the fourth component of complement (C4B)-BP. It has recently been suggested that β_2-glycoprotein-1, a phospholipid-binding protein, functions to inhibit binding of protein S by C4B-BP.[10]

FIGURE 1.2 — REGULATION OF THROMBIN ACTIVITY

To the left is heparan sulfate proteoglycan, to which antithrombin and thrombin bind. In the center, thrombomodulin (TM) binds thrombin, and the complex activates protein C, bound to its receptor (EPCR). Activated protein C (APC), with its cofactor, protein S, inactivates factors Va and VIIIa, limiting thrombin generation.

Simmonds RE, et al. In: *Thrombosis and Hemorrhage*. 3rd ed. Philadelphia, Pa: Lippincott Williams and Wilkins; 2003:36.

This would enhance the anticoagulant effect of protein S. Free protein S inhibits the tenase and prothrombinase complex by covering phospholipids on the cell membrane. In addition, the inactivation of VIIIa and Va by APC helps to limit thrombin generation.[11-13]

Fibrin Generation

Thrombin converts fibrinogen to fibrin and activates factor XIII (XIIIa) (**Figure 1.3**).[14] Fibrinogen is a 340-kd glycoprotein composed of a dimer of three polypeptide chains. Thrombin cleaves the amino-termini of the α- and β-chains, releasing fibrinopeptides A and B, converting fibrinogen to fibrin monomer. The monomers spontaneously aggregate, forming protofibrils. XIIIa cross-links the fibrils to solidify the clot.

Fibrinolysis

Circulating plasminogen binds to the fibrin clot and is converted to plasmin by tissue plasminogen activator (tPA) (**Figure 1.4**),[15] which is released from the endothelium and binds to fibrin. Fibrinolysis is also activated by the contact

FIGURE 1.3 — ENDOGENOUS FIBRINOLYSIS AND RELEASE OF D-DIMERS

Goldhaber SZ. *N Engl J Med.* 1998;339:93-104.

FIGURE 1.4 — COMPONENTS OF THE FIBRINOLYTIC SYSTEM

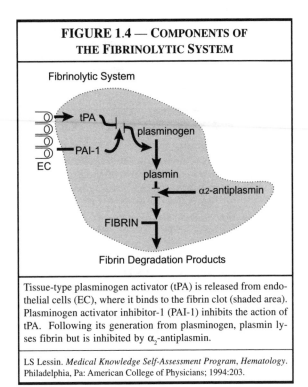

Tissue-type plasminogen activator (tPA) is released from endothelial cells (EC), where it binds to the fibrin clot (shaded area). Plasminogen activator inhibitor-1 (PAI-1) inhibits the action of tPA. Following its generation from plasminogen, plasmin lyses fibrin but is inhibited by α_2-antiplasmin.

LS Lessin. *Medical Knowledge Self-Assessment Program, Hematology.* Philadelphia, Pa: American College of Physicians; 1994:203.

activation system.[16] As noted previously, PK converts prourokinase to urokinase, which in turn activates plasminogen to plasmin. Plasmin dissolves fibrin, resulting in clot lysis. Activated platelets and endothelial cells release plasminogen activator inhibitor-1, and XIIIa cross-links α_2-antiplasmin to the fibrin clot. These two inhibitors act to control fibrinolysis. In addition, thrombin in the presence of TM activates a potent inhibitor of fibrinolysis, designated thrombin activatable fibrinolysis inhibitor (TAFI).[17,18]

Vascular Factors in Thrombus Formation

The hemostatic reactions described above occur in the setting of pulsatile blood flow, a vascular system lined by endothelium, and a milieu consisting of a variety of cells, cell fragments, and proteins.[19] Blood flow produces different shear stresses within the vasculature; on the arterial side of the circulation, platelets are driven against the vessel wall and are the principal component of thrombi (white thrombus), whereas on the venous side, thrombi consist mainly of fibrin and red cells, with platelets passively deposited. Under high shear stresses, adherence of platelets to the subendothelium is dependent on the binding of von Willebrand's factor (vWf) to platelet receptors. vWf is also critical for platelet aggregation. Another role of vWf is as a carrier protein for factor VIII. Factor VIII is resistant to inactivation by APC while it remains associated with the vWf.

The endothelium plays multiple roles in hemostasis, contributing factors that inhibit platelet aggregation, inactivate thrombin, and mediate clot lysis.[20] For example, endothelial cells are a rich source of prostacyclin and nitric oxide, which inhibit platelet aggregation and are potent vasodilators. Dermatan sulfate, a vessel-wall proteoglycan, binds heparin cofactor II, and the complex inactivates clotbound thrombin. The endothelium also releases tPA.[21]

Statins

"Statins" (3-hydroxy-3-methylglutaryl coenzyme A reductase inhibitors) not only decrease cholesterol, but also have important effects on hemostasis. Statins:

- Alter platelet aggregation, possibly by decreasing thromboxane A_2 synthesis and the cholesterol content of platelet membranes[22]
- Decrease tissue factor expression by monocytes, macrophages, and atheromatous plaques[23]
- Reduce factor VII activity
- Inhibit the activation of factor V and factor XIII (**Figure 1.5**).[24]

These anti-inflammatory and antithrombotic effects of statins enhance their salutary effects on atherosclerosis.

Summary

All coagulation reactions take place on a negatively charged surface; ie, the membrane of activated platelets. Thus platelets play a critical role in thrombin generation (see

21

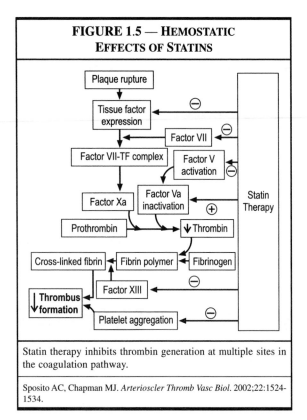

FIGURE 1.5 — HEMOSTATIC EFFECTS OF STATINS

Statin therapy inhibits thrombin generation at multiple sites in the coagulation pathway.

Sposito AC, Chapman MJ. *Arterioscler Thromb Vasc Biol.* 2002;22:1524-1534.

Chapter 2, *Role of the Platelet*).[25] Procoagulant complexes bind to specific platelet phospholipids, vWf adheres to membrane glycoproteins (GP) Ib and IIb/IIIa, and these glycoproteins are receptors for factor XI and prothrombin, respectively. Leukocytes adhere to activated platelets and secrete cytokines and expose tissue factor, which further amplifies hemostasis. Under pathologic conditions, the shedding of negatively charged membrane microparticles from erythrocytes and macrophages also enhances coagulation reactions. Modulating these processes are a vast number of physiologic antithrombotic mechanisms, which include circulating anticoagulants, such as proteins C and S, antithrombin, β_2-glycoprotein-1 and annexins; endothelium-derived factors, such as TFPI, TM, prostacyclin, and nitric oxide;

and fibrinolytic agents, including tPA, urokinase, and plasminogen. As Virchow noted more than 100 years ago, the vessel wall, the character of blood flow, and the composition of the blood all play a role in thrombus formation.[26]

REFERENCES

1. Mann KG, Gaffney D, Bovill EG. Molecular biology, biochemistry, and lifespan of plasma coagulation factors. In: Beutler E, Lichtmen MA, Coller VS, eds. *Williams Hematology.* 5th ed. New York, NY: McGraw-Hill, Inc; 1994:1206.

2. Broze GJ Jr. The tissue factor pathway of coagulation. In: Loscalzo J, Schafer AI, eds. *Thrombosis and Hemorrhage.* 2nd ed. Baltimore, Md: Williams and Wilkins; 1998:77-104.

3. Roberts HR, Monroe DM, Oliver JA, Chang JY, Hoffman M. Newer concepts of blood coagulation. *Haemophilia.* 1998;4:331-334.

4. Colman RW. Biologic activities of the contact factors in vivo. *Thromb Haemost.* 1999;82:1568-1577.

5. Walsh PN. Platelets and factor XI bypass the contact system of blood coagulation. *Thromb Haemost.* 1999;82:234-242.

6. Martincic D, Kravtsov V, Gailani D. Factor XI messenger RNA in human platelets. *Blood.* 1999;94:3397-3404.

7. Ilveskero S, Siljander P, Lassila R. Procoagulant activity on platelets adhered to collagen or plasma clot. *Arterioscler Thromb Vasc Biol.* 2001;21:628-635.

8. Heemskerk JW, Bevers EM, Lindhout T. Platelet activation and blood coagulation. *Thromb Haemost.* 2002;88:186-193.

9. Simmonds RE, Lane DA. Regulation of coagulation. In: Loscalzo J, Schafer AI, eds. *Thrombosis and Hemorrhage.* 2nd ed. Baltimore, Md: Williams and Wilkins; 1998:46.

10. Merrill JT, Zhang HW, Shen C, et al. Enhancement of protein S anticoagulant function by β_2-glycoprotein 1, a major target antigen of antiphospholipid antibodies. *Thromb Haemost.* 1999;81:748-757.

11. Smirnov MD, Safa O, Esmon NL, Esmon CT. Inhibition of activated protein C anticoagulant activity by prothrombin. *Blood.* 1999; 94:3839-3846.

12. Han X, Fiehler R, Broze GJ. Characterization of protein Z–dependent protease inhibitor. *Blood.* 2000;96:3049-3055.

13. Rezaie AR. Prothrombin protects factor Xa in the prothrombinase complex from inhibition by the heparin-antithrombin complex. *Blood.* 2001;97:2308-2313.

14. Goldhaber SZ. Pulmonary embolism. *N Engl J Med.* 1998;339:93-104.

15. Hemostasis and thrombosis. In: Lessin LS, ed. *Medical Knowledge Self-Assessment Program, Hematology.* Philadelphia, Pa: American College of Physicians; 1994:203.

16. Gaffney PJ, Edgell TA, Whitton CM. The haemostatic balance—Astrup revisited. *Haemostasis.* 1999;29:58-71.

17. Bajzar L, Manuel R, Nesheim ME. Purification and characterization of TAFI, a thrombin-activable fibrinolysis inhibitor. *J Biol Chem.* 1995;270:14477-14484.

18. Bouma BN, Meijers JCM. Fibrinolysis and the contact system: a role for factor XI in the down-regulation of fibrinolysis. *Thromb Haemost.* 1999;82:243-250.

19. Fuster V, Fayad ZA, Badimon JJ. Acute coronary syndromes: biology. *Lancet.* 1999;353(suppl 2):S5-S9.

20. Bombeli T, Mueller M, Haeberli A. Anticoagulant properties of the vascular endothelium. *Thromb Haemost.* 1997;77:408-423.

21. Rosenberg RD, Aird WC. Vascular-bed—specific hemostasis and hypercoagulable states. *N Engl J Med.* 1999;340:1555-1564.

22. Notarbartolo A, Davi G, Averna M, et al. Inhibition of thromboxane biosynthesis and platelet function by simvastatin in type IIa hypercholesterolemia. *Arterioscler Thromb Vasc Biol.* 1995;15:247-251.

23. Cortellaro M, Cofrancesco E, Arbustini E, et al. Atorvastatin and thrombogenicity of the carotid atherosclerotic plaque: the ATROCAP study. *Thromb Haemost.* 2002;88:41-47.

24. Sposito AC, Chapman MJ. Statin therapy in acute coronary syndromes: mechanistic insight into clinical benefit. *Arterioscler Thromb Vasc Biol.* 2002;22:1524-1534.

25. Beguin S, Keularts I. On the coagulation of platelet-rich plasma. *Haemostasis.* 1999;29:50-57.

26. Virchow RLK. *Thrombosis and Emboli* (1846-1856). Matzdorff AC, Bell WR, trans. Canton, Mass: Science History Publications; 1998:234.

2   Role of the Platelet

Platelets are recognized for their essential role in vascular hemostasis, but in addition they contribute directly to pathologic thrombosis, particularly events occurring within the arterial circulatory system in regions of high shear stress and at sites of either endothelial cell injury or atheromatous plaque disruption.

Platelet Physiology

Under normal physiologic conditions, platelets circulate freely within the cardiovascular system, avoiding meaningful interactions with other cells and the vessel wall. The circumstances are distinctly different following vascular injury, which elicits a rapid change in platelet behavior that can be either lifesaving or life-threatening, depending on the site of involvement, degree of response, and the functional capability of regulatory pathways.

The traditionally held view of platelets in arterial thrombosis is best appreciated in the context of five important physiologic steps (**Figure 2**.1):

- Platelet adhesion
- Platelet activation
- Platelet secretion
- Platelet aggregation
- Platelet support of coagulation.

■ Platelet Adhesion

For platelets to contribute meaningfully to the thrombotic process, they must first "stick" or adhere to sites of vessel-wall damage. This important initiating step is mediated by specific surface receptors that are recognized by adhesive proteins (ligands) residing on or near the vascular endothelial surface.[1] In the case of platelet adhesion, the critical components are:

- von Willebrand's factor (vWf)
- Glycoprotein (GP) Ib-IX-V complex.

FIGURE 2.1 — CHAIN OF EVENTS IN ARTERIAL THROMBOSIS

Abbreviations: Ca^{++}, calcium; Pl, phospholipid.

Chain of events in arterial thrombosis: 1) platelets *adhere* to sites of vessel-wall injury (via von Willebrand's factor bound to the GPIb/IX/V receptor complex); 2) *activation* elicits a conformational change that stimulates intracellular events and provokes microparticle release; 3) *secretion* of intracellular contents from α-granules, dense bodies, and lysosomes prepares the platelet for cellular events to follow; 4) *aggregation* is achieved through the fibrinogen-mediated binding of adjacent platelets via GPIIb/IIIa receptors; and; 5) the platelet aggregates provide a surface for *coagulation protease assembly*, thrombin generation, and fibrin formation.

Under high shear stress conditions, vWf can also bind the platelet GPIIb/IIIa receptors and participate in aggregation.

■ Platelet Activation

Following adhesion, platelets become *activated* in response to a wide variety of biochemical and mechanical stimuli.[2] Of physiologic relevance, many of the agonists are themselves a product of platelets that are released, initiating several strong and repetitive "positive-feedback" or "bioamplification" reactions.

Platelet agonists bind surface GPs and stimulate signal transduction across the membrane via specific messenger proteins that, in turn, trigger either one or two intracellular pathways—the phosphoinositide pathway (leading to calcium mobilization and surface expression of GPIIb/IIIa receptors) or the phospholipase A_2–arachidonate pathway (stimulating the production of thromboxane A_2 generation).

Platelet activation, in addition to its biochemical effects, results in physical changes that facilitate platelet–vessel-wall binding, platelet aggregation, and platelet-leukocyte interactions. The formation of microparticles expands the prothrombotic surface area substantially.

■ Platelet Secretion

Platelet activation stimulates intracellular calcium mobilization, surface receptor expression (ligand-receptive conformational change), and the secretion of contents from three distinct storage granules—lysosomes, α-granules, and dense bodies.[3]

Lysosomes contain a variety of acid hydrolases that digest endocytotic materials but do not play a pivotal role in arterial thrombosis. In contrast, dense bodies house adenosine diphosphate, serotonin, and calcium, each an important component of the thrombotic process. Similarly, platelet α-granules are an important storage site for platelet-specific proteins (platelet-derived growth factors), coagulation factors (factor V, fibrinogen), and GPs (thrombospondin, GPIIb/IIIa).

■ Platelet Aggregation

The adhered and activated platelets in essence are primed for aggregation and, in so being, provide a "plug" for localized vascular injury and a template for further thrombus growth. Platelet aggregation is mediated predominantly by fibrinogen (a dimeric GP found in abundance within plasma and α-granules) that binds surface GPIIb/IIIa receptors with high affinity (>40,000 molecules per cell), bridging adjacent platelets.

Sequences of the fibrinogen molecule that bind the platelet GPIIb/IIIa receptor have been identified on its Aα (RGDF) and δ (RGDS) chains. Other proteins that contribute to platelet aggregation, particularly under high shear stress conditions, include vWf, fibronectin, and vitronectin.

Because platelet aggregation is regulated by the GPIIb/IIIa receptor, it has been considered a favored target for pharmacologic therapies used in the management of acute coronary syndromes.[4-6] The importance of other targets are increasingly being recognized.

■ Platelet Support of Coagulation

A revised "cell-based" model of coagulation[7] proposes that blood clotting occurs not as a cascade, but in three overlapping stages:

- *Initiation*, which occurs on tissue factor–bearing cells
- *Amplification* or *priming*, in which platelets and co-factors are activated in preparation for large-scale thrombin generation
- *Propagation*, during which there is a "burst" of thrombin generation (**Figure 2.2**).

A cell-based model of coagulation provides a basis for other important cellular interactions occurring among platelets, leukocytes, and activated endothelial cells in the processes that underlie atherothrombosis (**Figure 2.3**).[8] In addition, it provides an explanation for differing thrombotic potential between individuals through the identification of coagulation protein binding sites on the surface of activated platelets (**Figure 2.4**).[9] Conceptually, the localization of coagulation to several cellular surfaces not only establishes an important mechanism for regulation but also expands the number of targets for therapeutic attenuation substantially.

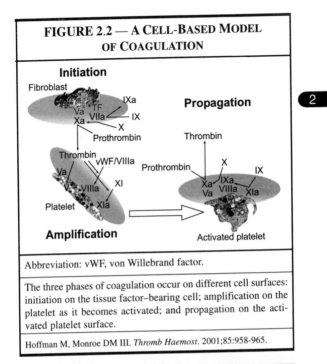

FIGURE 2.2 — A CELL-BASED MODEL OF COAGULATION

Abbreviation: vWF, von Willebrand factor.

The three phases of coagulation occur on different cell surfaces: initiation on the tissue factor–bearing cell; amplification on the platelet as it becomes activated; and propagation on the activated platelet surface.

Hoffman M, Monroe DM III. *Thromb Haemost*. 2001;85:958-965.

Summary

The platelet is a structurally and functionally complex component of both protective hemostasis and vascular thrombosis occurring at localized sites of injury. Platelet adherence, activation, secretion, and aggregation collectively define the primary phase of thrombosis, while assembly and initiation of the coagulation cascade and, ultimately, fibrin formation represent the second or growth phase. The defining steps for thrombosis are governed by several cell lines, including leukocytes, platelets, and activated endothelial cells. Specific surface receptors, coagulation protease binding sites, and adhesive proteins define individual thrombotic potential and provide potential targets for pharmacologic intervention designed to either prevent or, at the very least, attenuate the thrombotic response to vessel-wall injury.

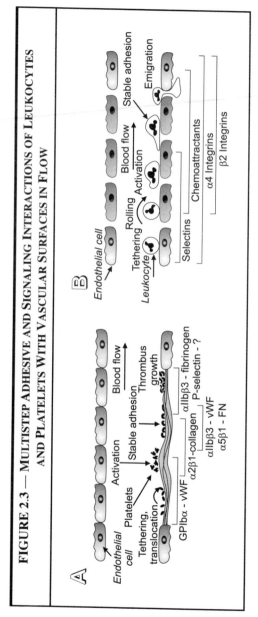

FIGURE 2.3 — MULTISTEP ADHESIVE AND SIGNALING INTERACTIONS OF LEUKOCYTES AND PLATELETS WITH VASCULAR SURFACES IN FLOW

Abbreviations: FN, fibronectin; GP, glycoprotein; vWF, von Willebrand factor.

(A) Adhesion of platelets to subendothelial surfaces. (B) Adhesion of leukocytes to activated endothelial cells. (C) Adhesion of platelets to activated platelets. (D) Adhesion of leukocytes to activated endothelial cells.

McEver RP. *Thromb Haemost.* 2001;86:746-756.

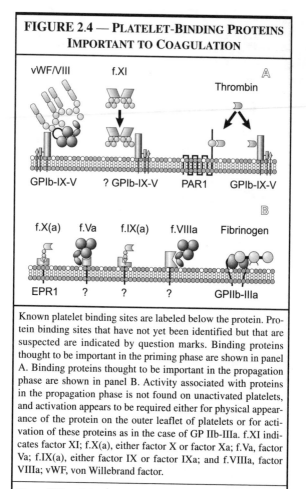

FIGURE 2.4 — PLATELET-BINDING PROTEINS IMPORTANT TO COAGULATION

Known platelet binding sites are labeled below the protein. Protein binding sites that have not yet been identified but that are suspected are indicated by question marks. Binding proteins thought to be important in the priming phase are shown in panel A. Binding proteins thought to be important in the propagation phase are shown in panel B. Activity associated with proteins in the propagation phase is not found on unactivated platelets, and activation appears to be required either for physical appearance of the protein on the outer leaflet of platelets or for activation of these proteins as in the case of GP IIb-IIIa. f.XI indicates factor XI; f.X(a), either factor X or factor Xa; f.Va, factor Va; f.IX(a), either factor IX or factor IXa; and f.VIIIa, factor VIIIa; vWF, von Willebrand factor.

Monroe DM, et al. *Arterioscler Thromb Vasc Biol.* 2002;22:1381-1389.

REFERENCES

1. Phillips DR, Agin PP. Platelet plasma membrane glycoproteins. Evidence for the presence of nonequivalent disulfide bonds using nonreduced-reduced two-dimensional gel electrophoresis. *J Biol Chem.* 1977;252:2121-2126.

2. Berridge MJ. Inositol triphosphate and diacylglycerol: two interacting second messengers. *Annu Rev Biochem.* 1987;56:159-193.

3. Stenberg PE, Shuman MA, Levine SP, Bainton DF. Redistribution of alpha-granules and their contents in thrombin-stimulated platelets. *J Cell Biol.* 1984;98:748-760.

4. Farrell DH, Thiagarajan P, Chung DW, Davie EW. Role of fibrinogen alpha and gamma chain sites in platelet aggregation. *Proc Natl Acad Sci USA.* 1992;89:10729-10732.

5. Byzova TV, Plow EF. Networking in the hemostatic system. *J Biol Chem.* 1997;272:27183-27188.

6. Lefkovits J, Plow EF, Topol EJ. Platelet glycoprotein IIb/IIIa receptors in cardiovascular medicine. *N Engl J Med.* 1995;332:1553-1559.

7. Hoffman M, Monroe DM 3rd. A cell-based model of hemostasis. *Thromb Haemost.* 2001;85:958-965.

8. McEver RP. Adhesive interactions of leukocytes, platelets, and the vessel wall during hemostasis and inflammation. *Thromb Haemost.* 2001;86:746-756.

9. Monroe DM, Hoffman M, Roberts HR. Platelets and thrombin generation. *Arterioscler Thromb Vasc Biol.* 2002;22:1381-1389.

2

3

Heparins, Selective Factor Xa Inhibitors, Direct Thrombin Inhibitors, and Warfarin

Heparin

Heparin is a highly charged polyanion consisting of chains of 18 to 50 saccharide units.[1] Since each saccharide has a molecular weight of about 300 d, the overall molecular weight of the compound ranges from 5000 to 30,000 d, with a mean of 15,000 d. About one third of the chains have a specific pentasaccharide sequence that binds antithrombin; the larger chains also bind thrombin, dramatically enhancing the ability of antithrombin to inactivate thrombin.

Heparin also binds to a variety of cells and plasma proteins. The former include macrophages and platelets, and the latter are fibrinogen, vitronectin, fibronectin, and von Willebrand's factor, among others. Heparin also has a strong affinity for platelet factor 4 exposed on the surface of activated platelets. As a consequence of these various interactions, there is dose-dependent absorption from subcutaneous injection sites and highly variable plasma levels, depending on the concentration of heparin-binding proteins. Furthermore, there is a dose-dependent half-life; as little as 56 minutes after a dose of 100 U/kg and as long as 156 minutes after 400 U/kg. Because of these pharmacologic characteristics, it is difficult to predict the dose of heparin that may be safe and effective in a given patient. Therefore, the dose must be titrated by trial and error, using the activated partial thromboplastin time (aPTT) as a guide (see Chapter 9, *Monitoring of Anticoagulants*).

By virtue of its ability to potentiate the anticoagulant effects of antithrombin, heparin promotes the inactivation of thrombin and activated clotting factors XI, X, IX, and the tissue factor–factor VIIa complex. This results in prolongation of the aPTT, prothrombin time (PT), and thrombin time. The most sensitive to the effects of heparin are the thrombin time and aPTT; the PT is affected by heparin concentrations >0.5 U/mL. Although heparin has a strong inhibitory effect on thrombin in plasma, the heparin-antithrombin complex is unable to inhibit thrombin bound to fibrin. This becomes important when lytic treatment is given; as thrombi lyse, fibrin-bound thrombin is able to continue converting fibrinogen to fibrin despite the presence of heparin, leading to rethrombosis.

Heparin has a number of other effects in addition to its binding of antithrombin. It impairs bone formation and enhances bone resorption; in susceptible persons, prolonged administration of the drug may lead to osteoporosis and fractures. Its binding to platelet factor 4 may stimulate antibody formation, resulting in heparin-induced thrombocytopenia (HIT). In concentrations >0.5 U/mL, it alters platelet function and increases vascular permeability. Heparin also has inhibitory activity toward aldosterone, manifest by a mildly increased serum potassium.

Low Molecular Weight Heparin

Low molecular weight heparin (LMWH) is prepared by the depolymerization of porcine heparin. A variety of proprietary processes are used, giving distinctive products whose molecular weights range from 4000 to 6500 d, and number of saccharide units, from 13 to 22.[2] As with unfractionated heparin (UFH), about one third of the LMWH chains have the pentasaccharide binding site for antithrombin, but unlike heparin, only chains having 18 or more saccharide units bind thrombin. Thus the LMWH-antithrombin complex has weak antithrombin activity but retains the ability to inactivate factor Xa. The ratio of anti-Xa activity to anti-IIa (antithrombin) activity varies from 2:1 to 4:1. Because of its weak effect on thrombin, LMWH only prolongs the aPTT when present in very high plasma concentrations. This raises the question of why LMWH is an effective anticoagulant. LMWH releases tissue factor pathway inhibitor (TFPI) from endothelium; TFPI binds factor Xa and inhibits the tissue factor–factor VIIa complex. In addition, complexes of LMWH and antithrombin are able to inactivate factor Xa bound to platelets. However, similar to heparin, LMWH is not able to inhibit thrombin bound to fibrin.[3]

When LMWH is given in either fixed or weight-adjusted doses by the subcutaneous route, >90% of the dose is absorbed. In contrast to heparin, LMWH has minimal binding to cells or plasma proteins, resulting in persistence of free drug in the circulation and a longer half-life of activity. While the half-life of UFH averages about 90 minutes, the half-lives of three LMWHs range from 108 to 252 minutes. Studies have also demonstrated that the effect of LMWH on factor Xa activity is linearly related to the dose administered. These pharmacologic characteristics mean that plasma levels are predictable and monitoring is unnecessary in most patients.[4] Anti-Xa activity can be detected in the plasma of most patients receiving LMWH, but the levels may not predict clinical efficacy. On the other hand, plasma anti-Xa concentrations >1.0 U/mL may be associated with bleeding. Therefore, it is prudent to monitor anti-Xa levels in patients in whom levels of drug may be less predictable. These include pregnant women and patients with renal failure; the former because their plasma volume of distribution changes as the pregnancy progresses, and the latter because LMWH is mainly excreted by the kidneys. One may also wish to measure anti-Xa levels in those weighing <50 kg or >120 kg receiving weight-adjusted doses, although a recent study of tinzaparin showed that anti-Xa levels were within the expected range in obese patients receiving weight-adjusted prophylactic or treatment doses.[5] Samples are usually obtained 4 to 6 hours after a dose (at peak plasma concentration).

Thrombocytopenia is infrequently associated with LMWH, but antibodies directed against complexes of LMWH and platelet factor 4 can be detected in some patients. On rare occasion, the full-blown syndrome of HIT occurs. Equally rare is necrosis at the site of skin injections with LMWH, which may be a form of local HIT. LMWH inhibits bone formation but does not enhance bone resorption in laboratory studies. Clinically, osteoporosis appears to be less frequent with LMWH than with UFH, based on investigation of bone density in pregnant women receiving these anticoagulants.

Bleeding is the major adverse effect of heparin and LMWH. It most commonly appears at the sites of trauma; for example, the inguinal area in patients having femoral vessel catheterization. The most feared complication is epidural bleeding and spinal hematoma following insertion or removal of an epidural catheter inserted to provide perioperative anesthesia.[6] The frequency of bleeding appears to be less with LMWH than with UFH, based on a meta-analysis of 13 studies comparing the two in the treatment of deep vein thrombosis (DVT).[7] The following factors increase the risk of bleeding:

- Low body weight
- Age >70 years
- Recent surgery or trauma
- Concomitant use of drugs that affect hemostasis, such as fibrinolytic agents or inhibitors of platelet function.

The latter include not only aspirin but also nonsteroidal anti-inflammatory agents. The antidote for bleeding due to UFH is protamine; this agent may also be used for bleeding associated with LMWH, but it is less effective.

A number of LMWHs are currently available or under development. The manufacturing process for each drug differs from that for the others, and each has pharmacologic properties that are modestly different. Whether these differences affect the safety and efficacy of an individual agent is unknown. However, based on the properties of their LMWH, manufacturers have recommended varying dosage regimens (**Tables 3.1** and **3.2**). For example, enoxaparin is administered in milligrams and given either once or twice daily, whereas dalteparin and tinzaparin are prescribed in units and usually given once daily. While some LMWHs are given in fixed doses for prophylaxis, tinzaparin is almost always given based on body weight. Because of their high degree of bioavailability, all LMWHs are given subcutaneously. The LMWHs and synthetic anti-Xa currently available for the prophylaxis of venous thromboembolism are shown in **Table 3.1**.

All LMWHs are given in higher doses for treatment indications such as the therapy of venous thrombosis or the management of unstable angina. Those currently available are shown in **Table 3.2**. In addition, many LMWHs have

TABLE 3.1 — CURRENTLY AVAILABLE LMWH PREPARATIONS AND SYNTHETIC FACTOR Xa ANTAGONISTS FOR THROMBOPROPHYLAXIS

Drug (Trade)	Dose	Indication
Low Molecular Weight Heparins		
Dalteparin (Fragmin)	2500 U q12h (5000 U daily)	Hip/abdominal surgery
Enoxaparin (Lovenox)	30 mg q12h (40 mg daily)	Medical inpatients; hip/knee/abdominal surgery
Tinzaparin (Innohep)	75 IU/kg daily	Hip/knee replacement surgery*
Synthetic Factor Xa Inhibitor		
Fondaparinux (Arixtra)	2.5 mg daily	Hip fracture/hip or knee replacement surgery

Abbreviations: LMWH, low molecular weight heparin.

* Not Food and Drug Administration (FDA) approved for this indication.

been used for a variety of other clinical conditions including stroke (both thromboprophylaxis and treatment), neurosurgery (prevention of postoperative thromboembolism), and thromboprophylaxis after trauma, including spinal cord injury and hip fracture.[8] They have also been used for the prevention of thrombi in vascular grafts and fistulae. Although these uses are not approved by the Food and Drug Administration (FDA) as yet, LMWH is gradually supplanting UFH because of its:

- Convenience (once or twice daily subcutaneous injections)
- Lack of need for routine monitoring
- Overall high degree of safety.[7,9]

TABLE 3.2 — CURRENTLY AVAILABLE LMWH PREPARATIONS FOR TREATMENT OF VENOUS AND/OR ARTERIAL THROMBOTIC DISORDERS*

Drug (Trade)	Dose	Indication
Dalteparin (Fragmin)	120 IU/kg q12h	Non–ST-segment elevation ACS
Enoxaparin (Lovenox)	1 mg/kg q12h (1.5 mg/kg daily)	Non–ST-segment elevation ACS; inpatient treatment of DVT (with or without PE); out-patient treatment of DVT
Tinzaparin (Innohep)	175 IU/kg daily	Treatment of DVT (with or without PE)

Abbreviations: ACS, acute coronary syndrome; DVT, deep vein thrombosis; LMWH, low molecular weight heparin; PE, pulmonary embolism.

* Administered subcutaneously.

Selective Factor Xa Inhibitors

Fondaparinux (Arixtra) is the first of a new class of antithrombotic drugs, the selective inhibitors of factor Xa. It is a sulfated pentasaccharide obtained totally by chemical synthesis, with no animal-source components. It has been designed to bind to a specific target, antithrombin, the fondaparinux-antithrombin complex selectively inhibits factor Xa.[10-12] Unlike heparins, fondaparinux does not inhibit thrombin directly. However, the inactivation of factor Xa via antithrombin results in strong inhibition of thrombin generation and thus thrombus formation and growth.[13,14] In addition, fondaparinux has no recognized effects on platelet aggregation.[15]

After subcutaneous dosing in healthy volunteers, fondaparinux is 100% bioavailable and absorption is rapid and complete (with C_{MAX} occurring within approximately 2 hours).[16] Fondaparinux is almost completely excreted in urine as unchanged compound. The terminal half-life is 17 hours (±3 hours) in young volunteers and 21 hours in elderly volunteers, allowing once-daily administration. Overall drug clearance is 25% lower in patients with mild renal impairment (creatinine clearance [CrCl] 50-80 mL/min), approximately 40% lower with moderate renal impairment (CrCl 30-50 mL/min), and 55% lower in those with severe renal impairment (CrCl <30 mL/min). Drug elimination is also reduced in patients weighing <50 kg. At recommended doses, coagulation tests, including the PT, aPTT, and activated clotting time (ACT), are not prolonged.

Fondaparinux underwent a large development program in orthopedic surgery for the prophylaxis of venous thromboembolism.[17-22] The program mainly consisted of four large, randomized, double-blind phase 3 studies comparing subcutaneous fondaparinux 2.5 mg once daily, starting 6 hours postoperatively, with the two enoxaparin regimens approved for use in orthopedic surgery, ie, 40 mg once daily starting 12 hours preoperatively and 30 mg twice daily starting 12 to 24 hours postoperatively. Its results showed greater efficacy of fondaparinux over enoxaparin in preventing venous thromboembolism in patients undergoing surgery for hip fracture, elective major knee surgery, and elective hip replacement surgery, with a highly significant overall relative reduction in risk of venous thromboembolism of 55.2% (13.7% vs 6.8%) and a 57.4% reduction in the risk of proximal DVT (2.9% vs 1.3%) in favor of fondaparinux, without increased risk of clinically relevant bleeding (**Figure 3.1**).[22]

Fondaparinux is currently being investigated for use in a variety of thrombotic disorders, such as:

- Long-term thromboprophylaxis in orthopedic surgery
- Prophylaxis of venous thromboembolic events in abdominal surgery and in acutely ill medical patients
- Treatment of DVT and pulmonary embolism (PE)
- HIT.

The efficacy and safety of three doses of fondaparinux were compared with those of the LMWH dalteparin 100 IU/kg/bid in patients with acute venous thromboembolism in a randomized, multicenter trial (REMBRANDT study).[23] There were 2.4% and 5.0% recurrent thromboembolic complications in the fondaparinux and dalteparin groups, respec-

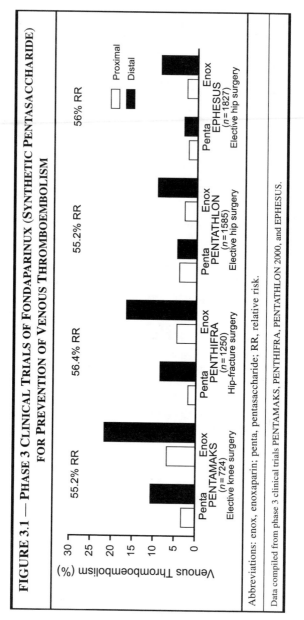

FIGURE 3.1 — PHASE 3 CLINICAL TRIALS OF FONDAPARINUX (SYNTHETIC PENTASACCHARIDE) FOR PREVENTION OF VENOUS THROMBOEMBOLISM

Abbreviations: enox, enoxaparin; penta, pentasaccharide; RR, relative risk.

Data compiled from phase 3 clinical trials PENTAMAKS, PENTHIFRA, PENTATHLON 2000, and EPHESUS.

tively. The incidence of bleeding was low and similar in the two groups. The MATISSE Trial examined the safety and effectiveness of fondaparinux in patients with acute DVT or PE.[24] More than 4000 patients were randomized to receive therapy with either fondaparinux 7.5 mg subcutaneously daily, or enoxaparin 1 mg/kg twice daily if they had DVT or intravenous (IV) heparin if they had PE. Patients assigned to fondaparinux who weighed <50 kg received 5 mg, and those weighing >100 kg received 10 mg. After 5 to 7 days of treatment, all patients were given warfarin for 3 months. Between 3% and 5% of patients in each group had recurrent PE or DVT and the frequency of major bleeding (1.1% to 1.3%) and other bleeding (2.6% to 5.2%) was low; none of the differences between groups was significant.

Fondaparinux has also been studied in arterial thrombotic disorders. In the Pentasaccharide as an Adjunct to Fibrinolysis in ST-Elevation Acute Myocardial Infarction (PENTALYSE) study, 333 patients with evolving ST-segment elevation myocardial infarction (MI) were treated with aspirin and tPA (alteplase) and randomized to UFH or to low-, intermediate-, or high-dose fondaparinux.[25] Thrombolysis in Myocardial Infarction (TIMI) flow grades at 90 minutes were similar in the four treatment groups; however, a trend toward reduced reocclusion 5 to 7 days after treatment was observed favoring fondaparinux (0.9% vs 7.0%; $P = 0.065$). The rates of major hemorrhage did not differ between groups (**Figure 3.2**). Promising preliminary results are also available in patients with acute coronary syndromes and in the setting of percutaneous transluminal coronary angioplasty.[26,27] However, large clinical trials are necessary before fondaparinux can be considered a standard therapeutic option in patients with arterial thrombotic disorders.

Direct Thrombin Inhibitors

Hirudin is a product of the medicinal leech, *Hirudo medicinalis*, but is currently prepared by recombinant DNA technology. Two forms have been examined clinically:

- Lepirudin
- Desirudin.

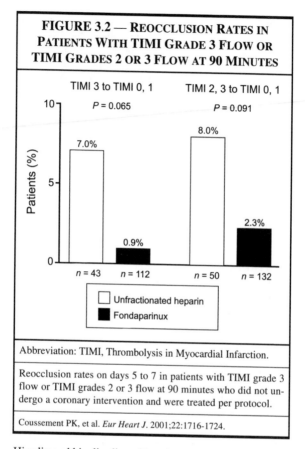

FIGURE 3.2 — REOCCLUSION RATES IN PATIENTS WITH TIMI GRADE 3 FLOW OR TIMI GRADES 2 OR 3 FLOW AT 90 MINUTES

Abbreviation: TIMI, Thrombolysis in Myocardial Infarction.

Reocclusion rates on days 5 to 7 in patients with TIMI grade 3 flow or TIMI grades 2 or 3 flow at 90 minutes who did not undergo a coronary intervention and were treated per protocol.

Coussement PK, et al. *Eur Heart J*. 2001;22:1716-1724.

Hirudin and bivalirudin, a 20 amino acid synthetic peptide, bind to both the catalytic site and the fibrinogen-binding exosite of thrombin.[28] Hirudin has been further modified by conjugation with polyethylene glycol (PEG-hirudin), which has a longer half-life than hirudin. The half-life of hirudin is 50 to 65 minutes, with a half-life of its effect on the aPTT of 2 hours.[29] Bivalirudin has a half-life of about 40 minutes. The pharmacologic advantages and disadvantages of the hirudins as compared with the heparins are shown in **Table 3.3**.

Hirudins and bivalirudin, bivalent direct thrombin inhibitors, form a tight complex with thrombin, inhibiting

TABLE 3.3 — PROPERTIES OF HEPARINS*, HIRUDIN, AND BIVALIRUDIN

Property	Heparins*	Hirudin	Bivalirudin
Thrombin inhibition	AT dependent	Direct	Direct
Clot-bound thrombin	Not inhibited	Inhibited	Inhibited
Thrombocytopenia	Yes	No	No
Immunogenicity	Yes	Yes (rare)	No
Effect on aPTT	Yes (weak with LMWH)	Yes	Yes
Effect on PT	Weak	Mild	Mild
Effect on ACT	Yes (weak with LMWH)	Yes	Yes
Metabolism	Liver, kidney	Kidney	Kidney (20%)
Antidote	Protamine†	None	None

Abbreviations: ACT, activated clotting time; aPTT, activated partial thromboplastin time; AT, antithrombin; LMWH, low molecular weight heparin; PT, prothrombin time.

* Unfractionated heparin and LMWH.
† 60% reversal with protamine.

thrombin conversion of fibrinogen to fibrin as well as thrombin-induced platelet aggregation.[30] These actions are independent of the presence of antithrombin, and also affect thrombin bound to fibrin. On the downside, the ability of thrombin to complex with thrombomodulin, activating protein C, is also inhibited. The hirudins do not bind to platelet factor 4 and do not elicit antibodies that induce platelet and endothelial cell activation; thus they may be safely administered to patients that have developed HIT. Hirudins do have weak immunogenicity, so that diminished (or rarely increased) responsiveness after repeated dosing is possible. The aPTT is prolonged and is used to monitor the effect of the hirudins. The PT is modestly prolonged, which may interfere with the monitoring of concomitant warfarin therapy. Hirudin rapidly increases to toxic levels in patients with renal failure; the doses must be halved or further reduced in such patients. While protamine effectively reverses the anticoagulant effect of UFH and is also partially effective in neutralizing LMWH, there is no antidote for hirudins except plasma exchange. Two preparations, a recombinant hirudin (lepirudin [Refludan]) and hirulog (bivalirudin [Angiomax]), have been licensed in the United States. Lepirudin is used for the management of HIT, and bivalirudin is indicated for patients with unstable angina undergoing percutaneous coronary intervention (PCI). In randomized clinical trials of patients undergoing PCI, the frequency of death, MI, and need for revascularization procedures was 6.2% in those treated with bivalirudin and 7.9% in those receiving heparin; the frequency of major hemorrhage was less with bivalirudin (3.5% vs 9.3%). The drug is always administered with aspirin; its safety in conjunction with platelet glycoprotein IIb/IIIa inhibitors has been demonstrated.[31]

Argatroban is a synthetic direct thrombin inhibitor derived from L-arginine that reversibly binds to the enzyme's active site. Accordingly, it is considered a univalent thrombin antagonist (**Table 3.3**). However, an important difference between argatroban and other direct thrombin inhibitors relates to its hepatic rather than renal metabolism. Therefore, the drug may be given without dose adjustment to patients with renal failure. The starting dose is 2 μg/kg/min; the aPTT is determined 2 hours later with dose adjustments until the target aPTT of 1.5 to 3.0 times the control is attained. The dose is decreased to 0.5 µg/kg/min if there is hepatic impairment. Argatroban is approved for the prophylaxis or treatment of thrombosis in HIT and as an anticoagulant in patients with or those at risk for HIT undergoing PCI.[32] Like the hirudins, argatroban can modestly prolong the prothrombin time, necessitating dose adjustments when warfarin is given concomitantly (see Chapter 18, *Complications of Antithrombotic Therapy*).

3

Melagatran, a small-molecule, monovalent inhibitor of the catalytic site of thrombin, has been modified to resist digestion by gastric secretions and undergo absorption by the intestine. This modified molecule (prodrug), ximelagatran, is an investigational drug not currently approved by the FDA. It has undergone study in three clinical trials of patients undergoing hip or knee arthroplasty.[33-35] The initial studies demonstrated that ximelagatran 24 mg bid by mouth is as safe and effective as dalteparin, enoxaparin, and warfarin, and does not require monitoring. Subsequently, a larger study using 36 mg twice daily demonstrated that ximelagatran is equally as effective as warfarin with no increase in bleeding.[36]

An open-label trial (Stroke Prevention Using Oral Thrombin Inhibition in Atrial Fibrillation [SPORTIF III]) examined the safety and efficacy of ximelagatran in patients with atrial fibrillation.[37] 3410 patients with atrial fibrillation and more than one additional risk factor for stroke were enrolled. Subjects received either ximelagatran 36 mg twice daily or standard warfarin therapy and were followed for 12 to 26 months. The event rate in the ximelagatran-treated patients was 1.6% vs 2.3% in those on warfarin, a relative risk reduction of 29%. There was no significant difference in major bleeding between groups, but there was more minor bleeding in those assigned to warfarin ($P = 0.007$). An important adverse event associated with ximelagatran was an increase in liver enzymes; elevation of alanine aminotransferase (ALT) greater than three times normal occurred in 6.5% of subjects, but returned to baseline when the drug was discontinued. It was concluded that ximelagatran is as safe and effective as warfarin but without the need for coagulation monitoring. These results were confirmed in the SPORTIF V trial.

47

A dose ranging study of ximelagatran in patients with recent ST-elevation or non–ST-elevation MI was recently concluded.[38] As compared with placebo, oral ximelagatran given for 6 months significantly reduced the risk of all-cause death, nonfatal MI, and severe recurrent ischemia (from 16.3% to 12.7%). While not a prespecified outcome, the risk of stroke was also decreased. All doses of the drug, from 24 mg to 60 mg twice daily, were equally effective. Major bleeding occurred in 1.8% of ximelagatran-treated patients and 0.9% of those on placebo. There was an increasing risk for hemorrhage with higher doses (>36 mg twice daily). Ximelagatran was associated with a fourfold excess in liver enzyme elevations, occurring in up to 16% of patients at higher doses.

The potential of ximelagatran to be used in the treatment of acute DVT was investigated in the Thrombin Inhibitor in Venous Thromboembolism (THRIVE) studies. THRIVE I was a randomized, controlled trial evaluating the safety and tolerability of ximelagatran (24, 36, 48, or 60 mg bid) compared with dalteparin followed by warfarin for 2 weeks. Evaluation of paired venograms from 295 of 350 patients showed regression of thrombus in 69% of patients in both groups. Change in thrombus size according to the Marder score and safety were also similar.[39]

Based on the encouraging results of THRIVE I, a large, multicenter, randomized, double-blind study (THRIVE Treatment Study) was performed. A total of 2489 patients with acute DVT (37% had confirmed PE) were assigned to receive either oral ximelagatran 36 mg bid for 6 months or enoxaparin 1 mg/kg subcutaneous, minimum 5 days, followed by warfarin (international normalized ratio [INR] 2 to 3). Recurrent venous thromboembolism occurred in 2.1% and 2.0% of patients, respectively. Major bleeding (on treatment analyses) was experienced in 1.3% and 2.2% of patients, respectively.[40]

The THRIVE III Study included 1233 patients with confirmed venous thromboembolism who had received standard anticoagulant therapy for 6 months. They were then randomized to either ximelagatran 24 mg bid or placebo for another 18 months. Recurrent events occurred in 12 patients receiving ximelagatran and in 71 patients on placebo (hazard ratio 0.16; P <0.0001). Six patients given active study

48

drug experienced a major hemorrhagic event (some were fatal or involved the central nervous system).[41]

Warfarin (Coumadin)

Coumarins inhibit the enzymatic reduction of vitamin K epoxide. Vitamin K (in the reduced state) is the coenzyme of a carboxylase responsible for the carboxylation of glutamic acid residues on factors II, VII, IX, and X and proteins C, S, and Z. The acarboxylated forms of these clotting proteins can be detected in the circulation of warfarin-treated patients but are inert with respect to coagulant activity.

Several coumarins have been developed for clinical use; acenocoumarol is available in Europe but not used in the United States, where warfarin is the most commonly used oral anticoagulant. Warfarin is rapidly absorbed from the gastrointestinal tract and has a half-life of 36 to 42 hours. After a dose of warfarin, the synthesis of carboxylated factors ceases, but the effects on coagulation will depend on the disappearance of carboxylated factors formed prior to warfarin exposure. The disappearance of these factors is a function of their half-life (factor VII and protein C: 6 to 7 hours; factors IX and X: 24 hours; prothrombin: 90 hours). Thus, after a dose of warfarin, factor VII and protein C will be 20% of normal at 48 hours, but prothrombin will not be reduced to this extent for 1 to 2 weeks. Since effective anticoagulation requires a decrease in clotting factors to 20% of normal, warfarin is considered a slow-acting anticoagulant.[42]

The effect of warfarin is monitored with the PT, which is sensitive to factors II, V, VII, and X. Although factor IX is not measured, it is usually reduced in parallel with factor X and therefore does not have to be separately quantitated. Clinical and laboratory studies suggest that prolongation of the PT to 1.5 to 2 times normal prevents the growth of a thrombus. The INR refers to the ratio of patient-to-control PT raised to a power—the international sensitivity index (ISI). For example, if the PT is 1.5 times longer than the control PT and the ISI (of the PT reagent) is 2, the INR is 2.25 (1.5 raised to the power of 2). Values of 2 to 3 are considered therapeutic. Therefore, the dose of warfarin is titrated to give an INR in this range.

Warfarin is subject to extensive binding by plasma proteins and is metabolized by the P450 detoxification system of the liver. Persons with genetic polymorphisms of the CYP 2C9 enzyme may have impaired metabolism of warfarin and may require doses of the drug that are substantially less than those in persons with the wild-type enzyme.[43] These polymorphisms occur in about one in ten white persons.[44] Drugs that alter protein binding or affect the liver may potentiate or inhibit the activity of warfarin (**Table 3.4**).[45] Acetaminophen has been shown to produce a dose-dependent increase in the INR of warfarin-treated patients, beginning with a dose as low as seven to thirteen 325-mg tablets per week.[46] Even herbal remedies such as ginkgo and ginseng, as well as numerous others, may alter warfarin metabolism.[47] Other factors found to affect warfarin were the dietary content of vitamin K, the ability to absorb vitamin K (altered by diarrheal disease), and advanced malignancy.

An important adverse reaction to warfarin therapy is tissue necrosis due to severely decreased levels of protein C or S. This complication occurs most often in the setting of acute thrombosis and is characterized by microvascular thrombosis involving the postcapillary venues. Susceptible patients either have congenital protein C or S defects or acquired deficiencies due to vitamin K deficiency, consumption of C and S, or HIT. When such individuals are exposed to warfarin, the sudden decline in proteins C and S leads to thrombus formation in venules with extensive skin and subcutaneous fat necrosis. Even more profound thrombosis, producing limb gangrene, occurs when warfarin is given to patients with HIT. The mechanism appears to be similar—an underlying deficiency in protein C that is exacerbated by the administration of warfarin.[48]

Other adverse effects attributed to warfarin are fetal embryopathy, especially with exposure to the drug from the sixth to twelfth weeks of gestation, and "purple toes," related to embolization of cholesterol-rich material from atheromatous aortic plaques.

A prolonged PT due to warfarin declines within 24 to 48 hours of drug discontinuation if the patient is eating. Vitamin K is the specific antidote: The dose is based on whether the patient is bleeding and the elevation of the INR, recognizing that the patient will be at risk for developing

TABLE 3.4 — LEVEL-1 EVIDENCE OF DRUG INTERACTIONS WITH WARFARIN

Interaction	Antibiotics	Cardiac	Anti-inflammatory	CNS	GI
Potentiate	Co-trimoxazole Erythromycin Fluconazole Isoniazid Metronidazole	Amiodarone Clofibrate Propafenone Propranolol Sulfinpyrazone	Phenylbutazone Piroxicam	Alcohol (with liver disease)	Cimetidine Omeprazole
Inhibit	Griseofulvin Nafcillin Rifampin	Cholestyramine	—	Barbiturates Carbamazepine Chlordiazepoxide	Sucralfate
No effect	Enoxacin	Atenolol Bumetanide Felodipine Metoprolol	Diflunisal Ketorolac Naproxen	Alcohol Fluoxetine Nitrazepam	Antacids Famotidine

Abbreviations: CNS, central nervous system; GI, gastrointestinal.

Wells PS, et al. *Ann Intern Med.* 1994;121:676-683.

new thrombotic events if the INR is overcorrected and will be refractory to warfarin for several days if too large a dose is given. The dose of vitamin K is 1.0 mg to 2.5 mg orally for an INR of 5 to 10 in a nonbleeding patient; inability to eat, bleeding, or higher INR is managed with doses of 1 to 10 mg subcutaneously.[49] A recent study observed that 1 mg of liquid phytonadione given orally is more rapidly effective than the same dose given subcutaneously.[50] The IV route is reserved for patients with major hemorrhage; because of the risk of anaphylaxis, vitamin K should be diluted in saline and administered slowly under constant supervision. In the event that bleeding is life-threatening, hemorrhage may be controlled by recombinant human factor VIIa concentrate, given in a dose of 15 to 20 µg/kg body weight.[51] While this agent is expensive, it is more reliable than fresh frozen plasma, which requires doses of at least 15 mL/kg and must be repeated every 4 to 6 hours to maintain correction of the PT.[52]

Anticoagulants Currently Under Development

A large variety of compounds are currently under development; these include inhibitors of factors VIIa, IXa, Xa, and XIIIa and direct thrombin inhibitors. In addition, other anticoagulants are being reformulated so that they may be given by mouth. For example, an oral formulation of heparin is currently in development and a long-acting form of fondaparinux, idraparinux, is in clinical trials. Idraparinux has an additional binding site for antithrombin, resulting in a prolonged half-life of 130 hours. In the PERSIST trial, idraparinux 2.5 mg subcutaneously once weekly was compared with warfarin.[53] Each drug was administered for 12 weeks and the frequency of recurrent thrombosis and bleeding recorded. No major bleeding or thromboembolism was observed with the idraparinux, whereas 2.5% of warfarin-treated patients had recurrences, and there were 10 major bleeds. In view of these very promising results, a larger trial is planned.

The rapid evolution of antithrombotic drugs requires careful evaluation of all phases of investigation before recommendations for use and potential changes in clinical practice are instituted. In addition, phase 4 (postmarketing) studies are a critical component of determining safety for patients with thrombotic disorders.

REFERENCES

1. Hirsh J. Heparin. *N Engl J Med.* 1991;324:1565-1574.

2. Hirsh J, Levine MN. Low molecular weight heparin. *Blood.* 1992;79:1-17.

3. Weitz JI. Low-molecular-weight heparins [published correction appears in *N Engl J Med.* 1997;337:1567]. *N Engl J Med.* 1997;337:688-698.

4. Laposata M, Green D, Van Cott EM, Barrowcliffe TW, Goodnight SH, Sosolik RE. College of American Pathologists Conference XXXI on Laboratory Monitoring of Anticoagulant Therapy: the clinical use and laboratory monitoring of low-molecular-weight heparin, danaparoid, hirudin and related compounds, and argatroban. *Arch Pathol Lab Med.* 1998;122:799-807.

5. Hainer JW, Barrett JS, Assaid CA, et al. Dosing in heavy-weight/obese patients with the LMWH, tinzaparin: a pharmacodynamic study. *Thromb Haemost.* 2002;87:817-823.

6. Wysowski DX, Talarico L, Bacsanyi J, Botstein P. Spinal and epidural hematoma and low-molecular-weight heparin. *N Engl J Med.* 1998;338:1774-1775.

7. Siguret V, Pautas E, Fevrier M, et al. Elderly patients treated with tinzaparin (Innohep) administered once daily (175 anti-Xa IU/kg): anti-Xa and anti-IIa activities over 10 days. *Thromb Haemost.* 2000;84: 800-804.

8. Green D, Hirsh J, Heit J, Prins M, Davidson B, Lensing AW. Low molecular weight heparin: a critical analysis of clinical trials. *Pharmacol Rev.* 1994;46:89-109.

9. Veiga F, Escriba A, Maluenda MP, et al. Low molecular weight heparin (enoxaparin) versus oral anticoagulant therapy (acenocoumarol) in the long-term treatment of deep venous thrombosis in the elderly: a randomized trial. *Thromb Haemost.* 2000;84:559-564.

10. Petitou M, Lormeau JC, Choay J. Chemical synthesis of glycosaminoglycans: new approaches to antithrombotic drugs. *Nature.* 1991;350(suppl):30-33.

11. van Boeckel CAA, Petitou M. The unique antithrombin III binding domain of heparin: a lead to new synthetic antithrombotics. *Angew Chem* [Int Ed Engl]. 1993;32:1671-1690.

12. Olson ST, Bjork I, Sheffer R, Craig PA, Shore JD, Choay J. Role of the antithrombin-binding pentasaccharide in heparin acceleration of antithrombin-proteinase reactions. Resolution of the antithrombin conformational change contribution to heparin rate enhancement. *J Biol Chem.* 1992;267:12528-12538.

13. Lormeau JC, Herault JP. The effect of the synthetic pentasaccharide SR 90107/ORG31540 on thrombin generation ex vivo is uniquely due to ATIII-mediated neutralization of factor Xa. *Thromb Haemost.* 1995;74:1474-1477.

14. Walenga JM, Bara L, Petitou M, Samama M, Fareed J, Choay J. The inhibition of the generation of thrombin and the antithrombotic effect of a pentasaccharide with sole anti-factor Xa activity. *Thromb Res.* 1988;51:23-33.

15. Herbert JM, Petitou M, Lormeau JC, et al. SR90107A/Org31540, a novel anti-factor Xa antithrombotic agent. *Cardiovasc Drug Rev.* 1997;15:1-26.

16. Donat F, Duret JP, Santoni A, et al. The pharmacokinetics of fondaparinux sodium in healthy volunteers. *Clin Pharmacokinet.* 2002;41(suppl 2):1-9.

17. Turpie AG, Gallus AS, Hoek JA, Pentasaccharide Investigators. A synthetic pentasaccharide for the prevention of deep-vein thrombosis after total hip replacement. *N Engl J Med.* 2001;344:619-625.

18. Bauer KA, Eriksson BI, Lassen MR, Turpie AG, Steering Committee of the Pentasaccharide in Major Knee Surgery Study. Fondaparinux compared with enoxaparin for the prevention of venous thromboembolism after elective major knee surgery. *N Engl J Med.* 2001;345: 1305-1310.

19. Eriksson BI, Bauer KA, Lassen MR, Turpie AG, Steering Committee of the Pentasaccharide in Hip-Fracture, Surgery Study. Fondaparinux compared with enoxaparin for the prevention of venous thromboembolism after hip-fracture surgery. *N Engl J Med.* 2001;345:1298-1304.

20. Lassen MR, Bauer KA, Eriksson BI, Turpie AG, European Pentasaccharide Elective Surgery Study (EPHESUS) Steering Committee. Postoperative fondaparinux versus preoperative enoxaparin for prevention of venous thromboembolism in elective hip-replacement surgery: a randomized double-blind comparison. *Lancet.* 2002; 359:1715-1720.

21. Turpie AG, Bauer KA, Eriksson BI, Lassen MR, PENTATHALON 2000 Study Steering Committee. Postoperative fondaparinux versus postoperative enoxaparin for prevention of venous thromboembolism after elective hip-replacement surgery: a randomized double-blind trial. *Lancet.* 2002;359:1721-1726.

22. Turpie AG, Bauer KA, Eriksson BI, Lassen MR. Fondaparinux vs enoxaparin for the prevention of venous thromboembolism in major orthopedic surgery: a meta-analysis of 4 randomized double-blind studies. *Arch Intern Med.* 2002;162:1833-1840.

23. The Rembrandt Investigators. Treatment of proximal deep vein thrombosis with a novel synthetic compound (SR90107A/ORG31540) with pure anti-factor Xa activity. *Circulation.* 2000;102:2726-2731.

24. The MATISSE Investigators. Fondaparinux (Arixtra) in comparison to (low molecular weight) heparin for the initial treatment of symptomatic deep venous thrombosis or pulmonary embolism — The MATISSE Clinical Outcome Studies. *Blood.* 2002;100:83a. Abstract #302.

25. Coussement PK, Bassand JP, Convens C, et al, for the PENTALYSE Investigators. A synthetic factor-Xa inhibitor (ORG31540/SR9017A) as an adjunct to fibrinolysis in acute myocardial infarction. *Eur Heart J.* 2001;22:1716-1724.

26. The Pentua trial. Hot line on the 74th Scientific Sessions of the American Heart Association, November 2001.

27. Vuillemenot A, Schiele F, Meneveau N, et al. Efficacy of a synthetic pentasaccharide, a pure factor Xa inhibitor, as an antithrombotic agent—a pilot study in the setting of coronary angioplasty. *Thromb Haemost.* 1999;81:214-220.

28. Coussement PK, Bassand JP, Convens C, et al. A synthetic factor-Xa inhibitor (ORG31540/SR9017A) as an adjunct to fibrinolysis in acute myocardial infarction. The PENTALYSE study. *Eur Heart J.* 2001;22:1716-1724

29. Verstraete M, Nurmohamed M, Kienast J, et al. Biologic effects of recombinant hirudin (CGP 39393) in human volunteers. European Hirudin in Thrombosis Group. *J Am Coll Cardiol.* 1993;22:1080-1088.

30. Verstraete M. Direct thrombin inhibitors: appraisal of the antithrombotic/hemorrhagic balance. *Thromb Haemost.* 1997;78:357-363.

31. Lincoff AM, Bittl JA, Harrington RA, et al. Bivalirudin and provisional glycoprotein IIb/IIIa blockade compared with heparin and planned glycoprotein IIb/IIIa blockade during percutaneous coronary intervention: REPLACE-2 randomized trial. *JAMA.* 2003;289:853-863.

32. Lewis BE, Wallis DE, Berkowitz SD, et al. Argatroban anticoagulant therapy in patients with heparin-induced thrombocytopenia. *Circulation.* 2001;103:1838-1843.

33. Eriksson BI, Arfwidsson AC, Frison L, et al. A dose-ranging study of the oral direct thrombin inhibitor, ximelagatran, and its subcutaneous form, melagatran, compared with dalteparin in the prophylaxis of thromboembolism after hip or knee replacement: METHRO I. Melaatran for Thrombin Inhibition in Orthopaedic Surgery. *Thromb Haemost.* 2002;87:231-237.

34. Heit JA, Colwell CW, Francis CW, et al, for the AstraZeneca Arthro-
    plasty Study Group. Comparison of the oral direct thrombin inhibitor
    ximelagatran with enoxaparin as prophylaxis against venous throm-
    boembolism after total knee replacement: a phase 2 dose-finding study.
    Arch Intern Med. 2001;161:2215-2221.

35. Francis CW, Davidson BL, Berkowitz SD, et al. Ximelagatran versus
    warfarin for the prevention of venous thromboembolism after total knee
    arthroplasty. A randomized, double-blind trial. *Ann Intern Med*.
    2002;137:648-655.

36. Francis DW, Berkowitz SD, Comp PC, et al. Randomized, double-
    blind comparison of ximelagatran, an oral direct thrombin inhibitor,
    and warfarin to prevent venous thromboembolism (VTE) after total
    knee replacement (TKR). *Blood*. 2002;100:82a. Abstract #300.

37. Olsson SB, the Executive Steering Committee on behalf of the
    SPORTIF III Investigators. Stroke prevention with the oral direct
    thrombin inhibitor ximelagatran compared with warfarin in patients
    with nonvalvular atrial fibrillation (SPORTIF III): randomised con-
    trolled trial. *Lancet*. 2003;362:1686-1687.

38. Wallentin L, Wilcox RG, Weaver WD, et al, for the ESTEEM Inves-
    tigators. Oral ximelagatran for secondary prophylaxis after myocar-
    dial infarction: the ESTEEM randomised controlled trial. *Lancet*.
    2003;362:789-797.

39. Eriksson H, Wahlander K. Gustafsson D, Welin LT, Frison L,
    Schulman S, Thrive Investigators. A randomized, controlled, dose-
    guiding study of the oral direct thrombin inhibitor ximelagatran com-
    pared with standard therapy for the treatment of acute deep vein
    thrombosis: THRIVE I. *J Thromb Haemost*. 2003;1:41-47.

40. Huisman MV, on behalf of the THRIVE II and V Investigators. Effi-
    cacy and safety of the oral direct thrombin inhibitor ximelagatran com-
    pared with current standard therapy for acute symptomatic deep vein
    thrombosis, with or without pulmonary embolism: a randomized,
    double-blind, multinational study. *J Thromb Haemost*. 2003;1(suppl
    1). Abstract OC 003.

41. Eriksson H, Wahlander K, Lundstrom T, et al, for the THRIVE III
    Investigators. Extended secondary prevention with the oral direct
    thrombin inhibitor ximelagatran for 18 months after 6 months of oral
    anticoagulation in patients with venous thromboembolism: a random-
    ized placebo-controlled trial. *J Thromb Haemost*. 2003;1(suppl 1).
    Abstract OC 005.

42. Hirsh J. Oral anticoagulant drugs. *N Engl J Med*. 1991;324:1865-1875.

43. Taube J, Halsall D, Baglin T. Influence of cytochrome P-450 CYP2C9
    polymorphisms on warfarin sensitivity and risk of over-anticoagula-
    tion in patients on long-term treatment. *Blood*. 2000;96:1816-1819.

44. Xie HG, Kim RB, Wood AJ, Stein CM. Molecular basis of ethnic differences in drug disposition and response. *Annu Rev Pharmacol Toxicol.* 2001;41:815-850.

45. Wells PS, Holbrook AM, Crowther NR, Hirsh J. Interactions of warfarin with drugs and food. *Ann Intern Med.* 1994;121:676-683.

46. Hylek EM, Heiman H, Skates SJ, Sheehan MA, Singer DE. Acetaminophen and other risk factors for excessive warfarin anticoagulation. *JAMA.* 1998;279:657-662.

47. Fugh-Berman A. Herb-drug interactions. *Lancet.* 2000;355:134-138.

48. Warkentin TE, Elavathil LJ, Hayward CP, Johnston MA, Russett JI, Kelton JG. The pathogenesis of venous limb gangrene associated with heparin-induced thrombocytopenia. *Ann Intern Med.* 1997;127:804-812.

49. Weibert RT, Le DT, Kayser SR, Rapaport SI. Correction of excessive anticoagulation with low-dose oral vitamin K1. *Ann Intern Med.* 1997;125:959-962.

50. Crowther MA, Douketis JD, Schnurr T, et al. Oral vitamin K lowers the international normalized ratio more rapidly than subcutaneous vitamin K in the treatment of warfarin-associated coagulpathy. A randomized, controlled trial. *Ann Intern Med.* 2002;137:251-254.

51. Deveras RA, Kessler CM. Reversal of warfarin-induced excessive anticoagulation with recombinant human factor VIIa concentrate. *Ann Intern Med.* 2002;137:884-888.

52. Makris M, Greaves M, Phillips WS, Kitchen S, Rosendaal FR, Preston EF. Emergency oral anticoagulant reversal: the relative efficacy of infusions of fresh frozen plasma and clotting factor concentrate on correction of the coagulopathy. *Thromb Haemost.* 1997;77:477-480.

53. Van Oers MHJ, the PERSIST Investigators. A novel, long-acting synthetic factor Xa inhibitor (idraparinux sodium) to replace warfarin for secondary prevention in deep vein thrombosis. A phase II evaluation. *Blood.* 2002;100:82a. Abstract #301.

4

Fibrinolytic Agents

Recognizing the impact of acute thrombotic coronary arterial occlusion has led to a new paradigm: rapid, complete, and sustained patency of an occluded artery and physiologic myocardial perfusion. Fibrinolytic agents promote the conversion of plasminogen to plasmin, which then proteolytically degrades fibrin, the structural meshwork of an arterial thrombus.

Overview of the Fibrinolytic System

The exogenous fibrinolytic system is an important component of natural vascular thromboresistance, preventing thrombus mass beyond that required for hemostasis. Plasminogen is converted to plasmin, an enzyme that proteolytically degrades fibrin (**Figures 4.1** and **4.2**). Circulating plasmin inhibitors, particularly α_2-antiplasmin, rapidly inactivate free plasmin; however, when the rate of generation of plasmin exceeds the rate of inhibition, a systemic lytic state may ensue, with depletion of clotting factors, including fibrinogen, factor V, and factor VIII.[1] The natural plasminogen activators tissue plasminogen activator (tPA) and single-chain urokinase plasminogen activator (scu-PA) have fibrin-specific properties, suggesting that physiologic fibrinolysis is clot selective.[2]

Tissue Plasminogen Activator

Tissue plasminogen activator, produced by vascular endothelial cells and released in response to developing thrombus, is a naturally occurring 70,000 dalton glycoprotein (GP) (**Figure 4.2**). The native molecule is a single-chain polypeptide, but is converted to the fully active two-chain enzyme by plasmin-mediated cleavage (**Figure 4.2** with an arrow). This unique structure, particularly the second kringle and the finger domain, confers high fibrin specificity.[2] Plasminogen activator inhibitor can rapidly inactivate circulating

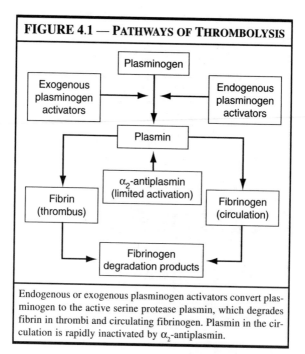

FIGURE 4.1 — PATHWAYS OF THROMBOLYSIS

Endogenous or exogenous plasminogen activators convert plasminogen to the active serine protease plasmin, which degrades fibrin in thrombi and circulating fibrinogen. Plasmin in the circulation is rapidly inactivated by α_2-antiplasmin.

tPA. In the absence of fibrin, tPA has weak enzymatic activity; however, when bound, tPA undergoes a conformational change that increases its plasmin-producing capacity by nearly 1000-fold. Thus plasmin is formed preferentially at the site of a developing thrombus (**Figure 4.3**).

Recombinant DNA technology was harnessed to produce alteplase, synthesized using the complementary DNA from natural human tPA. Alteplase is administered intravenously, starting with a bolus of 15 mg, followed by a rapid infusion of 50 mg over 30 minutes and a slower infusion of up to 35 mg over 60 minutes.[3,4] The rate of patency (Thrombolysis in Myocardial Infarction [TIMI] 2-3 flow) at 90 minutes is approximately 75% to 80%; full perfusion (TIMI-3 flow) occurs in approximately 55% of patients using a front-loaded regimen.[5] **Table 4.1** summarizes the pharmacokinetic profile of alteplase. The plasma half-life is short, on the order of 4 to 8 minutes, and has a high degree of clot selectivity, leading to sparing of physiologic

FIGURE 4.2 — CHEMICAL STRUCTURE OF TISSUE PLASMINOGEN ACTIVATOR

Domains and other molecular features: 1) finger domain, 2) growth factor domain, 3) kringle 1 domain, 4) kringle 2 domain, 5) peptide bond 275-276, 6) protease domain, 7) glycosylation sites, 8) carboxy terminus, 9) amino terminus.

Tissue plasminogen activator (tPA) is a serine protease containing 527 amino acids, with a finger and growth factor domain, 2 kringles, a protease domain, and numerous glycosylation sites and peptide bonds.

clotting mechanisms and a mild degree of fibrinogen depletion. Intracranial hemorrhage occurs in 0.5% to 1% of patients, and major (nonintracranial) bleeding in approximately 5%.[3] Clinical reocclusion occurs in approximately 10% of patients. Alteplase has been evaluated in randomized trials involving over 100,000 patients, with documented reductions in mortality and infarct size and improved left ventricular function. Antithrombotic therapy with intravenous (IV) unfractionated heparin (UFH) at a dose of 60 U/kg (maximum 4000 U) as a bolus, 12 U/kg/hr (maximum 1000 U) should be initiated simultaneously with tPA, with a target activated partial thromboplastin time (aPTT) of 50 to 70 seconds.[3] Antiplatelet therapy with aspirin (or clopidogrel in cases of true aspirin allergy) should also be given prior to IV infusion of alteplase. Enhanced antiplatelet therapy with GP IIb/IIIa receptor inhibitors has provided

FIGURE 4.3 — MECHANISM OF ACTION OF TISSUE PLASMINOGEN ACTIVATOR

Tissue plasminogen activator (tPA) preferentially binds to fibrin, undergoing a conformational change that increases its ability to convert plasminogen (PLGN) to plasmin (PLN) up to 1000-fold.

encouraging angiographic results with TIMI-3 flow rates of 80%.[6,7] The combined administration of tPA and enoxaparin is also an attractive alternative due to ease of use, consistency of antithrombotic effect, and improved clinical outcome.[3] A large phase 3 clinical trial (TIMI 25, the EXTRACT Trial) is under way to evaluate the combination of enoxaparin with fibrinolytic agents.

Streptokinase

Streptokinase (SK) is a bacterial protein secreted by group C β-hemolytic streptococci. It was the first fibrinolytic agent developed for clinical use, with reports of clinical benefit in lysing clots within the pleural space >50 years ago, and the first description of use for myocardial infarction (MI) was in 1954.[8] SK itself does not possess protease activity but must first bind to plasminogen, forming an activator complex, which can then convert plasminogen to plasmin (**Figure 4.4**). The circulating half-life of SK is approximately 20 minutes. Because SK possesses only a modest degree of fibrin specificity, it activates both clot-bound

TABLE 4.1 — CLINICAL FEATURES OF ESTABLISHED FIBRINOLYTIC AGENTS

Feature	SK	APSAC	tPA	rPA	TNKase
Half-life (minutes)	25	100	6	15	20
Method of administration	1-hr IV	Bolus	1.5-hr IV	2 boluses	Bolus
Dose	1.5 mU/60 min	30 mg in 5 min	15 mg bolus, up to 85 mg/90 min	10+10 MU over 30 min	0.55 mg/kg over 5-10 sec
Action	Indirect	Indirect	Direct	Direct	Direct
Fibrin specificity	NA	NA	++	+	+++
90 min patency rates (%)	~50	~65	~75	~75	~75
90-min TIMI 3 flow (%)	~30	~50	~60	~60	~60
Mortality rate* (%)	7.3	10.5	7.2	6.0	6.0
Allergic reactions[†]	Yes	Yes	No	No	No
ICH rates (%)	0.3	0.7	0.8	0.8	0.8
Cost ($US)	568	1700	2750	2750	2750

Abbreviations: APSAC, anisoylated plasminogen-streptokinase activator complex; ICH, intracranial hemorrhage; IV, intravenous; mU, milliunit; MU, megaunit; NA, not applicable; rPA, reteplase; SK, streptokinase; TIMI, Thrombosis in Myocardial Infarction; TNKase, tenecteplase; tPA, alteplase.

* In most recent comparative trials.
† Hypotension most common.

FIGURE 4.4 — THE STREPTOKINASE-PLASMINOGEN ACTIVATOR COMPLEX

Abbreviations: FBGN, fibrinogen; FDP, fibrinogen degradation product.

Streptokinase (SK) combines with plasminogen (PLGN) to form an activator complex that converts free plasminogen to plasmin (PLN).

plasminogen and circulating plasminogen. Free plasmin generated is rapidly inactivated by α_2-antiplasmin; however, once the capacity of this inhibitor is exhausted, residual plasmin continues to degrade circulating fibrinogen and other components of the clotting cascade, creating a systemic "lytic" state, which increases the risk of serious bleeding and complicates the performance of invasive procedures. On a more positive note, the systemic depletion of clotting factors provides a sustained (approximately 24 hours) anticoagulant effect that reduces the risk of coronary reocclusion. Regeneration of fibrinogen and other clotting factors through hepatic synthesis occurs over the subsequent 24 to 48 hours.[9]

Streptokinase is administered at a dose of 1.5 million U given IV over 1 hour. Patency (TIMI 2 or 3 flow) occurs in approximately 60% of patients at 90 minutes, increasing to 80% to 90% by 24 hours. Full reperfusion, TIMI-3 flow, occurs in 35% of patients at 90 minutes, as demonstrated in the Global Use of Strategies to Open Occluded Arteries (GUSTO) IIb angiographic substudy.[5] Numerous randomized clinical trials have demonstrated the ability of SK to reduce mortality, particularly when treatment is rendered within 6 hours of symptom onset. The landmark Gruppo Italiano per lo Studio della Streptochinasi nell'Infarcto Miocardio (GISSI) trial[10] demonstrated a 47% reduction in mortality when SK was administered within the first hour of symptom onset. Clinical benefits with SK are substantially enhanced with the addition of aspirin[3] at a dose of 160 mg to 325 mg daily, as demonstrated in the International Study of Infarct Survival (ISIS)-2 trial.[11] In patients at low risk for thromboemboli, antithrombotic therapy with subcutaneous heparin can be administered at a dose of 7500 to 15,000 U every 12 hours (see Chapter 13, *Acute Myocardial Infarction*), while patients at high risk for thromboemboli should receive IV heparin started 6 hours after SK therapy, when the aPTT declines to ≤60 seconds. The initial infusion rate should not exceed 1000 U/hr. After 48 hours, options include a change to subcutaneous heparin, warfarin, or aspirin alone.[3]

Adverse reactions to SK include bleeding, hypotension, and allergic reactions. Hemorrhage occurs in approximately 5% to 10% of patients who do not undergo invasive procedures and in 15% to 20% of those who do. Serious bleeding occurs in 2% of patients, and intracranial hemorrhage is observed at a rate of approximately 0.5%.[3,4,9] Transient hypotension occurs commonly (in 30% to 50% of patients) particularly when the SK infusion exceeds 750,000 U over 30 minutes. Because SK is a foreign protein, allergic reactions can and do occur in 2% to 5% of patients. Anaphylaxis, however, is rare (<0.3%).[9] Readministration of SK is not recommended between 5 days and 1 to 2 years of initial use or after recent streptococcal infection because of the high incidence of neutralizing antibodies, leading to reduced fibrinolytic activity or allergic reactions.[9]

Anistreplase

Anisoylated plasminogen-streptokinase activator complex (APSAC), also known as anistreplase, is a stoichiometric complex containing a 1:1 ratio of SK and human blood–derived lys-plasminogen to which a para-anisoyl group has been added to "mask" the active enzymatic site. When reconstituted, APSAC deanisoylates within 30 minutes to form SK-plasminogen activator, which itself degrades to SK and plasminogen, leading to a short (30-minute) shelf life.

Anistreplase is administered as a 30-U bolus given over 5 minutes, which corresponds approximately to 1.1 million U of SK. In the circulation, gradual hydrolysis of the anisoyl group exposes the catalytic site of the complex, leading to generation of plasmin from plasminogen (**Figure 4.5**). The circulating half-life is approximately 90 minutes. The inactive, acyl form of the drug is thought to attenuate the generation of bradykinin, largely responsible for the hypotension seen with SK.[12] Patency rates after anistreplase are slightly higher than with SK, in the range of 75%, with full perfusion (TIMI grade 3) in approximately 50% of patients. Several large randomized trials have demonstrated reduction in mortality, improvement in left ventricular ejection fraction, and reduction in infarct size with anistreplase.[12]

The largest comparative mortality trial, ISIS-3,[13] demonstrated similar mortality outcomes for SK and anistreplase. Adverse reactions, such as bleeding, hypotension, and allergic reactions, occur with similar frequency to those following SK administration. The recommendations for the conjunctive administration of aspirin and heparin parallel those for SK.

Third-Generation Fibrinolytics

Novel plasminogen activators have been designed with one or more of the following properties:
- Enhanced fibrin specificity
- A prolonged half-life, permitting bolus administration
- Resistance to natural inhibitors such as plasminogen-activator inhibitor-1 (PAI-1).

Reteplase (rPA), tenecteplase (TNK-tPA), lanoteplase, saruplase (single-chain urokinase plasminogen activator), and staphylokinase all represent third-generation fibrinolytic

FIGURE 4.5 — MECHANISM OF ACTION OF ANISTREPLASE

Abbreviations: APSAC, anisoylated plasminogen-streptokinase activator complex; FBGN, fibrinogen; FDP, fibrinogen degradation product; PLGN, plasminogen; PLN, plasmin; SK, streptokinase.

agents (**Tables 4.1** and **4.2**).[14] Lanoteplase, saruplase, and staphylokinase are not currently available in the United States.

■ Reteplase

Reteplase is a deletion mutant of tPA in which the finger and epidermal growth factor (EGF) domains and kringle 1 regions have been deleted, as have the carbohydrate side chains. Plasma clearance is prolonged to 18 minutes, due to reduced hepatic receptor binding and the lack of carbohydrate groups. Fibrin specificity is reduced because of the deletion of the finger domain. Reteplase is administered in two 10-MU boluses 30 minutes apart. In two large randomized trials, reteplase produced mortality results similar to those with SK in the International Joint Efficiency Comparison of Thrombolytics (INJECT) trial[15] and no benefit over alteplase in the GUSTO III trial.[16] There is evidence that reteplase is associated with a higher incidence of

TABLE 4.2 — CLINICAL FEATURES OF NEWLY DEVELOPED FIBRINOLYTIC AGENTS				
Feature	**Lanoteplase**	**Staphylokinase**	**Saruplase**	
Method of administration	Bolus	2 boluses	1-hr IV	
Dose	120 KU/kg	15 + 15 mg	20-mg bolus; 60 mg over 1 hr	
Half-life (min)	23	6	9	
Action	Direct	Indirect	Direct	
Fibrin specificity	+	++++	+	
Antigenicity	NA	+	NA	
PAI-1 resistance	NA	NA	+	
Full perfusion (TIMI grade 3)				
60 min (%)	47	68	—	
90 min (%)	57	68	—	
Patency (TIMI grade 2/3)				
60 min (%)	—	84	76	
90 min (%)	83	84	80	
Abbreviations: IV, intravenous; NA, not applicable; PAI-1, plasminogen-activator inhibitor-1; TIMI, Thrombolysis in Myocardial Infarction.				

reocclusion than alteplase, due to decreased fibrin specificity and greater platelet activation. Potent antiplatelet agents such as GPIIb/IIIa receptor antagonists may enhance the effectiveness of rPA.[17,18] The GUSTO V trial demonstrated similar 30-day mortality rates for full-dose rPA and half-dose rPA combined with abciximab (5.9% and 5.6%, respectively); however, reinfarction and urgent revascularization occurred less often with combination therapy.[19] Intracranial hemorrhage rates were particularly high in patients >75 years of age, suggesting that this combination (at least in the doses given) may not be optimal for all patients with acute MI (**Figure 4.6**).

■ Tenecteplase

Tenecteplase is a genetically engineered point-and-deletion mutant of tPA. The amino acid substitutions and altered glycosylation sites result in a 4-fold reduction in plasma clearance, a 14-fold increased fibrin specificity, and an 80-fold greater resistance to inactivation by PAI-1.[17] The long plasma half-life permits a single-push bolus (**Table 4.2**). Angiographic observations derived from the TIMI-10A and -10B trials suggested that tenecteplase achieved faster and more complete reperfusion than alteplase[18]; however, the Assessment of the Safety and Efficacy of a New Thrombolytic (ASSENT)-2 trial comparing TNK-tPA and alteplase in 16,000 patients demonstrated equivalent outcomes, with a lower risk of bleeding associated with TNK-tPA.[20]

The ASSENT 3[21] trial has further characterized the benefits of tenecteplase in acute MI. In this trial, 6095 patients were randomly assigned to full-dose TNK-tPA with weight-adjusted UFH,[3] TNK-tPA with enoxaparin, or reduced-dose TNK-tPA with abciximab. Mortality at 30 days was similar among the three treatment groups (6.6%, 5.4%, and 6%, respectively), with a trend toward lower mortality in the TNK-tPA plus enoxaparin group (**Figure 4.6**). There were significantly fewer cumulative efficacy end points in the enoxaparin and abciximab groups (11.4% and 11.1%) than in the UFH group (15.4%). Similar to observations made in GUSTO V, intracranial hemorrhage occurred more frequently in patients over the age of 75 who received the combination of a fibrinolytic agent and abciximab.

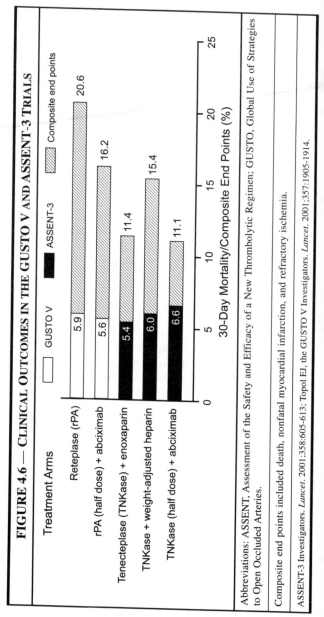

FIGURE 4.6 — CLINICAL OUTCOMES IN THE GUSTO V AND ASSENT-3 TRIALS

Treatment Arms

□ GUSTO V   ■ ASSENT-3   ▨ Composite end points

Treatment Arm	GUSTO V / ASSENT-3	Composite end points
Reteplase (rPA)	5.9	20.6
rPA (half dose) + abciximab	5.6	16.2
Tenecteplase (TNKase) + enoxaparin	5.4	11.4
TNKase + weight-adjusted heparin	6.0	15.4
TNKase (half dose) + abciximab	6.6	11.1

30-Day Mortality/Composite End Points (%)

Abbreviations: ASSENT, Assessment of the Safety and Efficacy of a New Thrombolytic Regimen; GUSTO, Global Use of Strategies to Open Occluded Arteries.

Composite end points included death, nonfatal myocardial infarction, and refractory ischemia.

ASSENT-3 Investigators. *Lancet.* 2001;358:605-613; Topol EJ, the GUSTO V Investigators. *Lancet.* 2001;357:1905-1914.

These data suggest that enhanced speed and extent of thrombolysis is achievable by combining more effective antiplatelet therapy with reduced doses of fibrinolytic drugs. They also show that benefits and risks of combined pharmacotherapy vary in patient subgroups. Thus, given the cost of combination therapy and the increased risk of bleeding for patients >75 years of age, the administration of abciximab and reteplase or tenecteplase with reduced-dose heparin may be a reasonable option in selected patients with anterior infarct location, age <75 years, and a low risk for bleeding.[3] On the other hand, combining tPA or TNK-tPA with anticoagulants like enoxaparin appears to be a promising reperfusion regimen that also offers ease of administration.

■ **Lanoteplase**

Lanoteplase is a deletion-and-point mutant of wild-type tPA, in which the glycosylation sites in kringle 1 have been modified and the EGF and finger domains have been removed. It has a prolonged half-life of 37 minutes, reduced fibrin affinity, and improved thrombolytic efficacy in animal models (**Table 4.2**).[17] TIMI-3 flow rates at 60 and 90 minutes compare favorably with those of alteplase. However, a large randomized trial, Intravenous nPA Treatment of Infarcting Myocardium Early II (InTIME-2), while demonstrating similar mortality outcomes to accelerated tPA, also revealed a higher rate of intracranial hemorrhage in patients receiving lanoteplase. Further development of the agent has not taken place.

■ **Saruplase**

Saruplase, also known as single-chain urokinase plasminogen activator or prourokinase, is a naturally occurring GP prodrug that is rapidly converted into urokinase by plasmin but has some intrinsic plasminogen activating properties as well.[22] The half-life is very short, in the range of 7 to 8 minutes (**Table 4.2**). Saruplase produces a systemic "lytic" state as demonstrated by decreases in fibrinogen and α_2-antiplasmin and increased fibrinogen degradation products.[17,23,24] Several trials have revealed similar patency rates between saruplase and a 3-hour infusion regimen of tPA[24] and slightly lower mortality than with SK but at a cost of increased intracranial hemorrhage.[25] Future modifications of the compound include chimeric variants consisting of the two kringle domains of tPA and the serine protease domain of saruplase, as well as chemical modification of saruplase with cross-linking with antifibrin and antiplatelet antibodies, with the aim of increasing drug concentration at the site of thrombus formation.[17]

■ Staphylokinase

Staphylokinase, a 136-amino acid protein produced naturally by strains of *Staphylococcus aureus*, is currently synthesized using recombinant techniques. Like SK, it must form a stoichiometric 1:1 complex with plasminogen, which must then be activated by plasminogen activators. This agent has high fibrin specificity and a unique mechanism of action.[17,26] Like SK, staphylokinase triggers antibodies in most patients within 2 weeks after initial administration. Allergic reactions were not reported in the early clinical trials, possibly due to the low molecular weight of the staphylokinase molecule. Although several small, comparative trials with tPA were promising,[27] large-scale randomized trials will be needed to determine its overall clinical potential and safety.

Selection of an Optimal Reperfusion Strategy

Reperfusion of an occluded infarct-related coronary artery within 12 hours of the onset of symptoms should be performed rapidly following presentation to the hospital, utilizing either fibrinolytic therapy or primary angioplasty, usually with coronary stenting. A number of clinical trials have compared a strategy of prompt (<30 minute door-to-needle time) pharmacologic reperfusion with primary angioplasty, demonstrating a modest clinical benefit for angioplasty if the door-to-balloon inflation time is ≤90 minutes and the procedure is performed by an experienced invasive cardiologist at a hospital performing a moderately high volume of these procedures.[3] If the anticipated door-to-balloon time exceeds the door-to-needle time by >60 minutes, fibrinolytic therapy should be administered unless contraindicated

(**Table 4.3**). Transfer of an acute MI patient to a hospital capable of immediately performing angioplasty has been shown to be an effective strategy, provided initial presentation-to-balloon times can be lowered to ≤90 minutes.[28]

An alternative strategy is facilitated percutaneous coronary intervention (PCI), where an initial reduced dose of fibrinolytic therapy, a platelet GPIIb/IIIa inhibitor, or both are administered, followed by relatively urgent angioplasty. This approach offers the advantages of earlier time to reperfusion, higher TIMI flow in the infarct-related coronary artery, greater procedural success rates, and improved survival, but with the limitations of increased cost and bleeding.[3] Several clinical trials are currently assessing this reperfusion strategy. For patients who have contraindications for fibrinolytic therapy (**Table 4.3**) or for those <75 years of age with cardiogenic shock, primary angioplasty is superior to fibrinolytic therapy.[3,29]

Goals for Future Development of Fibrinolytic Agents

Strategies to achieve optimal outcomes with fibrinolytic therapy include:

- Earlier administration
- Better and more easily administered compounds
- Better conjunctive antithrombotic therapies, such as low molecular weight heparin, direct antithrombins, and/or GPIIb/IIIa receptor antagonists
- Reduced reocclusion and reinfarction rates
- Better selection of patients for facilitated revascularization
- Reduced reperfusion damage through the use of microcirculatory "protective" agents, such as neutrophil chemotaxis or adhesion antagonists.

Long-term approaches to treatment will include:

- Plaque-stabilizing agents
- Lipid-modifying agents
- Inflammatory response–modulating agents
- Angiotensin-converting enzyme inhibitors or angiotensin receptor blockers to attenuate left ventricular remodeling

73

TABLE 4.3 — CONTRAINDICATIONS AND CAUTIONS FOR FIBRINOLYTIC USE IN STEMI*

Absolute Contraindications
- Any prior intracranial hemorrhage
- Known structural cerebral vascular lesion (eg, arteriovenous malformation)
- Known malignant intracranial neoplasm (primary or metastatic)
- Ischemic stroke within 3 months *except* acute ischemic stroke within 3 hours
- Suspected aortic dissection
- Active bleeding or bleeding diathesis (excluding menses)
- Significant closed head trauma within 3 months

Relative Contraindications
- History of chronic severe, poorly controlled hypertension
- Severe uncontrolled hypertension on presentation (systolic blood pressure >180 mm Hg or diastolic blood pressure >110 mm Hg)†
- History of prior ischemic stroke >3 months, dementia, or known intracranial pathology not covered in contraindications
- Recent trauma (within 2 to 4 weeks), including head trauma or traumatic or prolonged (>10 minutes) CPR or major surgery (<3 weeks)
- Recent (within 2 to 4 weeks) internal bleeding
- Noncompressible vascular punctures
- For streptokinase/anistreplase: prior exposure (especially within 5 days to 2 years) or prior allergic reaction to these agents
- Pregnancy
- Active peptic ulcer
- Current use of anticoagulants; the higher the INR, the higher the risk of bleeding

Abbreviations: CPR, cardiopulmonary resuscitation; INR, international normalized ratio; STEMI, ST-segment–elevation myocardial infarction.

* Viewed as advisory for clinical decision making and may not be all inclusive or definitive.
† Could be an absolute contraindication in low-risk patients with myocardial infarction.

Antman EM, et al. *J Am Coll Cardiol.* 2003. In press.

- Defined pharmacologic approaches to prevent late sudden death.[14]

Further refinement of currently available fibrinolytics, either alone or in combination with anticoagulants and platelet antagonists, will be required as we maximize treatments for the new millennium.

REFERENCES

1. Collen D, Verstraete M. Alpha$_2$-antiplasmin consumption and fibrinogen breakdown during thrombolytic therapy. *Thromb Res*. 1979;14: 631-639.

2. Stump DC, Collen D. The Fibrinolytic System: Implications for Thrombolytic Therapy. In: Califf R, Mark D, Wagner G, ed. *Acute Coronary Care in the Thrombolytic Era*. Chicago, Ill: Year Book Medical Publishers, Inc; 1988.

3. Antman EM, Smith SC, Anbe DT, et al. ACC/AHA guidelines for the management of patients with ST-elevation myocardial infarction. A report of the American College of Cardiology/American Heart Association Task Force on Practice Guidelines (Committee on Management of Acute Myocardial Infarction). *J Am Coll Cardiol*. 2003. In press.

4. The GUSTO Investigators. An international randomized trial comparing four thrombolytic strategies for acute myocardial infarction. *N Engl J Med*. 1993;329:673-682.

5. The GUSTO Angiographic Investigators. The effects of tissue plasminogen activator, streptokinase, or both on coronary-artery patency, ventricular function, and survival after acute myocardial infarction [published correction appears in *N Engl J Med*. 1994;330:516]. *N Engl J Med*. 1993;329:1615-1622.

6. Antman EM, Giugliano RP, Gibson CM, et al for the TIMI-14 Investigators. Abciximab facilitates the rate and extent of thrombolysis: results of the thrombolysis in myocardial infarction (TIMI)-14 trial. *Circulation*. 1999;99:2720-2732.

7. Brener S. Presentation of INTRO-AMI Data. AHA Scientific Sessions, November 1999.

8. Sherry S. Personal reflections on the development of thrombolytic therapy and its application to acute coronary thrombosis. *Am Heart J*. 1981;102:1134-1138.

9. Anderson J, Smith B. Streptokinase in acute myocardial infarction. In: Anderson J, ed. *Modern Management of Myocardial Infarction in the Community Hospital*. New York, NY: Marcel Dekker; 1991:187-215.

10. Gruppo Italiano per lo Studio della Streptochinasi nell'Infarto Miocardico (GISSI). Effectiveness of intravenous thrombolytic treatment in acute myocardial infarction. *Lancet.* 1986;1:397-402.

11. ISIS-2 (Second International Study of Infarct Survival) Collaborative Group. Randomised trial of intravenous streptokinase, oral aspirin, both, or neither among 17,187 cases of suspected acute myocardial infarction: ISIS-2. *Lancet.* 1988;2:349-360.

12. Anderson, J. Review of anistreplase (APSAC) for acute myocardial infarction. In: Anderson J, ed. *Modern Management of Myocardial Infarction in the Community Hospital.* New York, NY: Marcel Dekker; 1991:149-185.

13. ISIS-3 (Third International Study of Infarct Survival) Collaborative Group. A randomised comparison of streptokinase vs tissue plasminogen activator vs anistreplase and of aspirin plus heparin vs aspirin alone among 41,299 cases of suspected acute myocardial infarction: ISIS-3. *Lancet.* 1992;339:753-770.

14. White HD, Van de Werf FJ. Thrombolysis for acute myocardial infarction. *Circulation.* 1998;97:1632-1646.

15. International Joint Efficacy Comparison of Thrombolytics. Randomised, double-blind comparison of reteplase double-bolus administration with streptokinase in acute myocardial infarction (INJECT): trial to investigate equivalence. *Lancet.* 1995;346:329-336.

16. The Global Use of Strategies to Open Occluded Coronary Arteries (GUSTO III) Investigators. A comparison of reteplase with alteplase for acute myocardial infarction. *N Engl J Med.* 1997;337:1118-1123.

17. Ross AM. New plasminogen activators: a clinical review. *Clin Cardiol.* 1999;22:165-171.

18. The SPEED Study Group. Trial of abciximab with and without low-dose reteplase for acute myocardial infarction. Strategies for Patency Enhancement in the Emergency Department (SPEED) Group. *Circulation.* 2000;101:2788-2794.

19. Topol EJ, The GUSTO V Investigators. Reperfusion therapy for acute myocardial infarction with fibrinolytic therapy or combination reduced fibrinolytic therapy and platelet glycoprotein IIb/IIIa inhibition: the GUSTO V randomised trial. *Lancet.* 2001;357:1905-1914.

20. Cannon CP, Gibson MC, McCabe CH. TNK-tissue plasminogen activator compared with front-loaded alteplase in acute myocardial infarction: results of the TIMI 10B trial. *Circulation.* 1998;98:2805-2814.

21. The Assessment of the Safety and Efficacy of a New Thrombolytic Regimen (ASSENT)-3 Investigators. Efficacy and safety of tenecteplase in combination with enoxaparin, abciximab, or unfractionated heparin: the ASSENT-3 randomised trial in acute myocardial infarction. *Lancet.* 2001;358:605-613.

22. Presentation of ASSENT-2 data at the AHA Meeting; November 1999; Atlanta, GA.

23. de Munk GAW, Ryken DC. Fibrinolytic properties of single-chain urokinase-type plasminogen activator (pro-urokinase). *Fibrinolysis.* 1990;4:1-9.

24. PRIMI Trial Study Group. Randomised double-blind trial of recombinant pro-urokinase against streptokinase in acute myocardial infarction. *Lancet.* 1989;1:863-868.

25. Bar FW, Meyer J, Vermeer F, et al for the SESAM Study Group. Comparison of saruplase and alteplase in acute myocardial infarction. The Study in Europe with Saruplase and Alteplase in Myocardial Infarction. *Am J Cardiol.* 1997;79:727-732.

26. Tebbe U, Michels R, Adgey J, et al for the Comparison Trial of Saruplase and Streptokinase (COMPASS) Investigators. Randomized, double-blind study comparing saruplase with streptokinase therapy in acute myocardial infarction: the COMPASS equivalence trial. *J Am Coll Cardiol.* 1998;31:487-493.

27. Collen D, Lijnen HR. Staphylokinase, a fibrin-specific plasminogen activator with therapeutic potential? *Blood.* 1994;84:680-686.

28. Anderson HR, Nielsen TT, Rasmussen K, et al for the DANAMI-2 Investigators. A comparison of coronary angioplasty with fibrinolytic therapy in acute myocardial infarction. *N Engl J Med.* 2003;349:733-742.

29. Hochman JS, Sleeper LA, Webb JG, et al. Early revascularization in acute myocardial infarction complicated by cardiogenic shock. SHOCK Investigators. Should We Emergently Revascularize Occluded Coronaries for Cardiogenic Shock? *N Engl J Med.* 1999;341:625-634.

4

5   Aspirin

The development of oral and intravenous (IV) pharmacologic agents that selectively attenuate platelet function for clinical use in patients with atherosclerotic vascular disease has contributed greatly to improved outcomes worldwide.

Aspirin, considered the prototypic platelet antagonist, has been available for over a century and currently represents a mainstay, both in the prevention and treatment of vascular events that include stroke, myocardial infarction (MI), peripheral vascular occlusion, and sudden death.

Mechanism of Action

Aspirin irreversibly acetylates cyclooxygenase (COX), impairing prostaglandin metabolism and thromboxane A_2 (TXA_2) synthesis. As a result, platelet aggregation in response to collagen, adenosine diphosphate (ADP), thrombin (in low concentrations), and TXA_2 is inhibited.[1,2]

Because aspirin more selectively inhibits COX-1 activity (found predominantly in platelets) than COX-2 activity (expressed in tissues following an inflammatory stimuli), its ability to prevent platelet aggregation is seen at relatively low doses, compared with the drug's potential anti-inflammatory effects, which require much higher doses.[3] As a result, the benefit derived from aspirin therapy more than likely represents an antithrombotic effect.

Several alternative mechanisms of platelet inhibition by aspirin have been proposed:
- Aspirin facilitates the inhibition of platelet activation by neutrophils
- Inhibition of prostacyclin synthesis in endothelial cells enhances nitric oxide production.

In addition, aspirin may prevent the progression of atherosclerosis by protecting low-density lipoprotein (LDL) cholesterol from oxidation and scavenging hydroxyl radicals.

Pharmacokinetics

Following oral ingestion, aspirin is rapidly absorbed in the proximal gastrointestinal (GI) tract (stomach, duodenum), achieving peak serum levels within 15 to 20 minutes and platelet inhibition within 40 to 60 minutes. As would be expected, enteric-coated preparations are less well absorbed, causing a delay in peak serum levels and platelet inhibition to 60 and 90 minutes, respectively. The antiplatelet effect occurs even before acetylsalicylic acid is detectable in peripheral blood, owing to platelet exposure in the portal circulation.

The plasma concentration of aspirin decays rapidly with a circulating half-life of approximately 20 minutes. Despite the drug's rapid clearance, platelet inhibition persists for the platelet's life span (7 ± 2 days) due to aspirin's irreversible inactivation of COX-1. Because 10% of circulating platelets are replaced every 24 hours, platelet activity (bleeding time, primary hemostasis) returns toward normal (≥50% activity) within 5 to 6 days of the last aspirin dose.[4] A single dose of 100 mg aspirin effectively reduces the production of TXA_2 in normal individuals.

Adverse Effects

The adverse-effect profile of aspirin in general and its associated risk for major hemorrhage in particular are determined largely by:

- Dose
- Duration of administration
- Associated structural (peptic ulcer disease, *Helicobacter pylori* infection) and hemostatic (inherited, acquired) abnormalities
- Concomitant use of other antithrombotic agents.

Thus aspirin is usually well tolerated when given in low doses (≤325 mg) for brief periods of time (6 to 8 weeks) to patients at low risk for bleeding complications. Unfortunately, a majority of conditions for which aspirin is considered the standard of care persist over time (eg, atherosclerotic vascular disease) necessitating prolonged periods of exposure. For this reason, aspirin, like all antithrombotic drugs that can also compromise hemostatic capacity, should only be given after a comprehensive evaluation of an individual patient's thrombotic and hemorrhagic risk has been established.

Enteric coating of aspirin has *not* been shown to reduce the likelihood of adverse effects involving the GI tract. Patients with gastric erosions or peptic ulcer disease who require treatment with aspirin should concomitantly receive a proton pump inhibitor to minimize the risk of hemorrhage.[5]

The impact of aspirin use on the hemodynamic properties of angiotensin-converting enzyme (ACE) inhibitors is a subject of considerable clinical relevance. Because COX-1 participates in prostaglandin production, which in turn, influences vascular tone, drugs with preferential COX-1 activity would be expected to interact with ACE inhibitors to a greater extent than COX-2 antagonists. The available evidence, derived from retrospective analyses, suggests that the antihypertensive and hemodynamic benefits are attenuated when doses of aspirin in excess of 100 mg are administered daily. This effect may be particularly important in patients with poor ventricular performance and clinical heart failure. In these settings, alternative vascular/hemodynamic (eg, angiotensin II receptor antagonist) and antithrombotic (eg, clopidogrel) therapies should be considered.

The interaction of aspirin and ACE inhibitors does not influence short-term outcome following acute MI,[6] but must be considered with prolonged coadministration, particularly in patients with poor left ventricular function and moderate to severe congestive heart failure. In this setting, the aspirin dose should be limited to ≤100 mg.

Clinical Efficacy

Aspirin's beneficial effect is determined largely by the absolute risk of vascular events. Patients at low risk (healthy individuals without predisposing risk factors for vascular disease) derive minimal benefit, while those at high risk (unstable angina, prior MI, stroke) derive considerable benefit (**Figure 5.1**).[7] A risk-based approach to aspirin administra-

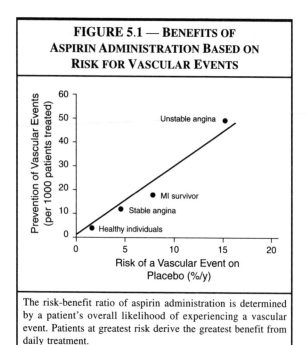

FIGURE 5.1 — BENEFITS OF ASPIRIN ADMINISTRATION BASED ON RISK FOR VASCULAR EVENTS

The risk-benefit ratio of aspirin administration is determined by a patient's overall likelihood of experiencing a vascular event. Patients at greatest risk derive the greatest benefit from daily treatment.

Patrono C, et al. *Chest.* 2001;119(suppl 1):49S.

tion is recommended to avoid subjecting individuals who are unlikely to benefit from aspirin administration to its potential adverse effects (**Table 5.1**).

Primary Prevention

Aspirin has been evaluated in three primary prevention trials involving over 30,000 healthy individuals.[8-10] A fourth trial confirmed the benefit of low-dose aspirin in patients with hypertension.[11] The Women's Health Initiative is evaluating the effects of low-dose aspirin prophylaxis (100 mg every other day) in 40,000 healthy women.

Considered collectively, the data show convincingly that aspirin reduces the likelihood of MI but at a cost of increased risk for hemorrhagic complications, including stroke. With increasing patient risk (for thrombotic events),

TABLE 5.1 — RECOMMENDATIONS FOR ASPIRIN ADMINISTRATION

Clinical Setting	Recommendation
Primary prevention	Not indicated unless risk factors exist*
Treatment of acute MI, unstable angina, ischemic stroke	Risk factors*: 75-162.5 mg/d; initial therapy: 162.5-325 mg; subsequent dose: 75-162.5 mg/d
Secondary prevention: chronic stable angina, MI, stroke, TIA	Daily therapy 75-325 mg

Abbreviations: MI, myocardial infarction; TIA, transient ischemic attack.

* Risk factors: men and women >50 years of age who have at least one major risk factor for coronary artery disease (cigarette smoking, hypertension, diabetes mellitus, high cholesterol level, history of parental MI).

additional benefit is gained, improving net clinical benefit. The potential role of clopidogrel as primary prevention for cardiovascular events is undergoing investigation.

Secondary Prevention

The Antiplatelet Trialist Collaboration update[12] included 287 studies involving 135,640 high-risk (acute or previous vascular disease or other predisposing condition) patients in comparisons of antiplatelet therapy vs control and 77,000 in comparisons of different antiplatelet regimens. The analysis extended the direct evidence of benefit from antiplatelet therapy to a much wider range of patients at high risk of occlusive vascular disease.[12]

Overall, 7705 (10.7%) serious vascular events were recorded among 71,912 high-risk patients allocated antiplatelet vs an adjusted total of 9502 (13.2%) among 72,139 allocated control (22% odds reduction; $P = 0.0001$). Antiplatelet therapy was associated with a highly significant 15% proportional reduction in vascular deaths ($P = 0.0001$)

(without heterogeneity between the high-risk groups); all-cause mortality (P <0.0001), nonfatal MI (34% odds reduction; I <0.001), nonfatal MI or death from coronary heart disease (26% odds reduction, P <0.001) and stroke (25% odds reduction, P <0.001). Overall, the proportional risk of experiencing a major intracranial hemorrhage was increased 50% with antiplatelet therapy (odds ratio 1.6). The proportional increase in fatal hemorrhage was not significantly different from that for nonfatal hemorrhage, although only the excess of nonfatal hemorrhagic events achieved statistical significance.

Among 18,788 patients with a history of MI, allocation to a mean duration of antiplatelet therapy of 27 months resulted in 36 fewer serious vascular events per 1000 patients (25% odds reduction; P <0.001). This benefit reflects large and highly significant reductions in nonfatal MI (18 fewer per 1000; P <0.0006), as well as a smaller, but still significant, reduction in nonfatal stroke (5 fewer per 1000; P <0.002). The overall benefits were larger than the excess risk of major extracerebral hemorrhage (3 per 1000 or 1 per 1000 patients per year) (**Figure 5.2**).

Data were available on 19,288 patients with suspected acute MI. Allocation to a mean treatment duration of 1 month of antiplatelet therapy led to a 30% odds reduction in vascular events (38 fewer serious vascular events per 1000 patients treated) (P <0.001). This reflects large and highly significant reductions in nonfatal reinfarction (13 fewer per 1000; P <0.0001) and in vascular death (23 fewer per 1000; P <0.0001), together with a smaller, but still significant, reduction in nonfatal stroke (2 fewer per 1000; P = 0.02). The risk of major extracranial bleeding was approximated at 1 to 2 per 100 patients treated.

Patients with prior aspirin use who experience an acute coronary syndrome, "aspirin failures," are at particularly high risk for MI and death over the ensuing weeks to months, suggesting a stimulus for thrombosis that overcomes the modest inhibitory potential of aspirin. Combination therapy that includes a platelet ADP antagonist (eg, clopidogrel) makes sound clinical sense in such individuals (**Figure 5.3**).[13]

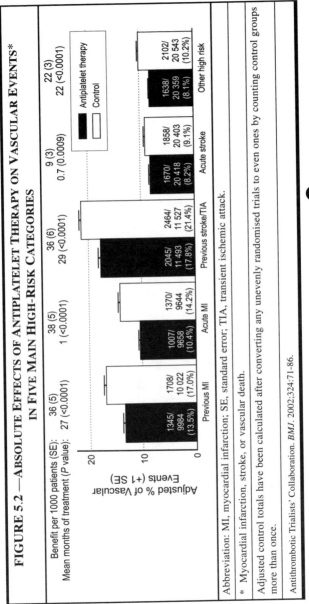

FIGURE 5.2 —ABSOLUTE EFFECTS OF ANTIPLATELET THERAPY ON VASCULAR EVENTS* IN FIVE MAIN HIGH-RISK CATEGORIES

Abbreviation: MI, myocardial infarction; SE, standard error; TIA, transient ischemic attack.

* Myocardial infarction, stroke, or vascular death.

Adjusted control totals have been calculated after converting any unevenly randomised trials to even ones by counting control groups more than once.

Antithrombotic Trialists' Collaboration. *BMJ.* 2002;324:71-86.

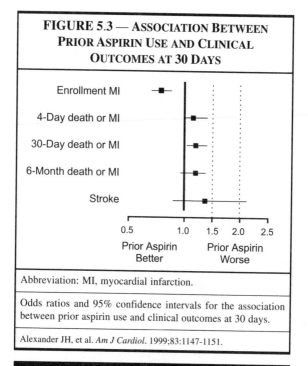

FIGURE 5.3 — ASSOCIATION BETWEEN PRIOR ASPIRIN USE AND CLINICAL OUTCOMES AT 30 DAYS

Enrollment MI

4-Day death or MI

30-Day death or MI

6-Month death or MI

Stroke

0.5 1.0 1.5 2.0 2.5

Prior Aspirin Better   Prior Aspirin Worse

Abbreviation: MI, myocardial infarction.

Odds ratios and 95% confidence intervals for the association between prior aspirin use and clinical outcomes at 30 days.

Alexander JH, et al. *Am J Cardiol.* 1999;83:1147-1151.

Aspirin Dosing

The updated meta-analysis[12] provides additional information on the effects of different doses of aspirin. Overall, among 3570 patients in three trials directly comparing aspirin (≥75 mg daily vs aspirin <75 mg daily), there were significant differences in vascular events (two trials compared 75 to 325 mg aspirin daily vs <75 mg daily and one trial compared 500 to 1500 mg aspirin daily vs <75 mg daily). Considering both direct and indirect comparisons of aspirin dose, the proportional reduction in vascular events was 19% with 500 to 1500 mg daily, 26% with 160 to 325 mg daily, and 32% with 75 to 150 mg daily. Whether the greater reductions observed with decreasing doses are clinically meaningful will require a large, randomized comparison of aspirin doses in patients with coronary heart disease. Similarly, the relative benefits for patients with non-ST–segment elevation ACS compared with other subsets must be more clearly defined through large-scale studies.

The effect of antiplatelet drugs other than aspirin (vs control) were assessed in 166 trials that included 81,731 patients. Indirect comparisons provided no clear evidence of differences in reducing serious vascular events (x^2 for heterogenicity between any aspirin regimen and other antiplatelet drugs = 10.8; NS). Most direct comparisons assessed the effects of replacing aspirin with another antiplatelet agent (**Figure 5.4**).

The effect of adding another antiplatelet drug to aspirin (vs aspirin alone) has been assessed in 43 trials including 39,205 patients. Overall, a 15% reduction in serious vascular events was observed ($P = 0.0001$). The benefit of combination therapy is supported by findings of the Clopidogrel in Unstable Angina to Prevent Recurrent Events (CURE) trial. The benefits of adding an IV glycoprotein (GP) IIb/IIIa receptor antagonist to aspirin were particularly evident among patients undergoing percutaneous coronary intervention (PCI).

Antiplatelet therapy is effective in reducing the number of vascular events in patients with evidence of atherosclerotic disease (acute MI, prior MI, unstable angina, stable angina, stroke, transient ischemic attack [TIA], or peripheral vascular disease). The benefits are consistent across all age ranges and risk profiles, with vascular events reduced by one fourth, nonfatal MI by one third, and vascular death by one fifth.

Coronary Artery Bypass Grafting

Patients undergoing coronary artery bypass surgery are unique for several reasons. First, a majority of patients have advanced coronary atherosclerosis. Second, many individuals have concomitant peripheral vascular and cerebrovascular disease. Last, new vascular conduits (bypass grafts) provide an additional nidus for atherothrombosis. Over the years, in excess of 20 clinical trials have been conducted to determine the effectiveness of antiplatelet therapy in preventing early (≤10 days) and late (6 to 12 months) saphenous vein graft occlusion. Ten of the trials investigated aspirin in doses ranging from 100 mg to 975 mg daily. Sev-

FIGURE 5.4 — INDIRECT COMPARISONS OF PROPORTIONAL EFFECTS OF DIFFERENT ANTIPLATELET REGIMENS ON VASCULAR EVENTS IN HIGH-RISK PATIENTS (EXCLUDING THOSE WITH ACUTE STROKE)

| Category of Trial Aspirin Alone (mg daily) | No of Trials With Data | No (%) of Vascular Events | | Observed-Expected | Variance | Odds Ratio (CI) Antiplatelet:Control | % Odds Reduction (SE) |
		Allocated Antiplatelet	Adjusted Control				
500-1500	34	1621/11,215 (14.5)	1930/11,236 (17.2)	-147.1	707.8		19 (3)
160-325	19	1526/13,240 (11.5)	1963/13,273 (14.8)	-219.9	742.6		26 (3)
75-150	12	366/3370 (10.9)	517/3406 (15.2)	-72.0	183.8		32 (6)
<75	3	316/1827 (17.3)	354/1828 (19.4)	-18.9	136.5		13 (8)
Any aspirin*	65	3829/29,652 (12.9)	4764/29,743 (16.0)	-452.3	1717.0		23 (2)
Other Antiplatelet Drugs							
Dipyridamole	15	392/2696 (14.5)	458/2734 (16.8)	-30.9	173.0		16 (7)
Sulfinpyrazone	19	315/2411 (13.1)	361/2416 (14.9)	-23.8	140.7		16 (8)
Ticlopidine	42	278/3435 (8.1)	385/3475 (11.1)	-50.5	132.3		32 (7)
Suloctidil	6	47/364 (12.9)	59/367 (16.1)	-5.6	20.5		24 (19)

	Trials	Antiplatelet	Control	O−E	Variance		% Odds reduction (SD)
Picotamide	4	41/1583 (2.6)	66/1602 (4.1)	−12.2	25.8		38(16)
Sulotroban	4	8/406 (2.0)	14/409 (3.4)	−3.2	5.3		45(33)
Triflusal	2	10/314 (3.2)	19/309 (6.1)	−4.7	6.7		50(28)
Other†	9	41/647 (6.3)	73/641 (11.4)	−16.1	25.6		47(15)
Any other single agent	101	1132/11,856 (9.5)	1435/11,953 (12.0)	−147.0	529.9		24(4)
Aspirin + Another Antiplatelet Drug							
Aspirin + dipyridamole	46	1036/9703 (10.7)	1393/9738 (14.3)	−172.6	488.7		30(4)
Aspirin + sulfinpyrazone	2	38/283 (13.4)	50/278 (18.0)	−6.5	18.5		30(20)
Any combination	48	1074/9986 (10.8)	1443/10,016 (14.4)	−179.1	507.2		30(4)
All Trials	**188**	**6035/51,494 (11.7)**	**7644/51,736 (14.8)**	**−715.7**	**2449.6**		**25(2)**

Treatment effect P <0.0001

0 0.5 1.0 1.5 2.0
Better ←— Antiplatelet —→ Worse

Only meta-analyses involving 500 or more high-risk patients are shown. Stratified ratio of odds of an event in treatment groups to that in control groups is plotted for each group of trials (*black square*) along with its 99% confidence interval (CI) (*horizontal line*). Meta-analysis of results for each main comparison and for all trials (and 95% CI) is represented by an *open diamond*. Adjusted control totals have been calculated after converting any unevenly randomized trials to even ones by counting control groups more than once, but statistical calculations are based on actual numbers from individual trials. Heterogeneity of odds reductions between: (1) different aspirin doses: $\chi^2 = 7.7$, df = 3; $P = 0.05$; (2) other antiplatelet vs any aspirin: $\chi^2 = 10.8$, df = 8; $P > 0.1$.

* Some trials contributed to more than one comparison.
† Includes indobufen, flurbiprofen, GR32191B, dazoxiben, and trapidil.

Antithrombotic Trialist's Collaboration. *BMJ.* 2002;324:71-86.

5

eral also evaluated patients receiving internal mammary coronary bypass grafts.[14-19]

Considered collectively, and aided by the Antiplatelet Trialists' Collaboration overview, the data reveal improved saphenous vein graft patency with aspirin administration. Although a direct benefit on internal mammary bypass grafts has not been established, treatment is recommended given the common coexistence of vascular disease (and the risk of thrombotic events). A majority of evidence supporting the use of aspirin after bypass grafting is based on clinical trials using a dose of at least 325 mg daily. Accordingly, the benefit derived from lower doses is less well established. Patients unable to take aspirin should be given clopidogrel 300 mg (loading dose) 24 hours after surgery followed by 75 mg daily.

Transient Ischemic Attacks/Stroke

The International Stroke Trial[20] and the Chinese Acute Stroke Trial[21] evaluated the efficacy and safety of aspirin given in a daily dose of 300 mg and 160 mg, respectively, in nearly 40,000 patients with acute ischemic stroke. Treatment was initiated within 48 hours of symptom onset and continued for 2 to 4 weeks. The combined results suggest an absolute benefit of 10 fewer deaths or nonfatal strokes per 1000 patients in the first month of treatment. The risk of hemorrhagic stroke was also increased (two excess events per 1000 patients).

Long-term aspirin administration reduces the likelihood of stroke (and other vascular events) in patients with TIAs and completed minor strokes.[22] Although there is an ongoing debate within the neurology community concerning the optimal daily dose, 75 mg to 325 mg is considered an acceptable range.

In the Clopidogrel versus Aspirin in Patients at Risk of Ischemic Events (CAPRIE) study, clopidogrel reduced the likelihood of ischemic strokes.

The ongoing Management of Atherothrombosis with Clopidogrel in High-Risk Patients with Recent Transient Ischemic Attack or Ischemic Stroke (MATCH) trial will evaluate combination (clopidogrel plus aspirin) versus mono (aspirin) therapy. A total of 9,600 patients will be followed for at least 18 months for a composite end point of ischemic stroke, MI, vascular death, or rehospitalization for an acute ischemic event. The patient population and trial design acknowledge the diffuse nature of atherothrombotic vascular disease and potential benefit of multi-targeted, platelet-directed therapy.

The combination of aspirin 25 mg and extended-release dipyridamole 200 mg bid is more effective than aspirin alone for the prevention of stroke. Patients unable to take aspirin should be treated with clopidogrel 75 mg daily.

Percutaneous Coronary Intervention

PCI, including standard balloon angioplasty, rotational atherectomy, and laser angioplasty, with or without stent placement, is associated with vascular injury, atheromatous plaque disruption, platelet activation, and at times, coronary thromboembolism. Several studies performed over the past decade have documented reduced periprocedural complications, including thrombus formation, abrupt closure, and MI, with antiplatelet therapy given prior to PCI (relative risk reduction, 60%).[23,24]

The current recommendations for PCI include aspirin 80 to 325 mg pretreatment followed by long-term administration 80 to 325 mg daily for secondary prevention of cardiovascular events; for patients unable to tolerate aspirin, pretreatment with clopidogrel 300 mg followed by 75 mg daily is suggested. Aspirin desensitization should be considered if true aspirin allergy is documented, given the potential for benefit.

The Importance of Aspirin Resistance

Aspirin's ability to inhibit platelet aggregation is discordant, and upward of 30% of individuals either are nonresponders or exhibit a paradoxic increase in platelet aggregation and activation following high-dose (325 mg) administration.

Nearly a century ago, Duke reported that patients with anemia and thrombocytopenia experienced a shortening of their bleeding time following transfusion, raising the possibility that platelet behavior is influenced directly by eryth-

91

rocytes.[25] *In vitro*, erythrocytes augment platelet activation through several mechanisms, including:

- Physical interactions
- ADP-mediated agonists
- Facilitated TXA_2 production.

The interplay between erythrocytes and platelets has important clinical implications with regard to aspirin dosing. Low-dose aspirin (80 mg) inhibits TXA_2 production; however, the relationship between TXA_2 concentration and platelet activation is nonlinear, suggesting one or more alternative pathways of platelet activation that include thrombin, serotonin, and platelet-activating factor. Erythrocytes can activate platelets in the presence of low-dose aspirin, but Santos and colleagues have shown that the acute administration of higher doses (500 mg) suppresses residual red blood cell–facilitated platelet function.[26]

Thromboxane A_2, a potent platelet agonist, must be suppressed by ≥90% for complete inhibition. Aspirin's ability to reduce COX activity varies considerably among individuals and, in addition, atherosclerosis is associated with increased tissue level expression due to cytokine-mediated induction. It is important to recognize an acquired form of aspirin resistance that is induced by concomitant administration of ibuprofen.[27] Genetic polymorphisms and resulting gene expression of COX and thromboxane synthase could limit aspirin effectiveness (**Figure 5.5**).[28] Last, the concomitant use of nonsteroidal anti-inflammatory agents, particularly ibuprofen, is a recognized cause for acquired aspirin resistance.

Clinical Impact of Aspirin Resistance and Failures

Despite its proven benefit, aspirin does have inherent limitations. A critical review of the existing literature reveals a sizable proportion of events in patients receiving aspirin. If one were to adopt a "half-empty" view toward aspirin, between 60% and 70% of patients experience MI, stroke, or cardiovascular death during periods of treatment (**Table 5.2**). Thus aspirin resistance has clear clinical relevance in current practice.[29]

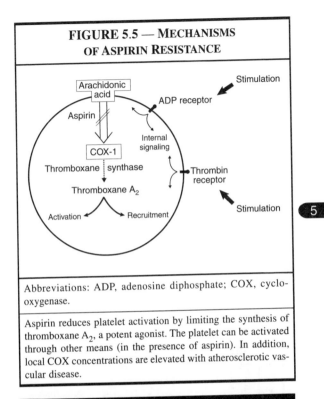

FIGURE 5.5 — MECHANISMS OF ASPIRIN RESISTANCE

Abbreviations: ADP, adenosine diphosphate; COX, cyclo-oxygenase.

Aspirin reduces platelet activation by limiting the synthesis of thromboxane A_2, a potent agonist. The platelet can be activated through other means (in the presence of aspirin). In addition, local COX concentrations are elevated with atherosclerotic vascular disease.

Summary

Aspirin is a time-tested platelet antagonist that is widely available, inexpensive, and well tolerated, even with long-term administration.[30] High-risk patients enjoy the greatest overall benefit, with a relative reduction in major vascular-event rates approaching 25% to 30%. The discordant effects of aspirin on platelet aggregation, aspirin resistance, aspirin failures, and the added benefit of combined pharmacotherapy must be investigated through large-scale clinical trials.

TABLE 5.2 — THE STRENGTHS AND WEAKNESSES OF ASPIRIN THERAPY			
Patient Group	Relative Risk Reduction (%)*	Absolute Risk Reduction (n)†	Majority of Patients Remain at Risk
Chronic stable angina	33	45	Yes
Unstable angina	39	50	Yes
Acute myocardial infarction	29	38	Yes
Post-myocardial infarction	25	36	Yes

* Effect on major vascular events.
† Per 1000 patients.

REFERENCES

1. Roth GJ, Majerus PW. The mechanism of the effect of aspirin on human platelets. I. Acetylation of a particulate fraction protein. *J Clin Invest.* 1975;56:624-632.

2. Burch JW, Stanford N, Majerus PW. Inhibition of platelet prostaglandin synthetase by oral aspirin. *J Clin Invest.* 1978;61:314-319.

3. Patrono C. Aspirin as an antiplatelet drug. *N Engl J Med.* 1994;330: 1287-1294.

4. O'Brien JR. Effects of salicylates on human platelets. *Lancet.* 1968;1:779-783.

5. Hawkey CJ, Karrasch JA, Szczepañski L, et al. Omeprazole compared with misoprostol for ulcers associated with nonsteroidal anti-inflammatory drugs. Omeprazole versus Misprostol for NSAID-induced Ulcer Management (OMNIUM) Study Group. *N Engl J Med.* 1998;338: 727-734.

6. Latini R, Tognoni G, Maggioni AP, et al. Clinical effects of early angiotensin-converting enzyme inhibitor treatment for acute myocardial infarction are similar in the presence and absence of aspirin: systemic overview of individual data from 96,712 randomized patients. Angiotensin-converting Enzyme Inhibitor Myocardial Infarction Collaborative Group. *J Am Coll Cardiol.* 2000;35:1801-1807.

7. Awtry EH, Loscalzo J. Aspirin. *Circulation.* 2000;101:1206-1218.

8. Steering Committee of the Physicians' Health Study Research Group. Final report on the aspirin component of the ongoing Physicians' Health Study. *N Engl J Med.* 1989;321:129-135.

9. The Medical Research Council's General Practice Research Framework. Thrombosis prevention trial: randomized trial of low intensity oral anticoagulation with warfarin and low-dose aspirin in the primary prevention of ischaemic heart disease in men at increased risk. *Lancet.* 1998;351:233-241.

10. Peto R, Gray R, Collins R, et al. Randomised trial of prophylactic daily aspirin in British male doctors. *Br Med J.* 1988;926:313-316.

11. Hansson L, Zanchetti A, Carruthers SG, et al. Effects of intensive blood-pressure lowering and low-dose aspirin in patients with hypertension: principal results of the Hypertension Optimal Treatment (HOT) randomised trial. HOT Study Group. *Lancet.* 1998;351:1755-1762.

12. Antiplatelet Trialists' Collaboration. Collaborative meta-analysis of randomised trials of antiplatelet therapy for prevention of death, myocardial infarction, and stroke in high risk patients. *BMJ.* 2002;324:71-86.

95

13. Alexander JH, Harrington RA, Tuttle RH, et al. Prior aspirin use predicts worse outcomes in patients with non-ST elevation acute coronary syndromes. PURSUIT Investigators. Platelet IIb/IIIa in Unstable angina: Receptor Suppression Using Integrilin Therapy. *Am J Cardiol.* 1999;83:1147-1151.

14. Lorenz RL, Schacky CV, Weber M, et al. Improved aortocoronary bypass patency by low-dose aspirin (100 mg daily). Effects of platelet aggregation and thromboxane formation. *Lancet.* 1984;1:1261-1264.

15. Hockings BE, Ireland MA, Gotch-Martin KF, Taylor RR. Placebo-controlled trial of enteric coated aspirin in coronary bypass graft patients. Effect on graft patency. *Med J Aust.* 1993;159:376-378.

16. Goldman S, Copeland J, Moritz T, et al. Improvement in early saphenous vein graft patency after coronary artery bypass surgery with antiplatelet therapy: results of a Veterans Administration Cooperative Study. *Circulation.* 1988;77:1324-1332.

17. Goldman S, Copeland J, Moritz T, et al. Internal mammary artery and saphenous vein graft patency. Effects of aspirin. *Circulation.* 1990;82(suppl):IV237-IV242.

18. van der Meer J, Brutel de la Riviere A, van Gilst WH, et al. Effects of low-dose aspirin (50 mg/day), low dose aspirin plus dipyridamole, and oral anticoagulant agents after internal mammary artery bypass grafting: patency and clinical outcome at 1 year. CABADAS Research Group of the Interuniversity Cardiology Institute of The Netherlands. Prevention of Coronary Artery Bypass Graft Occlusion by Aspirin, Dipyridamole and Acenocoumarol/Phenprocoumon Study. *J Am Coll Cardiol.* 1994;24:1181-1188.

19. Brown BG, Cukingnan RA, De Rouen T, et al. Improved graft patency in patients treated with platelet-inhibiting therapy after coronary bypass surgery. *Circulation.* 1985;72:138-146.

20. International Stroke Trial Collaborative Group. The International Stroke Trial (IST): a randomised trial of aspirin, subcutaneous heparin, both, or neither among 19,435 patients with acute ischaemic stroke. *Lancet.* 1997;349:1569-1581.

21. CAST (Chinese Acute Stroke Trial) Collaborative Group. CAST: randomised placebo-controlled trial of early aspirin use in 20,000 patients with acute ischaemic stroke. *Lancet.* 1997;349:1641-1649.

22. The SALT Collaborative Group. Swedish Aspirin Low-Dose Trial (SALT) of 75 mg aspirin as secondary prophylaxis after cerebrovascular ischaemic events. *Lancet.* 1991;338:1345-1349.

23. Barnathan ES, Schwartz JS, Taylor L, et al. Aspirin and dipyridamole in the prevention of acute coronary thrombosis complicating coronary angioplasty. *Circulation.* 1987;76:125-134.

24. Schwartz L, Bourassa MG, Lesperance J, et al. Aspirin and dipyridamole in the prevention of restenosis after percutaneous transluminal coronary angioplasty. *N Engl J Med*. 1988;318:1714-1719.

25. Duke WW. The relation of blood platelets to hemorrhagic disease. *JAMA*. 1983;250:1201-1209.

26. Santos MT, Valles J, Aznar J, Marcus AJ, Broekman MJ, Safier LB. Prothrombotic effects of erythrocytes on platelet reactivity. Reduction by aspirin. *Circulation*. 1997;95:63-68.

27. Catella-Lawson F, Reilly MP, Kapoor SC, et al. Cyclooxygenase inhibitors and the antiplatelet effects of aspirin. *N Engl J Med*. 2001;345:1809-1817.

28. Nair GV, Davis CJ, McKenzie ME, Lowry DR, Serebruany VL. Aspirin in patients with coronary artery disease: Is it simply irresistable? *J Thromb Thrombolysis*. 2001;11:117-126.

29. Eikelboom JW, Hirsch J, Weitz JI, Johnston M, Yi Q, Yusuf S. Aspirin-resistant thromboxane biosynthesis and the risk of myocardial infarction, stroke, or cardiovascular death in patients at high risk for cardiovascular events. *Circulation*. 2002;105:1650-1655.

30. Sixth American College of Chest Physicians. Conference on antithrombotic therapy. *Chest*. 2001;119(suppl 1):1S-370S.

5

6 Ticlopidine

Ticlopidine (Ticlid) is a thienopyridine derivative that is structurally and functionally distinct from most platelet antagonists.

In Vitro Effects

In vitro, ticlopidine is a weak inhibitor of platelet aggregation. Against low concentrations of collagen, arachidonic acid, or adenosine diphosphate (ADP), ticlopidine exhibits much less antiaggregative activity than aspirin.[1]

In addition to its modest *in vitro* platelet-inhibiting properties, ticlopidine:

- Attenuates endothelial cell growth
- Increases endothelial cell–associated von Willebrand's factor concentrations.[2]

Ex Vivo Effect on Platelet Function

After oral administration, ticlopidine becomes a concentration-dependent inhibitor of ADP-mediated platelet activation (granule release) aggregation.[3,4] With standard dosing, platelet inhibition is evident within 24 to 48 hours; however, peak effects are not produced for 3 to 6 days. The platelet-inhibiting effects of ticlopidine persist for 72 hours after the drug's discontinuation and progressive decline over the next 4 to 8 days. A synergistic effect on platelet inhibition has been reported with the combined administration of aspirin and ticlopidine.[5]

Although ticlopidine has lipophilic properties that can affect the fluidity of platelet membrane lipids, there is no evidence that it directly inhibits ADP binding. Ticlopidine does inhibit fibrinogen binding but does so without inducing a quantitative change in the surface glycoprotein (GP) IIb/IIIa receptor.[6]

Nonplatelet Effects

Ticlopidine binds to erythrocyte membranes and improves cellular deformability in response to shear stress. *In vitro*, ticlopidine dose-dependently inhibits platelet-mediated neutrophil activation, and in patients undergoing hemodialysis, reduces complement-mediated leukocyte trapping within the pulmonary circulation.[7]

Pharmacokinetics

Ticlopidine is well absorbed following oral administration, with peak plasma concentrations occurring within 1 to 3 hours. It is rapidly and extensively metabolized in the liver to one or more metabolites that are responsible for the drug's platelet-inhibiting properties.

Side Effects

Approximately 10% to 15% of patients receiving ticlopidine at the recommended dosage of 250 mg twice daily (taken with food) experience side effects, the most common of which are gastrointestinal complaints and skin rash. Bleeding is relatively uncommon but can occur. Cholestatic jaundice and hepatitis have also been reported.

Ticlopidine's hematologic side effects, including agranulocytosis, neutropenia, erythroleukemia, thrombocytopenia, and thrombotic thrombocytopenic purpura (TTP), are the most concerning and potentially life-threatening. The incidence of TTP peaks after 3 to 4 weeks of therapy, while neutropenia is most often seen following 4 to 6 weeks of exposure. Aplastic anemia has been reported 8 to 12 weeks after treatment initiation.

In an overview of 60 cases of TTP associated with ticlopidine administration, the drug had been taken for <1 month by 80% of patients and a normal platelet count was documented within 2 weeks of the disorder's onset.[8] A retrospective analysis of 43,322 patients undergoing coronary stenting at study sites participating in the Evaluation of Platelet GPIIb/IIIa Inhibitor for Stenting (EPISTENT) study disclosed an incidence of 1 case per 4,814 patients treated.[9]

Although an infrequent occurrence, the 0.02% incidence is noteworthy (and clinically relevant) when the estimated 0.0004% incidence in the general population is considered. Thus close monitoring of platelet counts is recommended, particularly if therapy is continued beyond 2 weeks.

Clinical Experience

The ability of ticlopidine to inhibit platelet aggregation in a dose-dependent manner, coupled with the synergistic effects observed when it is combined with aspirin, has led to a relatively large clinical experience that spans a variety of cardiovascular settings (**Tables 6.1** and **6.2**).

■ Coronary Artery Disease

Patients with coronary artery disease who are at risk for thrombotic events have been treated with ticlopidine, some for prolonged periods of time. A majority were either intolerant or allergic to aspirin. Despite an anecdotal experience, ticlopidine's use in the primary prevention of cardiovascular events has not been studied in large-scale randomized trials.

■ Stable Angina Pectoris

Several small-scale studies of patients with stable angina pectoris have been performed, each showing reduced platelet aggregation in response to ADP, collagen, and epinephrine following ticlopidine administration.[10] Despite a change in platelet responsiveness following exercise,[11] there was no clear impact on overall exercise tolerance or ischemic response.

■ Unstable Angina

In a multicenter trial of 652 patients admitted to the hospital with a diagnosis of unstable angina, conventional therapy (β-blocker, nitrates, calcium channel antagonists) plus ticlopidine 250 mg bid reduced the likelihood of vascular death or nonfatal myocardial infarction (MI) by nearly 50% compared with conventional therapy alone. The composite end point of fatal and nonfatal MI was reduced by >50%.[12]

TABLE 6.1 — RANDOMIZED CLINICAL TRIALS OF TICLOPIDINE IN PATIENTS WITH VASCULAR DISEASE

Trial/Investigator	Study Population	Patients (n)	Treatment
Stroke and TIA			
CATS	Recent stroke	1072	Ticlopidine 250 mg bid or placebo
TASS	Recent TIA or minor stroke	3069	Ticlopidine 250 mg bid or ASA 625 mg bid
TISS	Recent TIA, amaurosis fugax, or minor stroke	1632	Ticlopidine or indobufen (median doses, 250 and 200 mg bid, respectively)
PAOD			
Swedish Ticlopidine Multicentre Study	Intermittent claudication	687	Ticlopidine 250 mg bid or placebo
Arcan, et al	Chronic intermittent claudication	169	Ticlopidine 250 mg bid or placebo
EMATAP	Intermittent claudication	615	Ticlopidine 250 mg bid or placebo

Unstable Angina			
Balsano, et al	Unstable angina	652	Conventional therapy with or without ticlopidine 250 mg daily
SVG Patency			
Chevigne, et al	Coronary bypass surgery	77	Ticlopidine 250 mg bid (started 3 days before surgery) or placebo
Limet, et al	Coronary bypass surgery	173	Ticlopidine 250 mg bid (first dose on day 2) or placebo
Becquemin, et al	Femoropopliteal or femorofemoral bypass surgery	243	Ticlopidine 250 mg bid or placebo
Diabetic Retinopathy			
TMD	Nonproliferative diabetic retinopathy	435	Ticlopidine 250 mg bid or placebo

Abbreviations: ASA, aspirin; CATS, Canadian American Ticlopidine Study; EMATAP, Estudio Multicentrico Argentino de la Ticlopidine en las Arteriopatias Perifericas; PAOD, peripheral arterial occlusive disease; TASS, Ticlopidine Aspirin Stroke Study; TIA, transient ischemic attack; TISS, Ticlopidine Indobufen Stroke Study; TMD, Ticlopidine Microangiopathy of Diabetes; SVG, saphenous vein graft.

TABLE 6.2 — STUDY END POINTS OF RANDOMIZED CLINICAL TRIALS OF TICLOPIDINE IN PATIENTS WITH VASCULAR DISEASE

Study End Point	Follow-Up Duration	Ticlopidine Group Event Rate (%)	Comparison Group Event Rate (%)	P Value
Stroke, MI, or vascular death	Mean 2 years	11.3/y	14.8/y	0.02
Nonfatal stroke or death	3 years	17	19	0.048
Death, stroke, or MI at 1 year	—	2.9	5.8	0.004
MI, stroke, or TIA	Mean, 5.6 years	25.7	29.0	> 0.2
Cerebrovascular accident, TIA, or peripheral ischemia requiring surgery at 6 months	—	2.4	10.5	0.03
Death, MI, stroke, or cardiovascular intervention due to clinical deterioration	—	1.0	6.4	0.002
Vascular death or nonfatal MI at 6 months	—	7.3	13.6	0.009
Graft occlusion on angiography at 3 months	—	10.1	20.3	< 0.1
Graft occlusion at 360 days	—	15.9	26.1	< 0.01
Femoropopliteal or femorofemoral graft patency	2 years	82	63	0.002
Micronaneurysm progression	3 years	0.48/y	1.44/y	0.04

Abbreviations: MI, myocardial infarction; TIA, transient ischemic attack.

■ Myocardial Infarction

The administration of ticlopidine in the early hours following acute MI has received limited attention, perhaps because of the delayed onset (48 to 72 hours) of its antiplatelet effect. A study of patients treated with ticlopidine within 12 hours of symptom onset reported a lower peak creatine kinase concentration (suggesting reduced infarct size) compared with those not treated.[13]

■ Coronary Artery Bypass Grafting

Saphenous vein bypass conduits are prone to early occlusion that is predominantly a platelet-mediated thrombotic event. Ticlopidine 250 mg bid has been tested against placebo beginning on postoperative day 2 in a double-blind trial of 173 patients (475 grafts). Ticlopidine significantly reduced graft occlusion on day 10 (7.1% vs 13.4%; P <0.05), day 180 (15.0% vs 24.0%; P <0.02), and day 360 (15.9% vs 26.1%; P <0.01).[14]

■ Coronary Arterial Stenting

Since its introduction by Sigwart and colleagues in 1987,[15] coronary stent implantation has been hampered by two major complications: subacute stent thrombosis and hemorrhage (related to vascular access and antithrombotic therapy regimens).

An initial report generated by the French Multicenter Registry suggested that the combination of aspirin and ticlopidine was superior to strategies that included conventional anticoagulant therapy.[16] The rates of stent thrombosis, major cardiac events, and hemorrhage were reduced with antiplatelet therapy. In a randomized study of 257 patients, the combination of ticlopidine and aspirin reduced the incidence of cardiac death, MI, repeated angioplasty, and bypass surgery (composite end point) by 75% compared with unfractionated heparin followed by warfarin (plus aspirin).[17] Subacute stent thrombosis occurred in <1% of patients treated with the combination antiplatelet regimen (**Figure 6.1**). Hemorrhagic complications occurred only in the anticoagulant therapy group. The results of several multicenter trials have confirmed these observations. Evidence provided by the Full Anticoagulation Versus Aspirin and Ticlopidine (FANTASTIC) and Multicenter Aspirin and

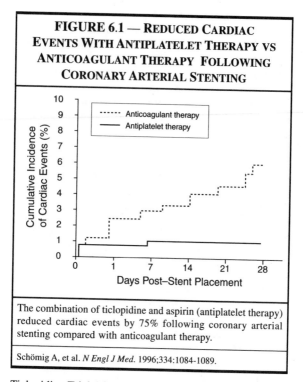

FIGURE 6.1 — REDUCED CARDIAC EVENTS WITH ANTIPLATELET THERAPY VS ANTICOAGULANT THERAPY FOLLOWING CORONARY ARTERIAL STENTING

The combination of ticlopidine and aspirin (antiplatelet therapy) reduced cardiac events by 75% following coronary arterial stenting compared with anticoagulant therapy.

Schömig A, et al. *N Engl J Med*. 1996;334:1084-1089.

Ticlopidine Trial After Coronary Stenting (MATTIS) trials suggest that antiplatelet strategies are superior to anticoagulant (or combined anticoagulant plus aspirin) strategies in terms of both efficacy and safety for both low- and high-risk patients.[18,19]

Although improved techniques of stent deployment, operator experience, and the development of less thrombogenic materials and design have contributed substantially to improved outcomes, the available evidence suggests that antithrombotic therapy is required for the initial 2 to 4 weeks. Whenever possible, treatment should be initiated 2 to 3 days prior to the procedure. In the EPISTENT trial,[20] ticlopidine pretreatment was associated with a significant decrease in the composite of death, MI, or target-vessel revascularization at 1 year. The benefit was most robust in patients who did not receive abciximab. Some low-risk patients may only require aspirin therapy; however, combination antiplatelet therapy represents the standard of care.[21]

■ Peripheral Vascular Disease

Patients with peripheral vascular disease are known to be at risk for vascular events including:
- Stroke
- MI
- Cardiovascular death.

In a multicenter trial, 169 patients with intermittent claudication due to obstructive peripheral vascular disease were randomized in a double-blind fashion to ticlopidine 250 mg bid or placebo.[22] At 6 months, a greater proportion of patients receiving ticlopidine had increased their walking distance and also experienced fewer cardiovascular events than those given placebo.

The Swedish Ticlopidine Multicenter Study[23] identified a nonsignificant trend favoring ticlopidine over placebo in preventing the composite clinical outcome of MI, stroke, and transient ischemic attack in patients with intermittent claudication. By "on-treatment" analysis, there was a significant benefit in favor of ticlopidine treatment.

■ Stroke

The Canadian-American Ticlopidine Study (CATS) identified a clinical benefit from ticlopidine, compared with placebo, in preventing the combined primary end point of stroke, MI, or vascular disease in patients with completed stroke.[24]

The Ticlopidine Aspirin Stroke Study[25] (TASS) was designed to determine the comparative benefits of ticlopidine 250 mg bid over aspirin 1300 mg/d in 3069 patients with recent transient or mild persistent focal cerebral or retinal ischemia. The 3-year event rate for nonfatal stroke or death (from any cause) was 17% for ticlopidine-treated and 19% for aspirin-treated patients (12% reduction; $P = 0.048$). The rates of fatal and nonfatal stroke at 3 years were 10% and 13%, respectively (21% risk reduction; $P = 0.024$).

The comparative benefit of ticlopidine (or clopidogrel) vs dipyridamole/aspirin combination therapy (Aggrenox) is currently unknown.

Summary

Ticlopidine is a thienopyridine derivative that inhibits ADP-mediated platelet aggregation. Because of its requirement for hepatic metabolism to an active compound, the platelet-inhibiting properties of ticlopidine (when given in currently recommended doses) are delayed for 2 to 3 days after treatment initiation. The available evidence suggests that ticlopidine offers benefit following coronary stenting, where in combination with aspirin, subacute stent thrombosis is reduced. Ticlopidine can also be used in patients with coronary artery disease who are unable to take aspirin (because of true allergy or an adverse reaction). Bone marrow suppression and TTP are ticlopidine's side effects that cause the most concern, and therefore careful monitoring is recommended when treatment is continued beyond 14 days. The more favorable safety profile of clopidogrel coupled with its proven benefit in a wide variety of patients with atherosclerotic vascular disease supports preferential use.

REFERENCES

1. Bruno JJ. The mechanism of action of ticlopidine. *Thromb Res.* 1983;4(suppl):59-67.

2. Piovella F, Ricetti MM, Almasioni P, Samaden A, Semino G, Ascari E. The effect of ticlopidine on human endothelial cells in culture. *Thromb Res.* 1984;33:323-332.

3. O'Brien JR, Etherington MD, Shuttleworth RD. Ticlopidine—an antiplatelet drug: effects in human volunteers. *Thromb Res.* 1978;13:245-254.

4. Ellis DJ, Roe RL, Bruno JJ, et al. The effects of ticlopidine hydrochloride on bleeding and platelet function in man. *Thromb Haemost.* 1981;46:176. Abstract.

5. De Caterina R, Sicari R, Bernini W, Lazzerini G, Buti Strata G, Giannessi D. Benefit/risk profile of combined antiplatelet therapy with ticlopidine and aspirin. *Thromb Haemost.* 1991;65:504-510.

6. De Minno G, Cerbone AM, Mattioli PL, Turco S, Iovine C, Mancini M. Functionally thromboasthenic state in normal platelets following the administration of ticlopidine. *J Clin Invest.* 1985;75:328-338.

7. Panak E, Blanchard J, Roe RL. Evaluation of the antithrombotic efficacy of ticlopidine in man. *Agents Actions Suppl.* 1984;15:148-166.

8. Bennett CL, Weinberg PD, Rozenberg-Ben-Dror K, Yarnold PR, Kwaan HC, Green D. Thrombotic thrombocytopenic purpura associated with ticlopidine. A review of 60 cases. *Ann Intern Med.* 1998; 128:541-544.

9. Steinhubl SR, Tan WA, Foody JM, Topol EJ for the EPISTENT Investigators. Incidence and clinical course of thrombotic thrombocytopenic purpura due to ticlopidine following coronary stenting. *JAMA.* 1999;281:806-810.

10. Berglund U, von Schenck H, Wallentin L. Effects of ticlopidine on platelet function in men with stable angina pectoris. *Thromb Haemost.* 1985;54:808-812.

11. Berglund U, Lassvik C, Wallentin L. Effects of the platelet inhibitor ticlopidine on exercise tolerance in stable angina pectoris. *Eur Heart J.* 1987;8:25-30.

12. Balsano F, Rizzon P, Violi F, et al. Antiplatelet treatment with ticlopidine in unstable angina. A controlled multicenter clinical trial. The Studio della Ticlopidina nell'Angina Instabile Group. *Circulation.* 1990;82:17-26.

13. Knudsen JB, Kjoller E, Skagen K, Gormsen J. The effect of ticlopidine on platelet functions in acute myocardial infarction. A double blind controlled trial. *Thromb Haemost.* 1985;53:332-336.

14. Limet R, David JL, Magotteaux P, Larock MP, Rigo P. Prevention of aorta-coronary bypass graft occlusion. Beneficial effect of ticlopidine on early and late patency rates of venous coronary bypass grafts: a double-blind study. *J Thorac Cardiovasc Surg.* 1987;94:773-783.

15. Sigwart U, Puel J, Mirkovitch V, Joffre F, Kappenberger L. Intravascular stents to prevent occlusion and restenosis after transluminal angioplasty. *N Engl J Med.* 1987;316:701-706.

16. Morice MC, Zemour G, Benveniste E, et al. Intracoronary stenting without coumadin: one month results of a French multicenter study. *Cathet Cardiovasc Diagn.* 1995;35:1-7.

17. Schömig A, Neumann FJ, Kastrati A, et al. A randomized comparison of antiplatelet and anticoagulant therapy after the placement of coronary-artery stents. *N Engl J Med.* 1996;334:1084-1089.

6

18. Bertrand ME, Legrand V, Boland J, et al. Randomized multicenter comparison of conventional anticoagulation versus antiplatelet therapy in unplanned and elective coronary stenting. The Full Anticoagulation Versus Aspirin and Ticlopidine (FANTASTIC) Study. *Circulation*. 1998;98:1597-1603.

19. Urban P, Macaya C, Rupprecht HJ, et al for the MATTIS Investigators. Randomized evaluation of anticoagulation versus antiplatelet therapy after coronary stent implantation in high risk patients: the Multicenter Aspirin and Ticlopidine Trial After Intracoronary Stenting (MATTIS). *Circulation*. 1998;98:2126-2132.

20. Steinhubl SR, Ellis SG, Wolski K, Lincoff AM, Topol EJ, for the EPISTENT Investigators. Ticlopidine pretreatment before coronary stenting is associated with sustained decrease in adverse cardiac events. *Circulation*. 2001;103:1403-1409.

21. Leon MB, Baim DS, Gordon P, et al. Clinical and angiographic results from the stent anticoagulation regimen study (STARS). *Circulation*. 1996;94(suppl I):I-685.

22. Arcan JC, Blanchard J, Boissel JP, Destors JM, Panak E. Multicenter double-blind study of ticlopidine in the treatment of intermittent claudication and the prevention of its complications. *Angiology*. 1988; 39:802-811.

23. Janzon L, Bergqvist D, Boberg J, et al. Prevention of myocardial infarction and stroke in patients with intermittent claudication: effects of ticlopidine. Results from STIMS, the Swedish Ticlopidine Multicenter Study. *J Intern Med*. 1990;227:301-308.

24. Gent M, Blakely JA, Easton JD, et al. The Canadian-American Ticlopidine Study (CATS) in thromboembolic stroke. *Lancet*. 1989;1:1215-1220.

25. Hass WK, Easton JD, Adams HP, et al. A randomized trial comparing ticlopidine hydrochloride with aspirin for the prevention of stroke in high risk patients. Ticlopidine Aspirin Stroke Study Group. *N Engl J Med*. 1989;321:501-507.

7   Clopidogrel

Clopidogrel is a novel platelet antagonist that is several times more potent than ticlopidine but associated with fewer adverse effects.

In Vitro and *Ex Vivo* Effect on Platelets

After repeated 75-mg oral doses of clopidogrel, plasma concentrations of the parent compound, which has no platelet inhibiting effect, are very low. Clopidogrel is extensively metabolized in the liver. The main circulating metabolite is a carboxylic acid derivative with a plasma elimination half-life of 7.7 ± 2.3 hours. Approximately 50% of an oral dose is excreted in the urine and the remaining 50% in feces over the following 5 days.

Dose-dependent inhibition of platelet aggregation is observed 2 hours after a single oral dose of clopidogrel, with significant inhibition achieved with loading doses ≥ 300 mg (**Figure 7.1**). Repeated doses of clopidogrel 75-mg per day inhibit adenosine diphosphate (ADP)–mediated aggregation on the first day, and inhibition reaches steady state between day 3 and day 7. At steady state, the average inhibition of ADP is between 40% and 60%.

Based on *ex vivo* studies, clopidogrel is approximately 100-fold more potent than ticlopidine. There are no cumulative antiplatelet effects with prolonged oral administration.

The combined administration of clopidogrel (300-mg loading dose) and aspirin yields a readily discernible antithrombotic effect within 90 to 120 minutes.[1,2]

Mechanism of Action

Clopidogrel selectively inhibits the binding of ADP to its platelet receptor ($P2Y_{12}$) and the subsequent G protein–linked mobilization of intracellular calcium and activation of the glycoprotein (GP) IIb/IIIa complex.[3,4] The specific receptor has been cloned and is abundantly present on the

FIGURE 7.1 — INHIBITION OF ADP-MEDIATED PLATELET AGGREGATION WITH CLOPIDOGREL VS TICLOPIDINE

Clopidogrel (375-mg load, 75 mg daily)

Ticlopidine (250 mg bid)

% Inhibition of ADP-Mediated Platelet Aggregation

Days

Inhibited adenosine diphosphate (ADP)–mediated platelet aggregation as a function of time with a "front-loaded" clopidogrel dosing strategy vs ticlopidine.

platelet surface.[5,6] Clopidogrel has no direct effect on cyclooxygenase, phosphodiesterase, or adenosine uptake.

Absorption

Clopidogrel is rapidly absorbed following oral administration, with peak plasma levels of the predominant circulating metabolite occurring 1 hour later. Administration with meals does not significantly modify the bioavailability of clopidogrel. No dose adjustment is required for elderly patients, women, or those with renal impairment.

Safety

The available information suggests that clopidogrel offers safety advantages over ticlopidine, particularly with regard to bone marrow suppression and other hematologic abnormalities. Although thrombotic thrombocytopenic purpura (TTP) has been reported with clopidogrel,[7] its occurrence

(11 cases per 3 million patients treated) is rare and has not been reported in clinical trials performed to date.

Clinical Experience

■ Vascular Disease

The well-documented benefit derived from platelet inhibition in patients with vascular disease, coupled with a concerning adverse-effect profile witnessed with aspirin and ticlopidine, fostered the rapid development of clopidogrel as a potential alternative to existing therapies. The Clopidogrel versus Aspirin in Patients at Risk for Ischemic Events (CAPRIE) study[8] was designed to test the hypothesis that clopidogrel 75 mg daily would reduce vascular events in high-risk patients by approximately 15% compared with aspirin 325 mg daily. The study population consisted of patients with atherosclerotic vascular disease manifested as recent ischemic stroke, recent myocardial infarction (MI), or symptomatic peripheral arterial occlusive disease. A total of 19,185 patients were enrolled in the international trial. The mean follow-up was 1.91 years. Patients treated with clopidogrel (by intention-to-treat analysis) had a 5.32% annual risk of ischemic stroke, MI, or vascular death compared with 5.83% among aspirin-treated patients (**Table 7.1** and **Figure 7.2**) (relative risk reduction 8.7%; 95% confidence interval [CI] 0.3 to 16.5; $P = 0.043$). A corresponding "on-treatment" analysis yielded a relative risk reduction of 9.4%.

Although CAPRIE was not powered to identify differences in specific subsets, for patients experiencing a stroke, the average event rate per year in the clopidogrel group was 7.15% compared with 7.71% in the aspirin group (relative reduction 7.3%; $P = 0.26$). For patients with MI, the average event rate per year was 5.03% in the clopidogrel group compared with 4.84% in the aspirin group (relative risk increase 3.7%; $P = 0.66$). In contrast, patients with peripheral vascular disease experienced a 3.71% annual event rate with clopidogrel and a 4.86% rate with aspirin (relative-risk reduction 23.8%; $P = 0.002$).

Although there were no major differences in safety between treatment groups, a greater proportion of patients receiving aspirin had the study drug permanently discontin-

TABLE 7.1 — CLINICAL OUTCOMES IN CAPRIE (INTENTION-TO-TREAT ANALYSIS)

| Outcome Event Cluster and Treatment Group | First Outcome Events | | | Event Rate (%/y) | RelativeRisk ↓ (95% CI) | P Value |
	Nonfatal	Fatal	Total			
Ischemic stroke, MI, or vascular death (primary cluster)						
Clopidogrel (nyrs = 17,636*)	631	308	939	5.32	8.7% (0.3-16.5)	0.043
Aspirin (nyrs = 17,519)	700	321	1021	5.83		
Ischemic stroke, MI, or vascular death						
Clopidogrel (nyrs = 17,594)	677	302	979	5.56	7.6% (−0.8-15.3)	0.076
Aspirin (nyrs = 17,482)	737	314	1051	6.01		
Vascular death						
Clopidogrel (nyrs = 17,482)	—	350	350	1.90	7.6% (6.9-20.1)	0.29
Aspirin (nyrs = 18,354)	—	378	378	2.06		

					% (−0.9-14.2)	
Any stroke, MI, or death from any cause†						
Clopidogrel (nyrs = 17,622)	643	490	1133	6.43	7.0% (−0.9-14.2)	0.081
Aspirin (nyrs = 17,501)	720	487	1207	6.90		
Death from any cause						
Clopidogrel (nyrs = 18,377)	–	560	560	3.05	2.2% (−9.9-12.9)	0.71
Aspirin (nyrs = 18,354)	–	571	571	3.11		

Abbreviations: CAPRIE, Clopidogrel versus Aspirin in Patients at Risk for Ischemic Events; CI, confidence interval; MI, myocardial infarction.

* Patient-years at risk for outcome cluster.
† Includes primary intracranial hemorrhage.

From: CAPRIE Steering Committee. *Lancet*. 1996;348:1329-1339.

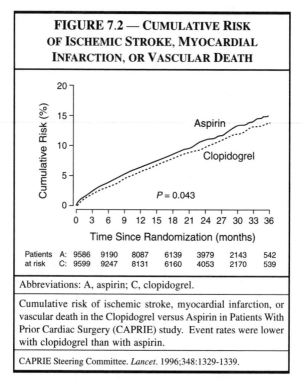

FIGURE 7.2 — CUMULATIVE RISK OF ISCHEMIC STROKE, MYOCARDIAL INFARCTION, OR VASCULAR DEATH

Patients							
at risk A:	9586	9190	8087	6139	3979	2143	542
C:	9599	9247	8131	6160	4053	2170	539

Abbreviations: A, aspirin; C, clopidogrel.

Cumulative risk of ischemic stroke, myocardial infarction, or vascular death in the Clopidogrel versus Aspirin in Patients With Prior Cardiac Surgery (CAPRIE) study. Event rates were lower with clopidogrel than with aspirin.

CAPRIE Steering Committee. *Lancet*. 1996;348:1329-1339.

ued because of gastrointestinal hemorrhage, indigestion, nausea, or vomiting. Approximately one out of every 1000 patients treated with clopidogrel experienced neutropenia ($<1.2 \times 10^9$/L) (similar to that which occurred with aspirin treatment); however, cases of TTP were not reported.

In the CAPRIE study, all-cause mortality, vascular death, MI, stroke, and rehospitalization were determined for 1480 patients who had previously undergone bypass grafting.[9] Those randomized to clopidogrel had a 31.2% relative risk reduction of events compared with aspirin treatment (**Figure 7.3**). Considering the composite end point used in the main CAPRIE trial—vascular death, MI, or ischemic stroke—a 36.3% relative reduction was seen with clopidogrel (5.8% per year) compared with aspirin (9.1% per year) ($P = 0.004$).

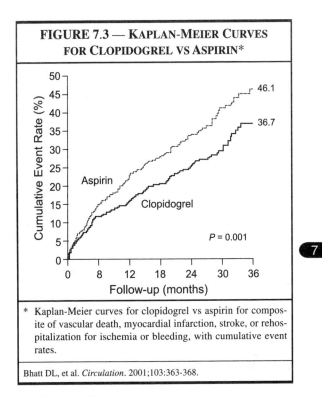

FIGURE 7.3 — KAPLAN-MEIER CURVES FOR CLOPIDOGREL VS ASPIRIN*

Aspirin

Clopidogrel

$P = 0.001$

46.1

36.7

Cumulative Event Rate (%)

Follow-up (months)

* Kaplan-Meier curves for clopidogrel vs aspirin for composite of vascular death, myocardial infarction, stroke, or rehospitalization for ischemia or bleeding, with cumulative event rates.

Bhatt DL, et al. *Circulation*. 2001;103:363-368.

■ **Coronary Stenting**

A multicenter, randomized, controlled trial, Clopidogrel Plus ASA vs Ticlodipine Plus ASA in Stent Patients Study (CLASSICS) included 1020 patients undergoing coronary stent placement who received either aspirin 325 mg qd plus ticlopidine 250 mg bid, aspirin plus clopidogrel 75 mg daily, or aspirin plus front-loaded clopidogrel 300 mg as an initial dose followed by 75 mg qd.[10] Treatment was continued for 28 days after stent placement. Intravenous (IV) GPIIb/IIIa antagonists were not administered to patients enrolled in the trial. The primary safety end point was a composite of neutropenia, thrombocytopenia, bleeding, and drug discontinuation for adverse events (noncardiac). The secondary efficacy end point was a composite of MI, target-vessel revascularization, and cardiovascular death.

The primary end point was experienced by 9.1% of ticlopidine-treated patients, 6.3% of clopidogrel-treated patients (75 mg), and 2.9% of front-loaded clopidogrel-treated patients. Early drug discontinuation occurred in 8.2%, 5.1%, and 2.0% of patients, respectively. The most commonly reported adverse effects prompting drug discontinuation were allergic reactions, gastrointestinal distress, and skin rashes. The secondary cardiovascular end points were reached by 0.9%, 1.5%, and 1.3% of patients, respectively.

In patients undergoing coronary arterial stent placement, clopidogrel (plus aspirin) compares favorably with ticlopidine in preventing thrombotic closure; however, it is associated with fewer noncardiac adverse events that cause discontinuation of treatment.[11]

The importance of adequate platelet inhibition both preceding and following percutaneous coronary intervention (PCI) (with stenting) was confirmed in the PCI-CURE study.[12] A total of 2658 patients undergoing PCI were randomized to double-blind treatment with clopidogrel or placebo (aspirin alone) for, on average, 6 days before the procedure followed by 4 weeks of open-label thienopyridine (after which study drug was resumed for 8 months). The primary end point (cardiovascular death, MI, or urgent target-vessel revascularization within 30 days) was reached in 4.5% of clopidogrel-treated patients and in 6.4% of placebo-treated patients (31% relative reduction) (**Figure 7.4**). Long-term administration of clopidogrel was associated with a lower rate of death, MI, or any revascularization with no increased bleeding complications (**Figure 7.5**).

The TARGET trial[13] investigated the safety and efficiency of two GPIIb/IIIa receptor antagonists in patients undergoing PCI (with the intent to perform stenting). All patients received aspirin and, when possible, clopidogrel 300 mg 2 to 6 hours before the procedure. Both antiplatelet agents were continued throughout the study period. Urgent target-vessel revascularization (<1.0%) and MI (CK >5 times normal) were low in both groups, as was major hemorrhage.

Intracoronary radiation therapy is an available means to treat in-stent restenosis; however, late total occlusion and thrombosis are serious complications, with rates approaching 10% to 15%. Accumulating evidence suggests that pro-

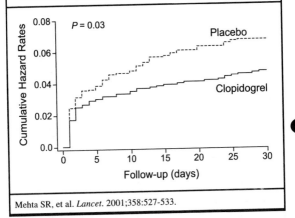

FIGURE 7.4 — KAPLAN-MEIER CUMULATIVE HAZARD RATES FOR PRIMARY OUTCOME OF CARDIOVASCULAR DEATH, MYOCARDIAL INFARCTION, OR URGENT TARGET-VESSEL REVASCULARIZATION AT 30 DAYS AFTER PERCUTANEOUS CORONARY INTERVENTION

Mehta SR, et al. *Lancet.* 2001;358:527-533.

longed treatment with clopidogrel and aspirin (≥6 months) is a more effective means to prevent late thrombosis than an abbreviated course (1 month).[14]

The duration of treatment following placement of drug-eluting stents requires investigation, however, several months of therapy may be warranted to allow endothelialization.

■ **Acute Coronary Syndromes**

The benefit of continued therapy with aspirin and clopidogrel was confirmed in the Clopidogrel in Unstable Angina to Prevent Recurrent Events (CURE) trial.[15] A total of 12,562 patients experiencing an acute coronary syndrome (ACS) without ST-segment elevation received clopidogrel 300 mg immediately, 75 mg daily plus aspirin 75 to 325 mg daily or aspirin alone for 3 to 12 months. The composite of death, MI, or stroke occurred in 9.3% and 11.4% of patients, respectively (relative risk reduction 20%). In hospital refractory ischemia, congestive heart failure and

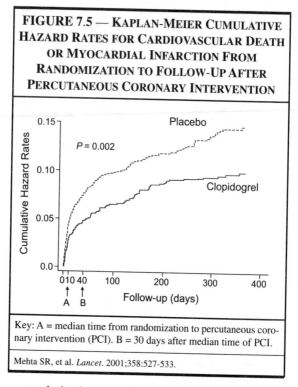

FIGURE 7.5 — KAPLAN-MEIER CUMULATIVE HAZARD RATES FOR CARDIOVASCULAR DEATH OR MYOCARDIAL INFARCTION FROM RANDOMIZATION TO FOLLOW-UP AFTER PERCUTANEOUS CORONARY INTERVENTION

Key: A = median time from randomization to percutaneous coronary intervention (PCI). B = 30 days after median time of PCI.

Mehta SR, et al. *Lancet.* 2001;358:527-533.

revascularization procedures were also less likely in clopidogrel-treated patients (**Figures 7.6** and **7.7**). Although there was a greater risk of major hemorrhage with combination therapy, life-threatening bleeding and hemorrhagic strokes occurred with similar frequency in the two groups.

The Clopidogrel for the Reduction of Events During Observation (CREDO) trial evaluated the long-term benefit (12 months) of treatment with clopidogrel after PCI as well as the potential benefit of initiating clopidogrel with a preprocedure loading dose (both in addition to aspirin therapy).[16] A total of 2116 patients scheduled to undergo elective PCI were randomly assigned to receive clopidogrel 300 mg or placebo 3 to 24 hours before PCI. All patients received aspirin 325 mg. Greater than two thirds of patients had either a recent MI or unstable angina as an indication for PCI. Thereafter, all patients received clopidogrel 75 mg

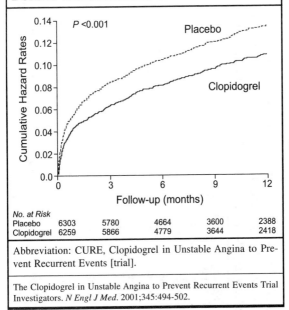

FIGURE 7.6 — CUMULATIVE HAZARD RATES FOR THE FIRST PRIMARY OUTCOME OF DEATH FROM CARDIOVASCULAR CAUSES, NONFATAL MYOCARDIAL INFARCTION, OR STROKE DURING THE 12 MONTHS OF THE CURE TRIAL

No. at Risk				
Placebo	6303	5780	4664	3600	2388
Clopidogrel	6259	5866	4779	3644	2418

Abbreviation: CURE, Clopidogrel in Unstable Angina to Prevent Recurrent Events [trial].

The Clopidogrel in Unstable Angina to Prevent Recurrent Events Trial Investigators. *N Engl J Med.* 2001;345:494-502.

daily through day 28. From day 29 through 12 months, patients in the loading-dose group receive clopidogrel 75 mg daily or placebo. Both groups continued to receive standard therapy, including aspirin 81 to 325 mg daily. Pretreatment with clopidogrel was associated with an 18.5% relative risk reduction for the combined end point of death, MI, or target-vessel revascularization at 28 days (6.8% vs 8.3%; 95% CI –14.2, 41.8; $P = 0.23$). Among patients receiving their clopidogrel loading dose 3 to <6 hours prior to PCI, no benefit was observed (relative risk reduction 13.4%; 95% CI 29.8, –83.3; $P = 0.60$). In contrast, among patients treated 6 to <12 hours prior to PCI and 12 to 24 hours before PCI, the relative risk reduction in the combined end point was 35.5% (95% CI 73.3, –55.6; $P = 0.32$) and 40.1% (95% CI

FIGURE 7.7 — RATES AND RELATIVE RISKS OF THE FIRST PRIMARY OUTCOME OF DEATH FROM CARDIOVASCULAR CAUSES, NONFATAL MYOCARDIAL INFARCTION, OR STROKE IN VARIOUS SUBGROUPS WITH CONSISTENCY OF BENEFIT WITH CLOPIDOGREL

Characteristic	No. of Patients	Patients With Event (%)	
		Placebo	Clopidogrel
Overall	12562	11.4	9.3
Associated myocardial infarction	3283	13.7	11.3
No associated myocardial infarction	9279	10.6	8.6
Male sex	7726	11.9	9.1
Female sex	4836	10.7	9.5
≤65 yr old	6354	7.6	5.4
>65 yr old	6208	15.3	13.3
ST-segment deviation	6275	14.3	11.5
No ST-segment deviation	6287	8.6	7.0
Enzymes elevated at entry	3176	13.0	10.7
Enzymes not elevated at entry	9386	10.9	8.8

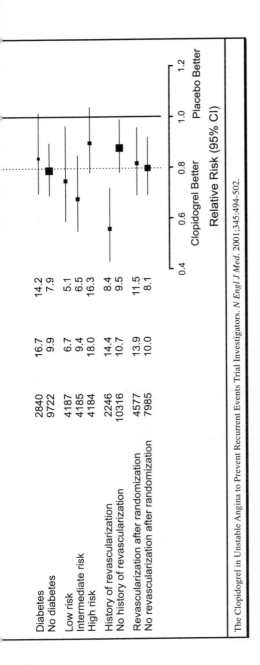

The Clopidogrel in Unstable Angina to Prevent Recurrent Events Trial Investigators. *N Engl J Med.* 2001;345:494-502.

67.6, −10.7; $P = 0.09$), respectively. Considered collectively, patients receiving a loading dose of clopidogrel at least 6 hours prior to PCI experienced a 38.6% relative risk reduction in the primary outcome (95%, CI −1.6, 62.9; $P = 0.051$) (**Figure 7.8**).

A total of 63% of patients in the clopidogrel group and 61% of patients in the control group completed the full 1-year course of study drug. Clopidogrel treatment was associated with a 26.9% reduction in the relative risk of death, MI, or stroke at 1 year (95% CI 3.9, 44.4; $P = 0.02$) (**Figure 7.9**). The benefits of clopidogrel were consistent across patient subgroups, including those receiving an IV GPIIb/IIIa receptor antagonist, those with diabetes, and ACS (27.6% reduction in the 1-year primary end point). There were no differences between groups in urgent target-vessel revascularization, any target-vessel revascularization, or any revascularization. By intention to treat, major bleeding occurred more often in clopidogrel-treated patients (8.8% vs 6.7%, $P = 0.07$), particularly in patients undergoing invasive procedures. Approximately two thirds of all major bleeding events were attributable to patients undergoing coronary artery bypass graft (CABG). Minor bleeding was similar between groups.

Minimizing Hemorrhagic Risk

The CURE trial employed an expanded definition to include life-threatening and non–life-threatening events. This is important to acknowledge when comparing rates from randomized trials in ACS. Thus the 38% increase in major bleeding in the CURE trial compares favorably to the 62% and 60% increases observed in trials of IV GPIIb/IIIa receptor antagonists and aspirin, respectively.

More than 2000 patients underwent CABG surgery after randomization in the CURE trial. Although the overall risk of major hemorrhage was not increased, patients receiving clopidogrel within 5 days of surgery had a trend toward higher rates (relative risk 1.53; $P = 0.06$). Although one must factor in the risks and benefits of interrupting therapy in high-risk patients, the likelihood of major hemorrhage will be lessened when clopidogrel is withheld for at least 5 days prior to surgery. Similarly, risk will be reduced when

FIGURE 7.8 — COMBINED END-POINT RESULTS AT 28 DAYS FOR CLOPIDOGREL VS PLACEBO

Pretreatment was associated with an 18.5% reduction in events. The benefit was most evident in patients receiving a loading dose of clopidogrel a minimum of 6 hours prior to percutaneous coronary intervention.

Steinhubl SR, et al. *JAMA.* 2002;288:2411-2420.

7

125

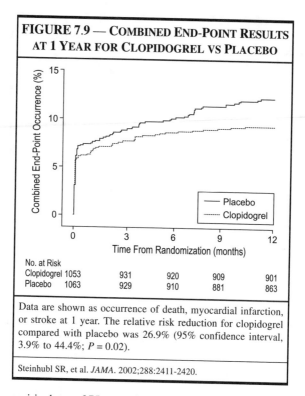

FIGURE 7.9 — COMBINED END-POINT RESULTS AT 1 YEAR FOR CLOPIDOGREL VS PLACEBO

No. at Risk					
Clopidogrel	1053	931	920	909	901
Placebo	1063	929	910	881	863

Data are shown as occurrence of death, myocardial infarction, or stroke at 1 year. The relative risk reduction for clopidogrel compared with placebo was 26.9% (95% confidence interval, 3.9% to 44.4%; *P* = 0.02).

Steinhubl SR, et al. *JAMA*. 2002;288:2411-2420.

aspirin doses of 75 mg to 100 mg are administered daily in conjunction with clopidogrel.

Summary

Clopidogrel (Plavix) is an effective inhibitor of ADP-mediated platelet aggregation. Like ticlopidine, clopidogrel must first be hepatically transformed to its active metabolite to exhibit platelet-inhibiting properties. With mounting clinical trial-based and clinical experience, clopidogrel appears to offer benefit in patients with atherothrombosis of the cardiovascular, peripheral vascular, and cerebrovascular systems where its administration reduces cardiac events to a greater degree than aspirin. Clopidogrel in combination with aspirin also represents the current standard of care following coronary stent placement and in patients with
126

ACS in whom benefits are seen within 24 hours of treatment initiation and persist for at least 12 months.

REFERENCES

1. Cadroy Y, Bossavy JP, Thalamas C, Sagnard L, Sakariassen K, Boneu B. Early potent antithrombotic effect with combined aspirin and a loading dose of clopidogrel on experimental arterial thrombogenesis in humans. *Circulation*. 2000;101:2823-2828.

2. Helft G, Osende JI, Worthley SG, et al. Acute antithrombotic effect of a front-loaded regimen of clopidogrel in patients with atherosclerosis on aspirin. *Arterioscler Thromb Vasc Biol*. 2000;20:2316-2321.

3. Gachet C, Stierlé A, Cazenave JP, et al. The thienopyridine PCR 4099 selectively inhibits ADP-induced platelet aggregation and fibrinogen binding without modifying the membrane glycoprotein IIb-IIIa complex in rat and in man. *Biochem Pharmacol*. 1990;40:229-238.

4. Gachet C, Savi P, Ohlmann P, Maffrand JP, Jakobs KH, Cazenave JP. ADP receptor induced activation of guanine nucleotide binding proteins in rat platelet membranes—an effect selectively blocked by the thienopyridine clopidogrel. *Thromb Haemost*. 1992;68:79-83.

5. Mills DC, Puri R, Hu CJ, et al. Clopidogrel inhibits the binding of ADP analogues to the receptor mediating inhibition of platelet adenylate cyclase. *Arterioscler Thromb*. 1992;12:430-436.

6. Hollopeter G, Jantzen HM, Vincent D, et al. Identification of the platelet ADP receptor targeted by antithrombotic drugs. *Nature*. 2001;409:202-207.

7. Bennett CL, Connors JM, Carwile JM, et al. Thrombotic thrombocytopenia purpura associated with clopidogrel. *N Engl J Med*. 2000;342:1773-1777.

8. CAPRIE Steering Committee. A randomised, blinded, trial of clopidogrel versus aspirin in patients at risk of ischaemic events (CAPRIE). *Lancet*. 1996;348:1329-1339.

9. Bhatt DL, Chew DP, Hirsch AT, Ringleb PA, Hacke W, Topol EJ. Superiority of clopidogrel versus aspirin in patients with prior cardiac surgery. *Circulation*. 2001;103:363-368.

10. Bertrand ME. Double-blind study of the safety of clopidogrel with and without a loading dose in combination with aspirin compared with ticlopidine in combination with aspirin after coronary stenting: the Clopidogrel Aspirin Stent International Cooperative Study (CLASSICS). *Circulation*. 2000;102:624-629.

11. Muller C, Buttner HJ, Peterson J, Roskamm H. A randomized comparison of clopidogrel and aspirin versus ticlopidine and aspirin after the placement of coronary-artery stents. *Circulation.* 2000;101: 590-593.

12. Mehta SR, Yusuf S, Peters RJ, for the CURE Investigators. Effects of pretreatment with clopidogrel and aspirin followed by long-term therapy in patients undergoing percutaneous coronary intervention: the PCI-CURE Study. *Lancet.* 2001;358:527-533.

13. Topol EJ, Moliterno DJ, Herrman HC, et al. Comparison of two platelet glycoprotein IIb/IIIa inhibitors, tirofiban and abciximab, for the prevention of ischemic events with percutaneous coronary revascularization. *N Engl J Med.* 2001;344:1888-1894.

14. Waksman R, Ajani AE, White RL, et al. Prolonged antiplatelet therapy to prevent late thrombosis after intracoronary γ-radiation in patients with restenosis: Washington Radiation for In-Stent Restenosis Trial plus 6 months of clopidogrel (WRIST PLUS). *Circulation.* 2001;103:2332-2335.

15. The Clopidogrel in Unstable Angina to Prevent Recurrent Events Trial Investigators. Effects of clopidogrel in addition to aspirin in patients with acute coronary syndromes without ST-segment elevation. *N Engl J Med.* 2001;345:494-502.

16. Steinhubl SR, Berger PB, Mann JT 3rd, et al. Early and sustained dual oral antiplatelet therapy following percutaneous coronary intervention. A randomized controlled trial. *JAMA.* 2002;288:2411-2420.

8 Platelet Glycoprotein IIb/IIIa Receptor Antagonists

The glycoprotein (GP) IIb/IIIa (αIIb/β_3) receptor, totaling 50,000 to 70,000 copies, represents a final common pathway for platelet aggregation in response to a wide variety of biochemical and mechanical stimuli. Accordingly, it represents an attractive target for pharmacologic therapies that can be applied to patients with acute coronary syndrome (ACS) in whom platelet activation is heightened substantially and represents the predominant pathobiologic substrate.

Intravenous Platelet GPIIb/IIIa Receptor Antagonists

The evolution of GPIIb/IIIa receptor antagonists represents a true "bench-to-bedside" metamorphosis that began with murine monoclonal antibodies and more recently has focused on small peptide or nonpeptide molecules that have structural similarities to fibrinogen and other circulating ligands. There are three intravenous (IV) platelet GPIIb/IIIa receptor antagonists that have been approved by the Food and Drug Administration:

- Abciximab (ReoPro)
- Tirofiban (Aggrastat)
- Eptifibatide (Integrilin).

■ Abciximab

Abciximab (ReoPro) is the Fab fragment of the chimeric human-murine monoclonal antibody c7E3.

Pharmacokinetics

Following an IV bolus, free plasma concentrations of abciximab decrease rapidly with an initial half-life of <10 minutes and a second-phase half-life of 30 minutes, representing rapid binding to the platelet GPIIb/IIIa receptor.

Abciximab remains in the circulation for ≥10 days in the platelet-bound state.

Pharmacodynamics

IV administration of abciximab in doses ranging from 0.15 mg/kg to 0.3 mg/kg produces a rapid dose-dependent inhibition of platelet aggregation in response to adenosine diphosphate (ADP). At the highest dose, 80% of platelet GPIIb/IIIa receptors are occupied within 2 hours and platelet aggregation, even with 20mM ADP, is completely inhibited. Sustained inhibition is achieved with prolonged infusions (12 to 24 hours), and low-level receptor blockade is present for up to 10 days following cessation of the infusion; however, platelet inhibition during infusions beyond 24 hours has not been well characterized. Platelet aggregation in response to 5 mM ADP returns to ≥50% of baseline within 24 hours in a majority of cases (**Figure 8.1**).

Clinical Experience

In nearly 2100 patients undergoing either balloon coronary angioplasty or atherectomy who were judged to be at high risk for ischemic (thrombotic) complications, a bolus of abciximab 0.25 mg/kg followed by a 12-hour continuous infusion of 10 µg/min was found to reduce the occurrence of death, myocardial infarction (MI), and the need for an urgent intervention (repeat angioplasty, stent placement, balloon pump insertion, or bypass grafting) by 35%.[1] At 6 months,[2] the absolute difference in patients with a major ischemic event or elective revascularization was 8.1%, comparing patients who received abciximab (bolus plus infusion) with those given placebo (35.1% vs 27.0%; 23% reduction). All patients received aspirin and unfractionated heparin during the procedure. At 3 years,[3] the composite end point occurred in:

- 41.1% of those receiving an abciximab bolus plus infusion
- 47.4% of those receiving an abciximab bolus only
- 47.2% of those receiving placebo.

The greatest benefit was observed in patients with refractory angina or evolving MI (**Table 8.1**).

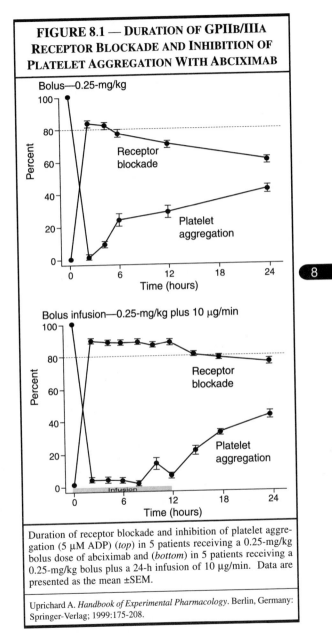

FIGURE 8.1 — DURATION OF GPIIb/IIIa RECEPTOR BLOCKADE AND INHIBITION OF PLATELET AGGREGATION WITH ABCIXIMAB

Duration of receptor blockade and inhibition of platelet aggregation (5 μM ADP) (*top*) in 5 patients receiving a 0.25-mg/kg bolus dose of abciximab and (*bottom*) in 5 patients receiving a 0.25-mg/kg bolus plus a 24-h infusion of 10 μg/min. Data are presented as the mean ±SEM.

Uprichard A. *Handbook of Experimental Pharmacology*. Berlin, Germany: Springer-Verlag; 1999:175-208.

End Point	Placebo (n = 696)	Bolus (n = 698)	Bolus + Infusion (n = 708)	P Value*	Odds Ratio (95% CI)*
Composite					
1 year	266 (38.6)	251 (36.3)	216 (30.8)	.002	0.75 (0.63-0.90)
2 years	290 (42.3)	290 (42.4)	253 (36.3)	.009	0.80 (0.68-0.95)
3 years	319 (47.2)	321 (47.4)	283 (41.1)	.009	0.81 (0.69-0.95)
Death					
1 year	31 (4.5)	29 (4.2)	30 (4.2)	.841	0.95 (0.58-1.57)
2 years	46 (6.6)	40 (5.8)	37 (5.2)	.277	0.79 (0.51-1.22)
3 years	59 (8.6)	54 (8.0)	47 (6.8)	.202	0.78 (0.53-1.14)

TABLE 8.1 — CLINICAL TRIALS OF ABCIXIMAB (REOPRO): LONG-TERM FOLLOW-UP IN THE EPIC STUDY

Myocardial infarction				
1 year	77 (11.2)	62 (9.0)	55 (7.9)	.032	0.69 (0.49-0.97)
2 years	84 (12.4)	73 (10.8)	64 (9.3)	.057	0.73 (0.53-1.01)
3 years	91 (13.6)	81 (12.2)	72 (10.7)	.075	0.76 (0.56-1.03)
Revascularization				
1 year	221 (32.6)	207 (30.4)	178 (25.6)	.004	0.75 (0.62-0.91)
2 years	242 (36.0)	237 (35.3)	207 (30.2)	.013	0.79 (0.66-0.95)
3 years	265 (40.1)	256 (38.6)	234 (34.8)	.021	0.81 (0.68-0.97)

Abbreviations: CI, confidence interval; EPIC, Evaluation of Platelet IIb/IIIa Inhibition for Prevention of Ischemic Complications [study].

* P values and odds ratio represent the comparison of bolus + infusion vs placebo. All values are No. (%) except where otherwise indicated.

From: Topol EJ, et al. *JAMA*. 1997;278:479-484.

The Evaluation in PTCA to Improve Long-term Outcome with Abciximab GPIIb/IIIa Blockade (EPILOG) study included 2792 patients undergoing elective or urgent percutaneous coronary revascularization.[4] They received either abciximab with standard, weight-adjusted unfractionated heparin (initial bolus 100 U/kg, target activated clotting time [ACT] $\geq$300 seconds); abciximab with low-dose, weight-adjusted heparin (initial bolus 70 U/kg, target ACT 200 seconds); or placebo with standard-dose, weight-adjusted heparin. At 30 days, the composite event rate was 5.4%, 5.2%, and 11.7%, respectively. The benefit was observed in both high-risk and low-risk patients.

The c7E3 Fab Antiplatelet Therapy in Unstable Refractory Angina (CAPTURE) study was uniquely designed to assess whether abciximab, given during the 18 to 24 hours before coronary angioplasty, could improve outcome in patients with refractory (myocardial ischemia despite nitrates, heparin, and aspirin) unstable angina.[5] A total of 1265 patients (of 1400 scheduled) were randomly assigned to abciximab or placebo. By 30 days, the primary end point (death, MI, urgent revascularization) occurred in 11.3% of abciximab-treated patients and in 15.9% of placebo-treated patients ($P = 0.012$). The rate of MI was lower *before* and *during* coronary interventions in those given abciximab.

Patients participating in the Global Use of Strategies to Open Occluded Arteries (GUSTO) IV-ACS trial had chest pain and either ST-segment depression or elevated troponin levels.[6] They were randomized to receive placebo, abciximab for 24 hours, or abciximab for 48 hours with recommended avoidance of revascularization during the initial 48 hours. Neither abciximab group fared better than the placebo group with respect to death or MI at 30 days. In fact, early mortality was increased with a 48-hour infusion. The overall event rates were low.

The Abciximab Before Direct Angioplasty and Stenting in Myocardial Infarction Regarding Acute and Long-Term Follow-up (ADMIRAL) trial included 300 patients with acute ST-segment elevation MI who underwent percutaneous coronary intervention (PCI) (plus stenting) and received either abciximab or placebo.[7] At 30 days, a composite of death, reinfarction, or urgent revascularization (target vessel) had occurred in 6% of abciximab-treated and

14.6% of placebo-treated patients; at 6 months, the corresponding figures were 7.4% and 15.9%, respectively. The early administration of abciximab improved coronary patency before stenting, the success rate of the procedures, and the rate of patency 6 months after the procedure.

Although clinical trials have differed in the timing of GPIIb/IIIa receptor antagonist administration, an overview of published studies suggests that the combined incidence of death, reinfarction, and urgent target-vessel revascularization can be reduced with abciximab[8]; however, mortality rates are not reduced, and one should anticipate an increased risk of thrombocytopenia and hemorrhagic complications (**Figure 8.2**).[9]

Arterial thrombi are composed of platelets and fibrin. Accordingly, the combined administration of GPIIb/IIIa receptor antagonists and fibrinolytics makes sound biologic sense and has been shown to improve both epicardial and microvascular coronary blood flow in the setting of acute MI (**Figure 8.3**).[10]

In the GUSTO V study, 16,588 patients with acute ST-segment elevation MI received either reteplase (standard dose) or half-dose reteplase plus abciximab.[11] Although the 30-day mortality rates did not differ significantly, there were fewer deaths or reinfarctions with combined therapy. Similarly, there was less need for urgent revascularization and fewer nonfatal ischemic complications of MI with reteplase plus abciximab compared with reteplase alone. Intracranial hemorrhage rates did not differ between treatments; however, moderate-to-severe bleeding was more likely with combined therapy and patients >75 years of age were at increased risk for hemorrhagic stroke (odds ratio 1.91). All patients in GUSTO V received unfractionated heparin and aspirin.

■ Tirofiban

Tirofiban (Aggrastat), a tyrosine derivative with a molecular weight of 495 kd, is a nonpeptide inhibitor (peptidomimetic) of the platelet GPIIb/IIIa receptor.

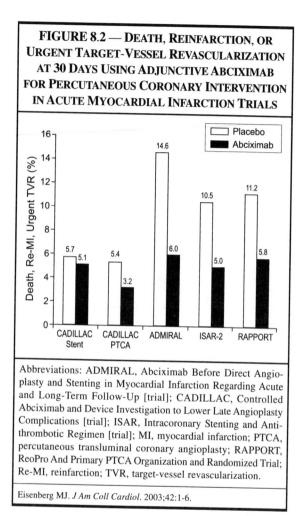

FIGURE 8.2 — DEATH, REINFARCTION, OR URGENT TARGET-VESSEL REVASCULARIZATION AT 30 DAYS USING ADJUNCTIVE ABCIXIMAB FOR PERCUTANEOUS CORONARY INTERVENTION IN ACUTE MYOCARDIAL INFARCTION TRIALS

Abbreviations: ADMIRAL, Abciximab Before Direct Angioplasty and Stenting in Myocardial Infarction Regarding Acute and Long-Term Follow-Up [trial]; CADILLAC, Controlled Abciximab and Device Investigation to Lower Late Angioplasty Complications [trial]; ISAR, Intracoronary Stenting and Antithrombotic Regimen [trial]; MI, myocardial infarction; PTCA, percutaneous transluminal coronary angioplasty; RAPPORT, ReoPro And Primary PTCA Organization and Randomized Trial; Re-MI, reinfarction; TVR, target-vessel revascularization.

Eisenberg MJ. *J Am Coll Cardiol*. 2003;42:1-6.

Pharmacodynamics

Tirofiban, like other nonpeptides, mimics the geometric, stereotactic, and change characteristics of the RGD sequence, thus interfering with platelet aggregation.

Three doses of tirofiban were studied in a phase 1 study of patients undergoing coronary angioplasty who received one of three graduated regimens intravenously with a bo-

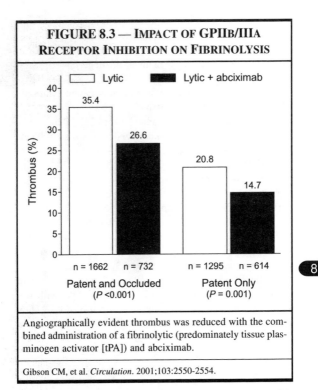

FIGURE 8.3 — IMPACT OF GPIIb/IIIa RECEPTOR INHIBITION ON FIBRINOLYSIS

Angiographically evident thrombus was reduced with the combined administration of a fibrinolytic (predominately tissue plasminogen activator [tPA]) and abciximab.

Gibson CM, et al. *Circulation.* 2001;103:2550-2554.

8

lus dose of 5, 10, or 15 μg/kg and a continuous (16- to 24-hour) infusion of 0.05, 0.10, or 0.15 μg/kg/min.[12] A dose-dependent inhibition of *ex vivo* platelet aggregation was observed within minutes of bolus administration and was sustained during the continuous infusion.

Clinical Trials and Experience

The Randomized Efficacy Study of Tirofiban Outcomes and Restenosis (RESTORE) trial was a randomized, double-blind, placebo-controlled trial of tirofiban in patients undergoing coronary intervention within 72 hours of hospital presentation with an ACS.[13]

Patients (n = 2139) received tirofiban as a 10-μg/kg IV bolus over a 3-minute period and a continuous infusion of 0.15 μg/kg/min over 36 hours. All patients received heparin and aspirin. The primary composite end point (death,

MI, angioplasty failure requiring bypass surgery or unplanned stent placement, recurrent ischemia requiring repeat angioplasty) at 30 days was reduced from 12.2% in the placebo group to 10.3% in the tirofiban group (16% relative reduction).

The Platelet Receptor Inhibition in Ischemic Syndrome Management (PRISM) trial included 3231 patients with unstable angina/non–ST-segment elevation MI.[14] All patients received aspirin and were randomized to treatment with either unfractionated heparin or tirofiban, given as a loading dose of 0.6 µg/kg/min over 30 minutes followed by a maintenance infusion of 0.15 µg/kg/min for 48 hours (angiography/revascularization was discouraged during the infusion period). The primary composite end point (death, MI, refractory ischemia) at 48 hours was 5.6% in tirofiban-treated patients and 3.8% in placebo (aspirin/heparin)–treated patients (risk reduction 33%). Benefit was maintained but overall was less impressive at 7 and 30 days.

The PRISM in Patients Limited by Unstable Signs and Symptoms (PLUS) trial included 1915 patients with unstable angina and non–ST-segment elevation MI.[15] They were treated with aspirin and heparin and randomized to either tirofiban (0.4 µg/kg/min × 30 min; then 0.1 µg/kg/min for a minimum of 48 hours and a maximum of 108 hours) or placebo (unfractionated heparin). Angiography and revascularization were performed at the discretion of the treating physician. Tirofiban-treated patients had a lower composite event rate at 7 days than the placebo group, 12.9% vs 17.9%, risk reduction 34%. The benefit was mainly due to a reduced incidence of MI (47% risk reduction) and refractory ischemia (30% risk reduction). The benefit was maintained at 30 days (22% risk reduction in composite event rate) and at 6 months (**Table 8.2**). The trial originally included a tirofiban-alone arm (no heparin) that was dropped because of excess mortality at 7 days.

The importance of early intervention among patients with non–ST-segment elevation ACS was emphasized in the Treat Angina With Aggrastat and Determine Cost of Therapy With an Invasive or Conservative Strategy (TACTICS)–Thrombolysis in Myocardial Infarction (TIMI) 18 trial, as was the benefit of aggressive pharmacologic therapy (GPIIb/IIIa receptor antagonists) in combination with PCI for patients at greatest risk for adverse ischemic outcomes (prior MI, ST-segment changes, elevated cardiac enzymes).[16]

■ Eptifibatide

Eptifibatide (Integrilin) is a nonimmunogenic cyclic heptapeptide with an active pharmacophore that is derived from the structure of barbourin, a platelet GPIIb/IIIa inhibitor from the venom of the southeastern pigmy rattlesnake.[17]

Pharmacokinetics

The plasma half-life of eptifibatide is 10 to 15 minutes and clearance is predominantly renal (75%) and to a lesser degree hepatic (25%). The antiplatelet effect has a rapid onset of action and is rapidly reversible.

Pharmacodynamics

In a pilot study of patients undergoing PCI, patients were randomized to one of four eptifibatide dosing schedules:

- 180-μg/kg bolus, 1-μg/kg/min infusion
- 135-μg/kg bolus, 0.5-μg/kg/min infusion
- 90-μg/kg bolus, 0.75-μg/kg/min infusion
- 135-μg/kg bolus, 0.75-μg/kg/min infusion.

All patients received aspirin and heparin and were continued on the study drug for 18 to 24 hours. The two highest bolus doses produced >80% inhibition of ADP-mediated platelet aggregation within 15 minutes of administration in a majority of patients (>75%). A constant infusion of 0.75 μg/kg/min maintained the antiplatelet effect, whereas an infusion of 0.50 μg/kg/min allowed gradual recovery of platelet function. In all dosing groups, platelet-function returned to >50% of baseline within 4 hours of terminating the infusion.[18]

Clinical Trials and Experience

The Integrilin to Minimize Platelet Aggregation and Coronary Thrombosis (IMPACT-II) trial enrolled 4010 patients undergoing elective, urgent, or emergency coronary interventions.[19] Patients were assigned to either placebo, a bolus of 135 μg/kg eptifibatide followed by an infusion of 0.5 μg/kg/min for 20 to 24 hours, or a 135-μg/kg bolus with a 0.75-μg/kg/min infusion. By 30 days, the composite end

TABLE 8.2 — CLINICAL TRIALS OF TIROFIBAN (AGGRASTAT): THE PRISM AND PRISM-PLUS STUDIES

Events (%)	PRISM			PRISM-Plus		
	Tirofiban	Heparin	Risk Ratio	Tirofiban + Heparin	Heparin	Risk Ratio
48 Hours						
Composite	3.8	5.6	0.67*	7.8	5.7	0.71
Refractory ischemia	3.5	5.3	0.65*	4.8	5.9	0.78
MI or death	1.2	1.6	0.76	0.9	2.6	0.34*
MI	0.9	1.4	0.64	0.8	2.4	0.32*
Death	0.4	0.2	1.48	0.3	0.1	0.51
7 Days						
Composite	10.3	11.2	0.90	12.9	17.9	0.68*
Refractory ischemia	9.1	9.9	0.91	9.3	12.7	0.70*
MI or death	3.3	4.2	0.77	4.9	8.3	0.57*
MI	3.6	3.1	0.84	3.9	7.0	0.53*
Death	1.0	1.6	0.63	1.9	1.9	1.01
30 Days						
Composite	15.9	17.1	0.92	18.5	22.3	0.78*

Refractory ischemia	10.6	10.8	0.98	10.6	13.4	0.76
MI or death	5.8	7.1	0.80	8.7	11.9	0.70*
MI	4.1	4.3	0.95	6.6	9.2	0.70
Death	2.3	2.6	0.62*	3.6	4.5	0.79
6 Months						
Composite	—	—	—	27.7	32.1	0.81*
Refractory ischemia	—	—	—	10.6	13.4	0.76
MI or death	—	—	—	12.3	15.3	0.78
MI	—	—	—	8.3	10.5	0.76
Death	—	—	—	6.9	7.0	0.97
Readmission for unstable angina	—	—	—	10.9	10.7	1.00

Abbreviations: MI, myocardial infarction; PRISM, Platelet Receptor Inhibition in Ischemic Syndrome Management; PRISM-Plus, Platelet Receptor Inhibition in Ischemic Syndrome Management in Patients Limited by Unstable Signs and Symptoms.

* $P < 0.05$.

point (death, MI, unplanned revascularization, stent placement for abrupt closure) occurred in 11.4%, 9.2%, and 9.9% of patients, respectively. Although the benefit of treatment was maintained at 6 months, the differences between groups were not statistically significant.

The IMPACT-After Myocardial Infarction (AMI) study was designed to determine the effect of eptifibatide on coronary arterial patency when used adjunctively with accelerated tissue plasminogen activator (tPA).[20] A total of 132 patients with MI received tPA, heparin, and aspirin and were randomized to receive a bolus and continuous infusion of one of six eptifibatide doses or placebo. The doses ranged from 36 to 180 μg/kg (bolus) to 0.2 to 0.75 μg/kg/min (infusion). Study drug was started within 30 minutes of tPA administration and continued for 24 hours. The highest dose eptifibatide groups had more complete reperfusion (TIMI grade 3 flow) and shorter mean time to ST-segment recovery than placebo-treated patients. The composite clinical event rate (death, reinfarction, revascularization, heart failure, hypertension, stroke) was relatively high in all groups: 44.8% in eptifibatide-treated patients and 41.8% in placebo-treated patients.

The Platelet Glycoprotein IIb/IIIa in Unstable Angina Receptor Suppression Using Integrilin Therapy (PURSUIT) trial included patients with unstable angina or non–ST-segment elevation MI with symptoms within 24 hours and electrocardiographic changes within 12 hours (of ischemia).[21] A total of 10,948 patients were randomized to eptifibatide: 180-μg/kg bolus plus 1.3-μg/kg/min infusion, or 180-μg/kg bolus plus 2.0-μg/kg/min infusion or placebo for up to 3 days (in addition to heparin [in most patients] and aspirin). The 30-day event rate of death or nonfatal MI was 14.2% with eptifibatide and 15.7% with placebo (1.5% absolute reduction) (**Figure 8.4**). A reduction in MI or death (composite) with eptifibatide was observed at 96 hours, 7 days, and 30 days in medically or interventionally treated patients; however, the benefit was less impressive at later time points.

The Enhanced Suppression of the Platelet GPIIb/IIIa Receptor With Integrilin Trial (ESPRIT) was designed to test the hypothesis that a minimum threshold of 80% GPIIb/IIIa receptor blockade was required for benefit.[22] A total of

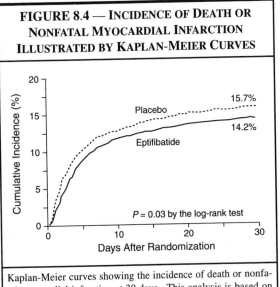

FIGURE 8.4 — INCIDENCE OF DEATH OR NONFATAL MYOCARDIAL INFARCTION ILLUSTRATED BY KAPLAN-MEIER CURVES

Kaplan-Meier curves showing the incidence of death or nonfatal myocardial infarction at 30 days. This analysis is based on end points as assessed by the central clinical events committee. The percentages shown are for the incidence at 30 days.

The PURSUIT Trial Investigators. *N Engl J Med.* 1998;339:436-443.

2064 patients received either eptifibatide (180-µg/kg boluses [× 2] 10 minutes apart, continuous infusion of 2.0 µg/kg/min for 18 to 24 hours) or placebo prior to PCI. The trial was terminated early for efficacy as patients receiving eptifibatide had a 4.0% absolute reduction in death, MI, urgent target-vessel revascularization, or "bailout" GPIIb/IIIa antagonist use within 48 hours compared with placebo. Major events were significantly lower at 30 days as well.

Similarities and Differences Between Intravenous GPIIb/IIIa Antagonists

Although considered collectively as GPIIb/IIIa receptor antagonists, abciximab, tirofiban, and eptifibatide differ at several levels, including their:

- Molecular size
- Binding characteristics

- Clearance
- Plasma
- Platelet-bound and biologic half-life
- Potential reversibility (**Table 8.3**).

The duration of platelet inhibition following drug discontinuation and the potential for reversing the pharmacologic effect are particularly important properties in cases of emergent surgery and major hemorrhagic complications. In general, a return of platelet function toward a physiologic state (≤50% inhibition) occurs within 4 hours following the cessation of tirofiban and eptifibatide. In contrast, 12 hours are required for abciximab (**Figure 8.5**). Some of the delayed return of physiologic platelet function following abciximab termination may be counterbalanced by its low free plasma concentration and drug-to-receptor ratio. These properties are responsible for the rapid return of hemostatic potential following platelet transfusions (and may also limit platelet-inhibiting potential with marked mobilization of GPIIb/IIIa receptors from intraplatelet storage pools). In contrast, the high plasma concentrations observed with the small-molecule inhibitors limit the effectiveness of platelet transfusions. Fibrinogen supplementation (fresh frozen plasma, cryoprecipitate) is the more logical choice for restoration of hemostatic potential, given the competitive nature of binding and relative availability of platelet GPIIb/IIIa receptors[23] (**Figure 8.6**).

Major Clinical End Points

The IV GPIIb/IIIa receptor antagonists have been shown to reduce cardiac event rates in patients with ACS who are treated by pharmacologic means alone or undergo PCI. The available data suggest that the greatest overall benefit occurs in high-risk patients, particularly those undergoing mechanical revascularization.

Methodologic differences between the major clinical trials make it difficult to compare the GPIIb/IIIa receptor antagonists; however, there is clear consistency among the agents with regard to efficacy and safety.[24] Meticulous attention to femoral arterial access, sheath care, and peri-

TABLE 8.3 — INDIVIDUAL CHARACTERISTICS OF THE GPIIB/IIIA RECEPTOR ANTAGONISTS				
Characteristic	Abciximab	Eptifibatide	Tirofiban
Type	Antibody	Peptide	Nonpeptide
Molecular weight (daltons)	~50,000	~800	~500
Platelet-bound half-life	Long (h)	Short (s)	Short (s)
Plasma half-life	Short (min)	Extended (2 h)	Extended (2 h)
Drug-to-GPIIb/IIIa receptor ratio	1.5–2.0	250–2500	> 250
50% return of platelet function (without transfusion)	12 h	~ 4 h	~ 4 h
Abbreviation: GP, glycoprotein.			

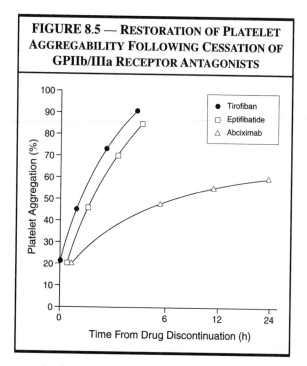

FIGURE 8.5 — RESTORATION OF PLATELET AGGREGABILITY FOLLOWING CESSATION OF GPIIb/IIIa RECEPTOR ANTAGONISTS

procedural heparin dosing has reduced vascular and major hemorrhagic complications substantially.

The Do Tirofiban And ReoPro Give Similar Efficacy Trial (TARGET) randomized 5308 patients to either tirofiban (RESTORE trial dosing strategy) or abciximab before PCI (with the intent to perform stenting). The primary end point, a composite of death, nonfatal MI, or urgent revascularization at 30 days, was reached in 7.6% and 6.0% of tirofiban-treated and abciximab-treated patients, respectively (hazard ratio 1.26).[25] The differences did not persist at 1-year follow-up. There were no differences in the rates of major bleeding complications or transfusions, but tirofiban was associated with a lower rate of minor bleeding episodes and thrombocytopenia (**Figure 8.7**).

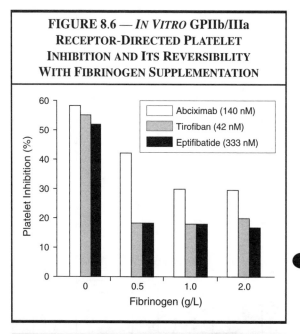

FIGURE 8.6 — *IN VITRO* **GPIIb/IIIa
RECEPTOR-DIRECTED PLATELET
INHIBITION AND ITS REVERSIBILITY
WITH FIBRINOGEN SUPPLEMENTATION**

Legend:
- Abciximab (140 nM)
- Tirofiban (42 nM)
- Eptifibatide (333 nM)

Y-axis: Platelet Inhibition (%)
X-axis: Fibrinogen (g/L)

Do Platelet GPIIb/IIIa Receptor Antagonists Reduce Mortality Rates?

When considering the potential benefits of treatment, a clinician must carefully consider the inherent risk for adverse outcomes. A meta-analysis of 19 randomized, placebo-controlled trials including over 20,000 patients with ACS (ST elevation and non-ST ACS) reported a 31% risk reduction (for mortality) at 30 days and 21% at 6 months in those receiving a platelet GPIIb/IIIa receptor antagonist (vs those not treated) in the setting of PCI.[26] Major bleeding was increased only in trials where anticoagulant therapy (unfractionated heparin) was continued after the procedure (relative risk 1.70).

Thrombocytopenia

The administration of GPIIb/IIIa receptor antagonists is associated with thrombocytopenia (platelet count

FIGURE 8.7 — MAJOR CLINICAL OUTCOMES IN THE TARGET TRIAL

End Point	P	Hazard Ratio	Tirofiban (%)	Abciximab (%)
Composite	0.038		7.6	6.0
Death	0.66		0.5	0.4
Nonfatal MI	0.04		6.9	5.4
Death or nonfatal MI	0.04		7.2	5.7
Urgent target vessel revascularization	0.49		0.8	0.7

Abbreviation: MI, myocardial infarction.

Hazard ratios for the individual end points in Tirofiban and ReoPro Give Similar Efficacy Outcomes Trial (TARGET).

Topol EI, et al. *N Engl J Med.* 2001;34:1888-1894.

$<100,000/mm^3$) in approximately 2% to 3% of patients.[27] A more marked reduction ($<50,000/mm^3$) is seen in <1% of patients and may be influenced by:

- Concomitant procedures (coronary interventions)
- Medications (unfractionated heparin)
- Age (>65 years)
- Pretreatment platelet count
- Duration of treatment
- Repeat administration (even with a different agent than the first exposure).

Acute, profound thrombocytopenia ($<2000/mm^3$) has been reported within 4 hours of abciximab treatment.[28] Whether preexisting or fibrin-induced antibodies, in addition to causing thrombocytopenia and hemorrhage, also cause platelet activation with attendant heightened thrombotic potential, is an area of active investigation.

Oral GPIIb/IIIa Receptor Antagonists

The success enjoyed by IV GPIIb/IIIa receptor antagonists, coupled with the recognized risk for recurrent cardiac events incurred by patients with atherosclerotic coronary artery disease, stimulated interest in the development of oral agents that would provide continued, low-level GPIIb/IIIa receptor inhibition.

To date, over 30,000 patients have been enrolled in four large-scale, double-blind, placebo-controlled clinical trials. Individually, each trial failed to identify a reduction in ischemic outcomes. Collectively, a significant excess in mortality with three different oral GPIIb/IIIa antagonists was observed (**Figure 8.8**).[29]

Clinician's Approach to GPIIb/IIIa Antagonist Therapy

A solid body of information derived from large-scale, randomized clinical trials allows several conclusions to be drawn regarding decision-making and patient care. First, the IV GPIIb/IIIa antagonists are an important component of medical and adjunctive therapy for ACS. Second, benefit

FIGURE 8.8 — MAJOR OUTCOMES IN TRIALS OF ORAL GPIIb/IIIa RECEPTOR ANTAGONISTS

Trial	No. in Study	Odds Ratio	Aspirin Alone (%)	GPIIb/IIIa Inhibitor (%)	P
EXCITE (xemilofiban)	7232	2.14	0.3	0.7	0.048
OPUS (orbofiban)	10288	1.40	1.4	2.0	0.049
SYMPHONY 1 (sibrafiban)	9169	1.14	1.8	2.0	0.420
SYMPHONY 2 (sibrafiban)	6637	1.55	1.3	2.1	0.038
Pooled	33,326	1.37	1.3	1.7	0.001

Abbreviations: EXCITE, Evaluation of Oral Xemilofiban in Controlling Thrombotic Events, OPUS; Orbofiban in Patients With Unstable Coronary Syndromes; SYMPHONY, Sibrafiban vs Aspirin to Yield Maximum Protection From Ischemic Heart Events Post-acute Coronary Syndromes.

Odds ratio and 95% confidence intervals for death beyond 30 days in trials of oral GPIIb/IIIa receptor antgonists.

Chew DP, et al. *Circulation*. 2001;103:201-206.

is evident for both ST and non-ST elevation ischemic syndromes, particularly when combined with early PCI. Third, a patient-specific threshold level of platelet inhibition must be achieved and maintained for maximum benefit. Fourth, combined pharmacotherapy with fibrinolytics requires further investigation to better define safe and effective dosing strategies, as will the role of facilitated PCI (**Table 8.4**). Fifth, the ideal adjunctive anticoagulant (low molecular weight heparin, very low molecular weight heparin, thrombin-directed antagonist, factor X inhibitor) can only be defined through carefully designed clinical trials. Last, future efforts in drug development must be mindful of pharmacokinetic and pharmacodynamic properties and patient-related differences in platelet-mediated thrombin generation that may strongly influence dosing and overall clinical benefit.

Summary

8

The GPIIb/IIIa receptor represents a final common pathway for platelet aggregation. The development of platelet GPIIb/IIIa receptor antagonists that can be administered intravenously represents a major step forward in the management of patients with ACS. The comparative and adjunctive role of multisite directed platelet-inhibiting therapy requires further investigation.

REFERENCES

1. Evaluation of Platelet IIb/IIIa Inhibition for Prevention of Ischemic Complications (EPIC) Investigators. Use of a monoclonal antibody directed against the platelet glycoprotein IIb/IIIa receptor in high-risk coronary angioplasty. *N Engl J Med*. 1994;330:956-961.

2. Topol EJ, Califf RM, Weisman HF, et al for the EPIC Investigators. Randomised trial of coronary intervention with antibody against platelet IIb/IIIa integrin for reduction of clinical restenosis: results at six months. *Lancet*. 1994;343:881-886.

3. Topol EJ, Ferguson JJ, Weisman HF, et al for the EPIC Investigator Group. Long-term protection from myocardial ischemic events in a randomized trial of brief integrin B_3 blockade with percutaneous coronary intervention. *JAMA*. 1997;278:479-484.

4. EPILOG Investigators. Platelet glycoprotein IIb/IIIa receptor blockade and low-dose heparin during percutaneous coronary revascularization. *N Engl J Med*. 1997;336:1689-1696.

TABLE 8.4 — INTRAVENOUS GPIIB/IIIA RECEPTOR ANTAGONISTS: STRATEGIES FOR CLINICAL PRACTICE

Agent	Medical Treatment ACS	PCI	PCI STEMI	Fibrinolytic Combination STEMI	Facilitated PCI
Abciximab	++*	+++	+++	+	++
Eptifibatide	+++	+++	+	+	+
Tirofiban	+++	++	+	+	+

Key: +++, marked benefit; ++, moderate benefit; +, risk-benefit not fully defined.

Abbreviations: ACS, acute coronary syndrome; GP, glycoprotein; PCI, percutaneous coronary intervention; STEMI, ST-elevation myocardial infartion.

* Refractory angina if PCI performed within 12 hours.

5. CAPTURE Investigators. Randomized placebo-controlled trial of abciximab before and during coronary intervention in refractory unstable angina: the CAPTURE study. *Lancet.* 1997;349:1429-1435.

6. The GUSTO IV Investigators. Effect of glycoprotein IIb/IIIa receptor blocker abciximab on outcome in patients with acute coronary syndromes without early coronary revascularization: the GUSTO IV-ACS randomised trial. *Lancet.* 2001;357:1915-1924.

7. Montalescot G, Barragan P, Wittenberg O, et al for the ADMIRAL Investigators. Platelet glycoprotein IIb/IIIa inhibition with coronary stenting for acute myocardial infarction. *N Engl J Med.* 2001;344:1895-1903.

8. Moliterno DJ, Chan AW. Glycoprotein IIb/IIIa inhibition in early intent-to-stent treatment of acute coronary syndromes: EPISTENT, ADMIRAL, CADILLAC, and TARGET. *J Am Coll Cardiol.* 2003;41 (suppl 4):49S-54S.

9. Eisenberg MJ, Jamal S. Glycoprotein IIb/IIIa inhibition in the setting of acute ST-segment elevation myocardial infarction. *J Am Coll Cardiol.* 2003;42:1-6.

10. Gibson CM, de Lemos JA, Murphy SA, et al. Combination therapy with abciximab reduces angiographically evident thrombus in acute myocardial infarction: a TIMI 14 substudy. *Circulation.* 2001; 103:2550-2554.

11. Topol EJ, for the GUSTO V Investigators. Reperfusion therapy for acute MI with fibrinolytic therapy or combination reduced fibrinolytic therapy and platelet glycoprotein IIb/IIIa inhibition: the GUSTO V randomised trial. *Lancet.* 2001;357:1905-1914.

12. Kereiakes DJ, Kleiman NS, Ambrose J, et al. Randomized, double-blind, placebo-controlled dose-ranging study of tirofiban (MK-383) platelet IIb/IIIa blockade in high risk patients undergoing coronary angioplasty. *J Am Coll Cardiol.* 1996;27:536-542.

13. Randomized Efficacy Study of Tirofiban for Outcomes and Restenosis (RESTORE) Investigators. Effects of platelet glycoprotein IIb/IIIa blockade with tirofiban on adverse cardiac events in patients with unstable angina or acute myocardial infarction undergoing coronary angioplasty. *Circulation.* 1997;96:1445-1453.

14. Platelet Receptor Inhibition in Ischemic Syndrome Management (PRISM) Study Investigators. A comparison of aspirin plus tirofiban with aspirin plus heparin for unstable angina. *N Engl J Med.* 1998; 338:1498-1505.

15. Platelet Receptor Inhibition in Ischemic Syndrome Management in Patients Limited by Unstable Signs and Symptoms (PRISM PLUS) Study Investigators. Inhibition of the platelet glycoprotein IIb/IIIa receptor with tirofiban in unstable angina and non-Q wave myocardial infarction. *N Engl J Med.* 1998;338:1488-1497.

8

153

16. Cannon CP, Weintraub WS, Demopoulos LA, et al for the TACTICS-TIMI 18 Investigators. Comparison of early invasive and conservative strategies for patients with unstable coronary syndromes treated with the glycoprotein IIb/IIIa inhibitor tirofiban. *N Engl J Med.* 2001;344:1879-1887.

17. Phillips DR, Scarborough RM. Clinical pharmacology of eptifibatide. *Am J Cardiol.* 1997;80:11B-20B.

18. Harrington RA, Kleiman NS, Kottke-Marchant K, et al. Immediate and reversible platelet inhibition after intravenous administration of a peptide glycoprotein IIb/IIIa inhibitor during percutaneous coronary intervention. *Am J Cardiol.* 1995;76:1222-1227.

19. Integrilin to Minimise Platelet Aggregation and Coronary Thrombosis (IMPACT)-II Investigators. Randomised placebo-controlled trial of effect of eptifibatide on complications of percutaneous coronary intervention: IMPACT-II. *Lancet.* 1997;349:1422-1428.

20. Ohman EM, Kleiman NS, Gacioch G, et al for the IMPACT-AMI Investigators. Combined accelerated tissue-plasminogen activator and platelet glycoprotein IIb/IIIa integrin receptor blockade with integrilin in acute myocardial infarction. Results of a randomized, placebo-controlled, dose-ranging trial. *Circulation.* 1997;95:846-854.

21. The Platelet Glycoprotein IIb/IIIa in Unstable Angina: Receptor Suppression Using Integrilin Therapy (PURSUIT) Trial Investigators. Inhibition of platelet glycoprotein IIb/IIIa with eptifibatide in patients with acute coronary syndromes. *N Engl J Med.* 1998;339:436-443.

22. The ESPRIT Investigators. Novel dosing regimen of eptifibatide in planned coronary stent implantation (ESPRIT): a randomised, placebo-controlled trial. *Lancet.* 2000;356:2037-2044.

23. Becker RC, Spencer FA, Liu T. Fibrinogen varying effects on GPIIb/IIIa receptor-directed platelet inhibition *in vitro. Am Heart J.* 2001;142:204-210.

24. Kong DF, Califf RM, Miller DP, et al. Clinical outcomes of therapeutic agents that block the platelet glycoprotein IIb/IIIa integrin in ischemic heart disease. *Circulation.* 1998;98:2829-2835.

25. Topol EJ, Moliterno DJ, Herrmann HC, et al, for the TARGET Investigators. Comparison of two platelet glycoprotein IIb/IIIa inhibitors, tirofiban and abciximab, for the prevention of ischemic events with percutaneous coronary revascularization. *N Engl J Med.* 2001; 344:1888-1894.

26. Karvouni E, Katritsis DG, Ioannidis JPA. Intravenous glycoprotein IIb/IIIa receptor antagonists reduce mortality after percutaneous coronary interventions. *J Am Coll Cardiol.* 2003;41:26-32.

27. Giugliano RP. Drug-induced thrombocytopenia—is it a serious concern for glycoprotein IIb/IIIa receptor inhibitors? *J Thromb Thrombolysis*. 1998;5:191-202.

28. Berkowitz SD, Harrington RA, Rund MM, Tcheng JE. Acute profound thrombocytopenia after c7E3 Fab (abciximab) therapy. *Circulation*. 1997;95:809-813.

29. Chew DP, Bhatt DL, Sapp S, Topol EJ. Increased mortality with oral platelet glycoprotein IIb/IIIa antagonists. *Circulation*. 2001;103:201-206.

8

9   Monitoring of Anticoagulants

Introduction

Because of the narrow therapeutic index of warfarin and unfractionated heparin (UFH), monitoring of the anticoagulant effect of these drugs is required. On the other hand, low molecular weight heparin (LMWH) and fibrinolytic agents need to be monitored only under certain specific circumstances, to be described subsequently. Laboratory control of anticoagulants adds a level of complexity to treatment; variations in procedures and reagents can complicate management, especially if different laboratories are involved in the care of a single patient. Efforts to standardize testing must be an ongoing process as new methods and reagents are continually being introduced.

Warfarin

The prothrombin time is used to monitor warfarin treatment. This test is sensitive to the plasma concentrations of clotting factors II (prothrombin), V, VII, and X. Warfarin affects the vitamin K–dependent factors: II, VII, IX, and X, as well as proteins C, S, and Z. Thus the prothrombin time does not reflect the effect of warfarin on some factors (IX, proteins C, S, and Z) and is sensitive to others (factor V), which are not vitamin K–dependent. Therefore, the prothrombin time is not the ideal test of warfarin treatment, but its simplicity and widespread availability have enshrined it in clinical practice.

By convention, prothrombin times are now reported as international normalized ratio (INR). This is the ratio of the patient's prothrombin time to a control prothrombin time, raised to a power—the international sensitivity index (ISI). The latter reflects the calibration of the thromboplastin used for the prothrombin time testing to an internationally agreed upon standard. In many laboratories, the reagent currently used is a recombinant thromboplastin which has an ISI of

1, whereas in the past, the most commonly used reagents had ISIs of 2. In a laboratory with a control prothrombin time of 10 seconds, a prothrombin time of 15 seconds using a thromboplastin with ISI of 2 would have a calculated INR of 2.25 (15/10).[1] The same INR could be achieved with a recombinant thromboplastin (ISI of 1), but the prothrombin time would be 22.5 seconds (22.5/10).[2] Thus, the INR standardizes test values across laboratories using different reagents.

An INR in the range of 2 to 3 has been found to be optimal for patients with thrombotic disease; this was best exemplified in the Stroke Prevention in Atrial Fibrillation (SPAF) studies.[1,2] In these trials of oral anticoagulation in atrial fibrillation, INR values of <2 were most often associated with thrombotic events, while most hemorrhagic events occurred when the INR exceeded 3. Similar results have been obtained in patients with deep vein thrombosis and pulmonary embolism. INRs of 2 to 3 have also been recommended for the prevention of thromboembolism in patients undergoing high-risk surgery (joint replacement), and in those with valvular heart disease.[3] On the other hand, higher INRs have been suggested for patients with the lupus anticoagulant/antiphospholipid antibody (APA) syndrome and for those with prosthetic heart valves. With regard to the APA syndrome, retrospective studies indicated that INR values of 3 to 4 were more effective in thrombus prevention than lower ranges. However, prospective studies randomizing patients to INRs of 2 to 3 vs 3 to 4 are currently under way and should establish whether the higher range is necessary. Mechanical prosthetic heart valves pose a high risk of thromboembolism. The recommendations of the Sixth American College of Chest Physicians (ACCP) Consensus Conference on Antithrombotic Therapy with regard to the various types of valves are summarized in **Table 9.1**.[4]

There are a few cautions in interpreting the results of prothrombin time tests.[5] Since the test is sensitive to the level of factor V in the plasma, improper sample storage or delayed testing may cause loss of factor V and give prothrombin time values outside the expected range. High concentrations of heparin may also prolong the prothrombin time; this usually occurs when the sample is obtained within a few minutes of administering a bolus dose of heparin.

TABLE 9.1 — INTENSITY OF ORAL ANTICOAGULANT THERAPY IN PATIENTS WITH PROSTHETIC HEART VALVES (ACCP RECOMMENDATIONS)

Type of Valve	Location	Recommended INR
Mechanical		
Bileaflet	Aortic	2.0-3.0
Bileaflet with AF	Aortic	2.5-3.5 or 2.0-3.0 plus ASA 80-100 mg/day
Bileaflet	Mitral	2.5-3.5 or 2.0-3.0 plus ASA 80-100 mg/day
Tilting disk	Mitral	2.5-3.5 or 2.0-3.0 plus ASA 80-100 mg/day
Caged ball	Any	2.5-3.5 plus ASA 80-100/day
Bioprosthetic		
No AF	Aortic/mitral	2.0-3.0: first 3 mo postop
AF, atrial thrombus, prior thromboembolism	Aortic/mitral	2.0-3.0: indefinitely

Abbreviations: ACCP, American College of Chest Physicians; AF, atrial fibrillation; ASA, aspirin; INR, international normalized ratio.

Proceedings of the ACCP 6th Consensus Conference on Antithrombotic Therapy. *Chest.* 2001;119(suppl 1):220S-227S.

9

Neutralizing heparin prior to sample testing may allow one to overcome this problem. Direct thrombin inhibitors, such as hirudin and argatroban, may also prolong the prothrombin time to a modest degree. Some thromboplastins are sensitive to the lupus anticoagulant; the prolonged prothrombin times reported under these circumstances may deceive the clinician into thinking that the patient is adequately anticoagulated. In patients known to have a lupus anticoagulant, prothrombin times should be performed with thromboplastins that are insensitive to lupus anticoagulant, or other tests, such as factor X assay, should be obtained.

Heparin

Unfractionated heparin is monitored with the activated partial thromboplastin time (aPTT) test. In contrast to the prothrombin time, there is no generally agreed upon standardization for the aPTT. Different laboratories use reagents with varying sensitivities to the effects of UFH. Therapeutic anticoagulation requires heparin concentrations of 0.2 to 0.4 U/mL; in most laboratories this would correspond with aPTT values 1.5 to 2.5 times control values. However, each laboratory should calibrate its particular aPTT reagents against plasma containing a known amount of heparin, usually measured by the protamine titration method.[6]

Studies by Hull and colleagues demonstrated the importance of rapidly achieving a therapeutic aPTT.[7] Patients whose aPTT failed to reach therapeutic levels by 24 hours after the start of therapy were at increased risk of subsequent recurrent venous thrombosis. Several methods for rapidly achieving therapeutic aPTTs have been published; these are summarized in **Table 9.2**.[8-10] Hull and associates[9] make an adjustment for clinical history of increased bleeding risk, and the nomogram of Raschke and colleagues[10] is based on body weight. All of the methods were successful in having the aPTTs of the majority of patients exceed the lower limit of the therapeutic range at 24 hours. However, bleeding occurred more frequently in patients managed with the Hull nomogram than in those treated according to the Raschke method. At our institution, we prefer the weight-based nomogram because of its simplicity, safety, and effectiveness.

TABLE 9.2 — REGIMENS USING UNFRACTIONATED HEPARIN FOR THE TREATMENT OF VENOUS THROMBOEMBOLISM

Cruikshank 5000 U* (1280 U/h)		Hull 5000 U* (1680 U/h); High Risk[†] = 1240 U/h		Raschke 80 U/kg* (18 U/kg/h)	
aPTT (s)	Rate Change (U/h)	aPTT (s)	Rate Change (U/h)	aPTT (s)	Rate Change (U/kg/h)
<50	+120	<45	+240	<35	+4
50-59	+120	46-54	+120	35-45	+2
60-85	0	55-85	0	46-70	0
86-95	–80	86-110	–120	71-90	–2
95-120	–80	>110	–240	>90	–3
>120	–160	—	—	—	—

Abbreviation: aPTT, activated partial thromboplastin time.

* Bolus followed by continuous infusion.
† Patients having surgery within past 2 weeks, history of peptic ulcer, gastrointestinal or genitourinary tract bleeding, thrombotic stroke within past 2 weeks, platelet count <150,000/ mL, high risk of bleeding.

Cruikshank MK, et al. *Arch Intern Med.* 1991;151:333-337; Hull RD, et al. *Arch Intern Med.* 1992;152:1589-1595; Raschke RA, et al. *Ann Intern Med.* 1993;119:874-881.

9

Low molecular weight heparin does not require laboratory monitoring in clinically stable patients, whether given for prophylaxis or as treatment.[11] Monitoring is recommended in the following patients:

- Pediatric patients and those who weigh <50 kg
- Those weighing >120 kg
- Pregnant patients, initially and during the third trimester
- Those with renal failure (creatinine >2 mg/dL)
- Those at high risk for bleeding.

The usual test selected for monitoring is the chromogenic anti-factor Xa (anti-Xa) assay, obtained 4 hours after the dose of LMWH. Levine and colleagues studied patients receiving LMWH prophylaxis for hip replacement.[12] Wound hematoma occurred in 5.3% when the anti-Xa level was ≤0.2 U/mL but increased to 24.5% when levels exceeded 0.2 U/mL. Conversely, thrombosis was 6.3% if minimum anti-Xa levels exceeded 0.1 U/mL but increased to 14.6% when they were ≤0.1 U/mL. These differences were all statistically significant. One should recognize, however, that LMWHs have a variety of effects on hemostasis that are not assessed by the anti-Xa test; this measurement provides only an approximation of the antithrombotic activity of these agents. The anti-Xa assay in patients receiving therapeutic, as opposed to prophylactic, doses of the drug are much less predictive of bleeding or thrombosis. Values >1 U/mL appear to be associated with an increased risk of bleeding. A novel point-of-care enoxaparin-specific coagulation test is undergoing evaluation in the setting of percutaneous coronary intervention (PCI).

Direct Thrombin Inhibitors

Monitoring is required when the currently available direct thrombin inhibitors (lepirudin, bivalirudin, and argatroban) are administered.[11] **Table 9.3** shows the tests that are used, the therapeutic range needed, and the conditions requiring dose adjustments for each agent. When lepirudin is used for cardiopulmonary bypass, the ecarin clotting time, titrated to the lepirudin plasma level, appears to be the most reliable monitoring assay. Levels of 3.5 to

TABLE 9.3 — MONITORING DIRECT THROMBIN INHIBITORS

Agent	Test	Therapeutic Range	Dose Adjustment
Lepirudin	aPTT at 4 h*	1.5-2.5[†] (not to exceed 70s)	Renal failure
Bivalirudin	ACT at 45 min	300-350s[‡]	Renal failure
Argatroban	aPTT at 2 h	1.5-3.0[†] (not to exceed 100s)	Liver failure

Abbreviations: ACT, activated clotting time; aPTT, activated partial thromboplastin time.

* Ecarin clotting time at 15-minute intervals for cardiopulmonary bypass.
† Above mean normal control.
‡ During percutaneous coronary intervention.

9

4.5 U/mL are optimal.[13] The adaptation of whole-blood thrombin-generation tests to point-of-care technology may have a role in the monitoring of anticoagulant therapy, but further investigation must be undertaken.

Fibrinolytic Agents

Monitoring plays a limited role in the management of thrombolytic therapy. Prior to initiating fibrinolytics, a careful clinical assessment should be conducted to evaluate the potential for serious bleeding. Hemorrhagic stroke or ischemic stroke within the past year, intracranial neoplasm, aortic dissection, recent surgery or trauma (<2 to 4 weeks), pregnancy, and active peptic ulcer are some of the conditions that would preclude thrombolysis except under the most dire circumstances.[14] Obtaining baseline tests of hemostasis, such as a platelet count, aPTT, prothrombin time, thrombin time, and fibrinogen level, will detect underlying hemostatic abnormalities.[15]

To assess the systemic effects of therapy, the reduction in fibrinogen, generation of fibrin degradation products, or depletion of plasminogen or α_2-antiplasmin may be examined.[16] If signs of excessive bleeding or oozing become apparent, measuring the fibrinogen level is helpful; values <100 mg/dL may be associated with increased hemorrhagic risk.[17]

REFERENCES

1. Stroke Prevention in Atrial Fibrillation (SPAF) Investigators. Adjusted-dose warfarin versus low-intensity, fixed-dose warfarin plus aspirin for high-risk patients with atrial fibrillation: Stroke Prevention in Atrial Fibrillation III randomised clinical trial. *Lancet*. 1996;348:633-638.

2. Stroke Prevention in Atrial Fibrillation (SPAF) Investigators. Bleeding during antithrombotic therapy in patients with atrial fibrillation. *Arch Intern Med*. 1996;156:409-416.

3. Hirsh J, Dalen JE, Anderson DR, et al. Oral anticoagulants: mechanism of action, clinical effectiveness, and optimal therapeutic range. *Chest*. 1998;114(suppl):445S-469S.

4. Stein PD, Alpert JS, Dalen JE, Horstkotte D, Turpie AG. Antithrombotic therapy in patients with mechanical and biological prosthetic heart valves. *Chest*. 1998;114(suppl):602S-610S.

5. Fairweather RB, Ansell J, van den Besselaar MHP, et al. College of American Pathologists Conference XXXI on laboratory monitoring of oral anticoagulant therapy. *Arch Pathol Lab Med*. 1998;122:768-781.

6. Brill-Edwards P, Ginsberg JS, Johnston M, Hirsh J. Establishing a therapeutic range for heparin therapy. *Ann Intern Med*. 1993;119: 104-109.

7. Hull RD, Raskob GE, Brant RF, Pineo GF, Valentine KA. Relation between the time to achieve the lower limit of the aPTT therapeutic range and recurrent venous thromboembolism during heparin treatment for deep vein thrombosis. *Arch Intern Med*. 1997;157:2562-2568.

8. Cruikshank MK, Levine MN, Hirsh J, Roberts R, Siguenza M. A standard heparin nomogram for the management of heparin therapy. *Arch Intern Med*. 1991;151:333-337.

9. Hull RD, Raskob GE, Rosenbloom DR, et al. Optimal therapeutic level of heparin therapy in patients with venous thrombosis. *Arch Intern Med*. 1992;152:1589-1595.

10. Raschke RA, Reilly BM, Guidry JR, Fontana JR, Srinivas S. The weight-based heparin dosing nomogram compared with a "standard care" nomogram. *Ann Intern Med*. 1993;119:874-881.

11. Laposata M, Green D, Van Cott EM, Barrowcliffe TW, Goodnight SH, Sosolik RC. The clinical use and laboratory monitoring of low-molecular-weight heparin, danaparoid, hirudin and related compounds, and argatroban. *Arch Pathol Lab Med*. 1998;122:799-807.

9

12. Levine MN, Planes A, Hirsh J, Goodyear M, Vochelle N, Gent M. The relationship between anti-factor Xa level and clinical outcome in patients receiving enoxaparin low molecular weight heparin to prevent deep vein thrombosis after hip replacement. *Thromb Haemost.* 1989;62:940-944.

13. Poetzsch B, Madlener K. Management of cardiopulmonary bypass anticoagulation in patients with heparin-induced thrombocytopenia. in: Warkentin TE, Greinacher A, eds. *Heparin-Induced Thrombocytopenia.* New York, NY: Marcel Dekker; 2000:355-369.

14. Leopold JA, Keaney JF Jr, Loscalzo J. Pharmacology of thrombolytic agents. In: Loscalzo J, Schafer AI, eds. *Thrombosis and Hemorrhage.* 2nd ed. Baltimore, Md: Williams and Wilkins; 1998:1236.

15. van Breda A, Katzen BT. Radiologic aspects of intra-arterial thrombolytic therapy. In: Comerota AJ, ed. *Thrombolytic Therapy.* Orlando, Fla: Grune & Stratton; 1988:113.

16. Nora RE, Bell WR. Practical aspects of thrombolytic therapy for deep vein thrombosis. In: Comerota AJ, ed. *Thrombolytic Therapy.* Orlando, Fla: Grune and Stratton; 1988:35-36.

17. Loscalzo J. Fibrinolytic therapy. In: Beutler E, Lichtmann MA, Coller BS, Kipps TJ, eds. *Williams Hematology.* 5th ed. New York, NY: McGraw-Hill, Inc; 1995:1589.

10   Monitoring of Platelet Activity

Despite the well-recognized benefits of platelet inhibition for the prevention and treatment of acute coronary syndromes, studies using traditional monitoring tools have not successfully achieved "proof of concept" in determining the degree of inhibition that is both safe and effective. In addition, measurements that are capable of assessing underlying atherosclerotic disease activity, prothrombotic potential, and response to treatment have not been developed for routine daily practice nor do they consider individual variability in prothrombotic potential. The advent of near-patient, whole-blood assays and point-of-care technology may change management substantially, facilitating a more targeted and comprehensive approach.

Assessing Hemostatic Potential

Traditionally, platelet function studies have been employed in the evaluation of patients with unexplained bleeding where they have contributed greatly to the understanding, diagnosis, and management of hereditary abnormalities such as von Willebrand's disease, Glanzmann's thrombasthenia (platelet glycoprotein [GP] IIb/IIIa receptor deficiency), and Bernard-Soulier disease (platelet GPIb/IX receptor deficiency). Although conventional platelet function studies (eg, turbidimetric aggregometry) have technical limitations that preclude their routine use for gauging antithrombotic therapy, they may provide guidance when hemorrhagic complications arise and when determining pretreatment risk in individuals suspected of having an intrinsic platelet abnormality.

Bleeding Time

The bleeding time, considered an indicator of primary hemostasis (platelet plug formation), is defined as the time between making a small standardized skin incision and the precise moment when bleeding stops. The test is performed with a template, through which the medial surface of the forearm is incised under 40-mm Hg standard pressure. A normal bleeding time is between 6 and 10 minutes. Although considered a "standardized" test of platelet function, the bleeding time can be influenced by a variety of factors, including platelet count, qualitative abnormalities, and features intrinsic to the blood vessel wall.[1]

Platelet Adhesion Tests

Platelet adhesion is the initiating step in primary hemostasis. Although platelet binding is an important component of this process, there are many others, including blood flow rate, endothelial cell function, adhesive proteins, and the subendothelial matrix. The original platelet adhesion (or platelet retention) test was based on adherence to glass-bead columns.

Platelet Aggregometry

The current laboratory evaluation of platelet function is based predominantly on *turbidimetric platelet aggregometry* (also known as light-transmission aggregometry). This test is performed by preparing platelet-rich plasma (with platelet-poor plasma as a control) and eliciting an aggregation response with adenosine diphosphate (ADP), epinephrine, collagen, arachidonic acid, and ristocetin.[2]

Impedance platelet aggregometry has been introduced as an alternative to turbidimetric methods, with the potential physiologic advantage of using whole-blood samples.[3] The reproducibility of platelet aggregometry is influenced by a variety of factors that include:

- Concentration of sodium citrate in the collecting tubes
- Adjustment of the platelet count
- Storage time
- Stirring rate
- Temperature
- pH of the blood sample.

Hereditary (Congenital) Abnormalities Affecting Platelet Function

Abnormal platelet function (qualitative defect) is capable of causing clinical hemorrhage that, at times, can be life-threatening. The common congenital thrombocytopathies for which *in vitro* testing may be diagnostic are summarized in **Table 10.1**.

Acquired Platelet Defects

Quantitative or, more commonly, qualitative platelet abnormalities are encountered frequently in clinical practice and in most cases represent a desired effect from drug therapy (**Figure 10.1**). A variety of systemic disorders can also influence platelet function (**Table 10.2**).

Flow Cytometry

Although not routinely available, flow cytometry offers a wide range of diagnostic capabilities for determining hemostatic potential, thrombotic potential, and response to platelet-inhibiting therapies. Whole-blood samples are used and must be processed rapidly to maintain the "physiologic" environment.[4-6]

Bedside Assays and Instruments

Bedside assays, near-patient testing, and point-of-care monitoring instruments are attractive for several reasons. First, they provide a rapid, reliable, and reproducible means to assess hemostatic potential and treatment response. Second, the techniques involved require minimal training, reagent handling, calibration, and physical space. Third, emerging technology will offer a full complement of coagulation and platelet tests that can be used for management in the home, ambulatory clinic, emergency department, angioplasty suite, coronary care unit, and operating room.[7]

10

TABLE 10.1 — HEREDITARY PLATELET DISORDERS

Disease	Genetic Transmission	Specific Deficiency	Defect/Effect	Diagnosis
Glanzmann's thrombasthenia	Autosomal recessive	GPIIb/IIIa	Inability to bind fibrinogen and thus form platelet-to-platelet bridges	BT prolonged; abnormal aggregation response with all agonists; normal aggregation with ristocetin
Storage pool disease	Autosomal recessive and dominant	Storage and release of platelet granules	Important proteins for activation and aggregation inaccessible	Impaired aggregation response to various agonists
Bernard-Soulier disease	Autosomal recessive	GPIb/IX	Missing ligand for vWf leads to inability of platelets to bind to subendothelium	BT may exceed 20 min; thrombocytopenia; abnormal aggregation response with ristocetin
von Willebrand's disease	—	—	—	Reduced vWf antigen
Type I	Autosomal dominant	vWf-factor VIII	Decreased adhesion	Decreased response to RIPA; decreased ristocetin cofactor activity

Type IIa	Autosomal dominant in vWf	Qualitative defect	Increased clearance of multimers	Reduced vWf; high molecular weight multimers
Type IIb	Autosomal dominant	Increased affinity of vWf for GPIb/IX receptor	Decreased adhesion	Reduced vWf; high molecular weight multimers; ↑ RIPA at low levels*
Type III	Autosomal dominant	Very low or absent vWf	Decreased adhesion	Similar to type I; severe bleeding common
Platelet type or pseudo vWd	Autosomal dominant	vWf receptor	Enhanced avidity for vWf leads to platelet consumption and low plasma vWf	RIPA with patient's platelets and normal plasma reproduce the defect; this differentiates from type IIb vWd

Abbreviations: BT, bleeding time; GP, glycoprotein; RIPA, ristocetin-induced platelet aggregation; vWd, von Willebrand's disease; vWf, von Willebrand's factor.

* Aggregation in response to very low concentrations of ristocetin (<0.6 mg/mL).

10

FIGURE 10.1 — PHARMACOLOGIC CONTROL OF THROMBUS FORMATION

Abbreviations: AA, arachidonic acid; ADP, adenosine diphosphate; AMP, adenosine monophosphate; ATP, adenosine triphosphate; cAMP, cyclic adenosine monophosphate; GPIIb/IIIa, glycoprotein IIb/IIIa; PD, phosphodiesterase.

The available platelet antagonists "target" specific receptors and/ or biologic events rendering the platelet "unfit" for participation in thrombus formation.

■ **Platelet Function Analyzer–100**

The platelet function analyzer (PFA)-100 simulates primary hemostasis under high shear stress conditions. Citrated whole blood is drawn by capillary action through a membrane coated with either collagen and epinephrine or collagen and ADP.[8] An aperature in the membrane occludes following platelet adhesion and aggregation and the test results are recorded as closure time.

The assay is most useful in detecting primary hemostasis abnormalities (primary platelet function disorders and von Willebrand's disease) and in determining response to replacement therapy.[9]

■ **Clot Retraction Assay**

The strength of clot retraction can serve as a measure of platelet function,[10] and a hemostasis analyzer has been

TABLE 10.2 — CAUSES OF ACQUIRED DEFECTS IN PLATELET FUNCTION

Drugs
- Aspirin
- Ticlopidine
- Clopidogrel
- Cilostazol
- Glycoprotein (GP) IIb/IIIa antagonists (abciximab, tirofiban, eptifibatide)

Systemic Disorders and Disease States
- Chronic renal failure
- Myeloproliferative disorders
- Paraproteinemias
- Cardiopulmonary bypass
- Hemodialysis
- Disseminated intravascular coagulation

developed for this purpose. Citrated whole blood or platelet-rich plasma is placed in a sample chamber where calcium and thrombin are added to stimulate clot formation. As platelets bind, undergo cellular contraction, and polymerize with fibrin strands, the force developed by the platelets is measured by a probe transducer that produces an electrical output (a voltage signal converted to force reported in dynes) proportional to the amount of force generated.

The clot retraction assay provides information on the functional contribution of platelets to clot formation, and can use whole blood or plasma obtained from standard citrated blood collection tubes. Potential uses include the evaluation of hemostatic defects in uremia and following bypass surgery.[11]

■ Rapid Platelet Function Assay

The Rapid Platelet Function Assay is a semiautomated turbidimetric system that is based on the ability of activated platelets to interact with fibrinogen, yielding macroscopically visible agglutination.

Fibrinogen-coated polystyrene beads, buffers, and a modified thrombin receptor-activating peptide (iso-TRAP) are incorporated into a disposable cartridge and exposed to samples of citrated whole blood. The instrument detects agglutination between the fibrinogen-coated beads and activated platelets, providing a quantitative digital display. Because agglutination is proportional to the proportion of unblocked GPIIb/IIIa receptors, this device is well suited for determining platelet inhibitory response to currently available GPIIb/IIIa receptor antagonists (**Figure 10.2**).[12] The time required to obtain results is 2 minutes.

The semiautomated system is easy to use and correlates closely with traditional measurements of platelet function, turbidimetric platelet aggregation ($r^2 = 0.95$) and the percentage of free GPIIb/IIIa molecules ($r^2 = 0.96$).[13] The use of whole blood and duplicate analysis eliminates variables in sample preparation and minimizes random errors. Results can be reported as an absolute rate of aggregation or as a percentage of the baseline aggregation.

A rapid bedside assay that provides a reliable measurement of GPIIb/IIIa receptor blockade offers a broad range of medical, interventional, and surgical applications. Dose titration with intravenous agents may be performed, achieving a safe and effective degree of platelet inhibition.[14]

The intensity or level of platelet inhibition (achieved with GPIIb/IIIa antagonist therapy) required to prevent thrombotic complications following percutaneous coronary intervention (PCI) was determined in 485 patients participating in the GOLD study.[15] One quarter of all patients did not achieve ≥95% inhibition (rapid platelet function assay) 10 minutes after the initiation of treatment and experienced a significantly higher incidence of death, myocardial infarction (MI), or urgent target-vessel revascularization (14.4% vs 6.4%). Those with <70% inhibition at 8 hours were also at increased risk (25% vs 8.1%) (**Figures 10.3** and **10.4**).

A reliable and readily available means to assess inhibitory response to GPIIb/IIIa receptor antagonists may also provide guidance for dose titration in patients at risk for bleeding complications, including those with thrombocytopenia, prior hemorrhagic events, and known coagulopathies (**Table 10.3**).[16]

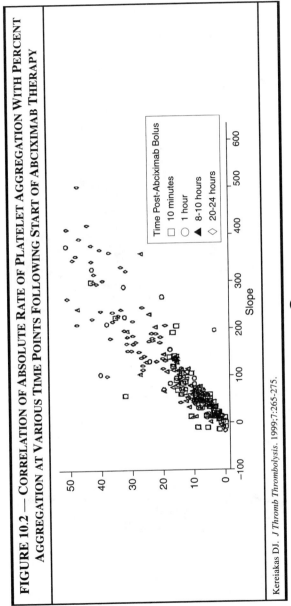

FIGURE 10.2 — CORRELATION OF ABSOLUTE RATE OF PLATELET AGGREGATION WITH PERCENT AGGREGATION AT VARIOUS TIME POINTS FOLLOWING START OF ABCIXIMAB THERAPY

Kereiakas DJ. *J Thromb Thrombolysis.* 1999;7:265-275.

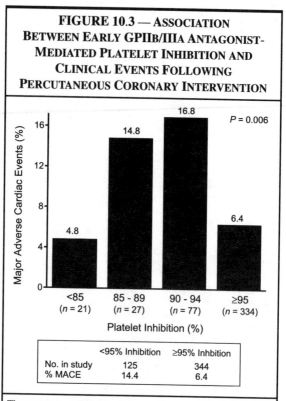

FIGURE 10.3 — ASSOCIATION BETWEEN EARLY GPIIb/IIIA ANTAGONIST-MEDIATED PLATELET INHIBITION AND CLINICAL EVENTS FOLLOWING PERCUTANEOUS CORONARY INTERVENTION

$P = 0.006$

	<95% Inhibition	≥95% Inhbition
No. in study	125	344
% MACE	14.4	6.4

The occurrence of major adverse cardiac events (MACE), death, myocardial infarction, and urgent target-vessel revascularization, correlated with the intensity of platelet inhibition 10 minutes after initiation of glycoprotein (GP) IIb/IIIa antagonist therapy.

Steinhubl SR, et al. *Circulation*. 2001;103:2572-2578.

Assessing the Contribution of Platelets to Thrombin Generation

Platelet activation, aggregation, and coagulation are complementary, mutually dependent processes in hemostasis and thrombosis. It has become clear that platelets differ in their capacity to support thrombin generation, creating a

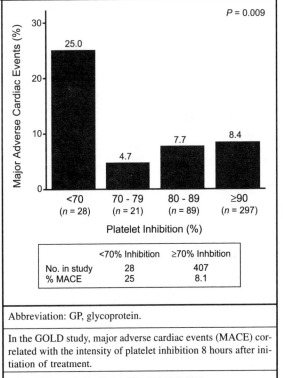

FIGURE 10.4 — THE THRESHOLD LEVEL OF PLATELET INHIBITION REQUIRED TO ACHIEVE OPTIMAL OUTCOME WITH GPIIb/IIIa RECEPTOR ANTAGONISTS IN PERCUTANEOUS CORONARY INTERVENTION

$P = 0.009$

	<70% Inhibition	≥70% Inhbition
No. in study	28	407
% MACE	25	8.1

Abbreviation: GP, glycoprotein.

In the GOLD study, major adverse cardiac events (MACE) correlated with the intensity of platelet inhibition 8 hours after initiation of treatment.

Steinhubl SR, et al. *Circulation.* 2001;103:2572-2578.

10

complex situation for assessing response to pharmacologic therapy (**Figure 10.5**).[17]

Summary

The recognized role of platelets as the initiating step in arterial thrombosis provides a strong basis for their tar-

TABLE 10.3 — CLINICAL SETTINGS IN WHICH PLATELET MONITORING MIGHT BE USEFUL

Patient-Related (confirm target inhibition)
- Prior to percutaneous coronary intervention
- Patients with refractory ischemia or recurrent symptoms despite receiving glycoprotein (GP) IIb/IIIa receptor antagonist therapy
- Interruption of infusion
- Thrombocytopenia
- Qualitative platelet abnormality
- Renal insufficiency
- Low or high body weight

Clinically Related
- Bleeding:
  - Confirm intensity of inhibition
  - Confirm reversal of inhibition following replacement therapy
- Emergent surgery:
  - Guidance to reverse platelet inhibition (if clinically necessary)
- Transition from one GPIIb/IIIa receptor antagonist to another

geted inhibition in the primary and secondary prevention of cardiovascular events. Traditionally, the assessment of platelet activity has been viewed as a diagnostic tool for evaluating patients with hemorrhage. The development of potent antagonists, coupled with a long-standing absence of information correlating treatment response, disease activity, and pharmacologic platelet inhibition, has fostered point-of-care technology that changes the focus of patient care from "one size fits all" to pathobiology-based, targeted, patient-specific antithrombotic intervention.

REFERENCES

1. George JN, Shattil SJ. The clinical importance of acquired abnormalities of platelet function. *N Engl J Med.* 1991;324:27-39.

2. Born GVR. Qualitative investigations into the aggregation of blood platelets. *J Physiol* (London). 1962:67:162.

FIGURE 10.5 — INDIVIDUAL VARIABILITY IN PLATELET PROCOAGULANT FUNCTION

Data for this figure were taken from Sumner WT, et al (*Thromb Res.* 1996;81:533-543). Platelets from 14 normal individuals were activated with thrombin. Thrombin generation (IIase activity) was measured with factor Xa supplied by the platelets. Factor Xa generation (Xase activity) was measured with factor IXa, factor VIIIa, and factor X. There was no significant correlation between thrombin generation and factor Xa generation. Note that neither the X axis nor the Y axis goes to zero.

Monroe DM, et al. *Arterioscler Thromb Vasc Biol.* 2002;22:1381-1389.

3. Cardinal DC, Flower RJ. The electronic aggregometer: a novel device for assessing platelet behavior in blood. *J Pharmacol Methods.* 1980;3:135-158.

4. Becker RC, Tracy RP, Bovill EG, Mann KG, Ault K for the TIMI-III Thrombosis and Anticoagulation Study Group. The clinical use of flow cytometry for assessing platelet activation in acute coronary syndromes. *Coronary Artery Dis.* 1994;5:339-345.

5. Becker RC, Bovill EG, Corrao JM, et al for the TIMI III Thrombosis and Coagulation Study Group. Platelet activation determined by flow cytometry persists despite antithrombotic therapy in patients with unstable angina and non-Q-wave myocardial infarction. *J Thromb Thrombolysis.* 1994;1:95-100.

6. Becker RC, Bovill EG, Corrao JM, et al. Dynamic nature of thrombin generation, fibrin formation, and platelet activation in unstable angina and non-Q-wave myocardial infarction. *J Thromb Thrombolysis.* 1995;2:57-64.

7. Becker RC. Exploring the medical need for alternate site testing. A clinician's perspective. *Arch Pathol Lab Med.* 1995;119:894-897.

8. Mammen EF, Comp PC, Gosselin R, et al. PFA-100 system: a new method for assessment of platelet dysfunction. *Semin Thromb Hemost.* 1998;24:195-202.

9. Jennings LK, White MM. Expression of ligand induced binding sites on glycoprotein IIb/IIIa complexes and the effect of various inhibitors. *Am Heart J.* 1998;135(suppl, pt 2):S179-S183.

10. Greilich PE, Carr ME, Carr SL, Chang AS. Reductions in platelet force development by cardiopulmonary bypass are associated with hemorrhage. *Anesth Analg.* 1995;80:459-465.

11. Carr ME, Zekert SL, Hantgan RR, Braaten J. Glycoprotein IIb/IIIa blockade inhibits platelet-mediated force development and reduces gell elastic modulus. *Thromb Haemost.* 1995;73:499-505.

12. Coller BS, Scudder LE, Beer J, et al. Monoclonal antibodies to platelet glycoprotein IIb/IIIa as antithrombotic agents. *Ann NY Acad Sci.* 1991;614:193-213.

13. Smith JW, Steinhubl SR, Lincoff AM, et al. Rapid platelet-function assay: an automated and quantitative cartridge-based method. *Circulation.* 1999;99:620-625.

14. Kereiakes DJ, Mueller M, Howard W, et al. Efficacy of abciximab induced platelet blockade using a rapid point of care assay. *J Thromb Thrombolysis.* 1999;7:265-276.

15. Steinhubl SR, Talley JD, Braden GA, et al. Point-of-care measured platelet inhibition correlates with a reduced risk of an adverse cardiac event after percutaneous coronary intervention: results of the GOLD (AU-Assessing Ultegra) multicenter study. *Circulation.* 2001;103:2572-2578.

16. Mukherjee D, Chew DP, Robbins M, et al. Clinical application of procedural platelet monitoring during percutaneous coronary intervention among patients at increased bleeding risk. *J Thromb Thrombolysis.* 2001;11:151-154.

17. Sumner WT, Monre DM, Hoffman M. Variability in platelet procoagulant activity in healthy volunteers. *Thromb Res.* 1996;81:533-543.

11 Inherited/Acquired Coagulation and Platelet Disorders (Thrombophilia)

Introduction

Thrombophilia is the term used to describe a tendency toward developing thrombosis. This tendency may be inherited, involving polymorphisms in gene coding for platelet or clotting factor proteins, or acquired due to alterations in the constituents of the blood or blood vessels. An example of a thrombophilic state that is both inherited and acquired is hyperhomocysteinemia; persons may have a genetic mutation leading to a modest defect in homocysteine metabolism, as well as a diet deficient in folate, with both contributing to an increase in plasma homocysteine and thrombosis.

When to Investigate for Thrombophilia

A complete history and physical examination are mandatory in patients presenting with either venous or arterial thrombosis. Inherited thrombophilia is likely if there is a history of repeated episodes of thrombosis or a family history of thromboembolism. One should also consider an inherited thrombophilia when there are no obvious predisposing factors for thrombosis or when clots occur in a patient under the age of 45. Repeated episodes of thromboembolism occurring in patients over the age of 45 raise suspicion of an occult malignancy. On the other hand, deep vein thrombosis (DVT) complicating joint replacement surgery occurs in persons without other risk factors, and a search for inherited thrombophilia usually is not warranted. Recurrence or extension of thrombus in a leg previously affected by DVT often indicates permanent damage to the involved venous structures and is a manifestation of the postphlebitic syndrome.

Inherited Thrombophilia

Some causes of inherited thrombophilia are shown in **Table 11.1**. This list is by no means complete, as new genetic polymorphisms are regularly being discovered and linked to a tendency to venous or arterial thrombosis.

Incidence

The prevalence of the more common thrombophilias is shown in **Figure 11.1**. Note that the factor V Leiden (FVL) mutation and hyperhomocysteinemia are present in nearly 5% of the general population and are often found in patients with venous thrombosis, while deficiencies of antithrombin (AT), protein C (PC), and protein S (PS) are relatively uncommon. Elevated levels of factor VIII (FVIII) are frequently noted in the general population and in patients with thrombosis. This is not surprising as FVIII is an acute-phase reactant that increases rapidly after surgery or trauma. However, prospective studies have shown that the increases in FVIII in some patients cannot be attributed to a stress reaction and probably indicate mutations in the genes controlling FVIII synthesis or release.[1]

The relative risks for thrombosis in patients with inherited thrombophilia have been examined. While AT mutations are the least common, they are associated with high frequencies of venous thrombosis (8%); similar risk is seen with PC and PS deficiency. In contrast, the lifetime risk of having a thromboembolic event in an individual heterozygous for FVL is only 2.2%.[2] Incidence rates markedly increase with age,[3] and are highest in those with AT deficiency, then PC and PS, and least with FVL.[4] FVL occurs with the highest frequency in persons of Northern European ancestry (3% to 8%), followed by Southern European (0.6% to 2.9%), and is rare in Asians and Africans. In the United States, the prevalence is 4% to 6%.[5]

Etiology

Mutations in the genes for either clotting factors or their inhibitors may increase the risk of thrombosis. A gene

TABLE 11.1 — CAUSES OF THROMBOPHILIA

Inherited
- Factor V Leiden mutation
- Prothrombin 20210A mutation
- MTHFR 677, CS mutations
- Mutations in protein C gene
- Mutations in protein S gene
- Mutations in antithrombin gene
- Mutations in TM and TFPI genes
- Increased factors VIII, IX, X, ?vWF
- Mutations in fibrinogen genes
- Mutations in plasminogen gene
- Platelet GPIIIa (β_3) mutation
- Increased PAI-1
- Mutant heparin cofactor II

Acquired
- Hyperhomocysteinemia
- Antiphospholipid antibody
- Pregnancy, estrogens, oral contraceptives
- Hyperlipidemias
- Nephrotic syndrome
- Malignancy
- Trauma
- Immobilization
- Myeloproliferative disorders
- Thrombotic microangiopathies
- Heparin-induced thrombocytopenia
- Endotoxemia

Abbreviations: GP, glycoprotein; MTHFR, 5,10-methylenetetrahydrofolate reductase; PAI, plasminogen activator inhibitor; TFPI, tissue factor pathway inhibitor; TM, thrombomodulin; vWf, von Willebrand factor.

11

mutation may result in increased production of a procoagulant protein, such as FVIII or prothrombin, or lead to a mutated factor that is resistant to inactivation by its natural inhibitor (factor V and activated PC). An alteration in the amino acid sequence of antithrombin may prevent heparin from binding to and activating this anticoagulant. Mutant fibrinogens may be resistant to profibrinolytic

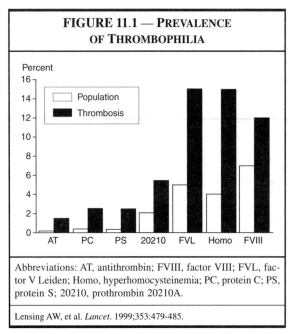

FIGURE 11.1 — PREVALENCE OF THROMBOPHILIA

Abbreviations: AT, antithrombin; FVIII, factor VIII; FVL, factor V Leiden; Homo, hyperhomocysteinemia; PC, protein C; PS, protein S; 20210, prothrombin 20210A.

Lensing AW, et al. *Lancet.* 1999;353:479-485.

enzymes.[6] Last, patients may have more than one mutation, greatly increasing their risk of thrombosis.

Factor V Leiden is a mutant factor V that has an arginine-to-glutamic acid substitution at position 506, rendering the activated factor V partially resistant to inactivation by activated protein C (aPC).[7] The FVL also alters the ability of aPC to inactivate FVIII.[8] The impaired inactivation of activated factors V and VIII enhances blood coagulability. Persons may be either heterozygous or homozygous for the FVL mutation; thrombosis occurs much more frequently in those who are homozygous. In heterozygotes, the first episode of thrombosis usually occurs when there are superimposed risk factors such as surgery, trauma, immobilization, or exposure to oral contraceptives. The latter increases the risk of thrombosis more than 5-fold.[9] Persistence of this trait in the population has been attributed to a decreased risk of intrapartum bleeding.[10] However, FVL is associated with recurrent fetal loss.[11,12] Other mutations in factor V may also contribute to the risk of thrombosis. For example, the

HR2 haplotype, a mutation predicting two amino acid changes is not in itself a risk factor for thrombosis. However, when coinherited with FVL, the risk of thrombosis is increased three- to fourfold.[13]

Prothrombin G20210A has a mutation in a regulatory sequence of the prothrombin gene leading to an increased synthesis of the prothrombin protein. Heterozygotes for the mutation have prothrombin concentrations that are increased about 1.3-fold,[14] and this is associated with an odds ratio of 2 to 3 for thrombosis.[15] An association of the prothrombin mutation with cerebral venous thrombosis has been reported.[16] As with FVL, there is also an increased frequency of thrombosis with this mutation in women who take oral contraceptives.[17]

Hyperhomocysteinemia may be congenital or acquired (**Table 11.2**).[18] In clinical practice, most patients with hyperhomocysteinemia are either homozygous for the C677T polymorphism of the methylenetetrahydrofolate reductase (MTHFR) gene, and/or have nutritional folate deficiency. Thrombosis is associated with raised homocysteine levels but not the C677T mutation, and may occur in either the venous or arterial circulation. The usual manifestations are DVT, stroke, myocardial infarction (MI), and peripheral vascular disease. In one series, hyperhomocysteinemia was found in 13% of venous and 19% of arterial disease, and the risk for occlusive disease was increased 1.7-fold. Occlusive disease occurs at a younger age and there is a significantly higher recurrence rate.[19,20] Furthermore, the mortality associated with coronary heart disease is increased in proportion to the plasma homocysteine concentration.[21] The mechanism by which elevated levels of homocysteine promote thrombosis is unclear. There is experimental evidence of injury to the endothelium, decrease in nitric oxide (NO) production, induction of oxidation of low-density lipoprotein cholesterol, and increased affinity of lipoprotein (a) (Lp[a]) for plasmin-modified fibrin surfaces, thereby inhibiting lysis of thrombi.[22-24] Plasma homocysteine concentrations decline when folate is taken, even in doses as low as 1 mg daily. In other patients, however, folate must be given along with vitamins B_6 and B_{12} in order to affect homocysteine levels. Clinical trials are in progress to deter-

11

TABLE 11.2 — CAUSES OF HYPERHOMOCYSTEINEMIA

- Genetic mutations:
  - Cystathione synthase
  - Methylenetetrahydrofolate reductase (MTHFR)
- Nutritional:
  - Deficiencies of folate, vitamin B_6, and vitamin B_{12}
- Diseases:
  - Kidney
  - Pernicious anemia
  - Hypothyroidism
  - Acute lymphocytic leukemia
  - Carcinoma of the breast, ovary, pancreas
  - Severe psoriasis
- Medications:
  - Folate antagonists
  - Oral contraceptives
  - Theophylline
- Miscellaneous:
  - Older age
  - Male sex
  - Menopause
  - Smoking

Adapted from: Martinelli I, et al. *Arterioscler Thromb Vasc Biol.* 1999; 19:700-703.

mine whether a reduction in homocysteine levels actually alters thrombosis frequency.

Proteins C, S, and AT are natural anticoagulant factors. Homozygosity for AT deficiency is lethal in utero, and for PC and PS, it leads to widespread thrombosis at birth (purpura fulminans) and death unless the protein is replaced by transfusion. Persons with one mutant gene (heterozygotes) develop thromboses in early adulthood, although some may not experience blood clots until later in life. Thrombi are usually venous in location and may affect mesenteric, cerebral, and other veins in addition to those in the legs and pelvis. In general, thrombosis occurs when there are risk factors in addition to the inherited mutations; these include surgery, cigarette smoking, pregnancy, and oral contraceptive use and any illness that results in the need for bed rest, dehydration, and increases in stress-related proteins such as FVIII, fibrinogen, and plasminogen activator inhibitor-1.

Heparin cofactor II is a protease inhibitor like AT, but it is activated by dermatan sulfate rather than heparin. Thrombosis occurs only in persons with homozygous deficiency. Other causes of inherited thrombophilia include abnormalities in clot lysis. Cases have been reported where fibrin, the principal component of the blood clot, is altered so that it resists lysis, or there are mutations in the gene for plasminogen required for clot dissolution. Other components of the clotting pathway, such as thrombomodulin, which is necessary for PC activation, and tissue factor pathway inhibitor, an anticoagulant, may be abnormal and increase susceptibility to clotting.

Factor VIII has been found to be increased in one third of persons with thrombosis, as well as in their relatives, suggesting that mutations in the FVIII gene that give rise to increased FVIII activity will be important in thrombosis risk.[25] However, such mutations have not yet been discovered.[26] In addition, increased concentrations of fibrinogen and levels of factors IX and XI above the 90th percentile have been demonstrated to be risk factors for venous thrombosis.[27-29]

Location of Thrombi

In patients with inherited thrombophilia, thrombi are usually located in the venous circulation, with a few important exceptions. Patients with hyperhomocysteinemia may have early-onset arterial as well as venous thrombosis.[19] A study in Japan reported that the frequency of the MTHFR gene mutation (homozygous) was more than twice as high in stroke patients as in controls.[30] FVL and prothrombin 20210A are associated with a risk of MI in young women who smoke, and in male smokers, but not in nonsmokers.[31-33] The prothrombin mutation 20210A and FVL are both associated with an increased odds ratio for MI in male smokers, as well as in those with hypertension, hypercholesterolemia, and diabetes. The prothrombin mutation was also found to be overrepresented in persons who had a stroke prior to the age of 50.[34] As mentioned earlier, prothrombin 20210A is also associated with cerebral vein thrombosis. Inherited thrombophilia may lead to thrombosis of placental vessels. As previously noted, recurrent pregnancy losses occur in patients with FVL, and this is also the case for persons with the prothrombin mutation[35] and inherited deficiencies of AT, PC, and PS, and there is an eightfold risk of thrombosis in pregnancy.[36,37]

Platelet Abnormalities

A number of mutations in the genes controlling the formation of platelet proteins are being discovered; some of them may increase the tendency for thrombosis. For example, the platelet surface protein, glycoprotein (GP) Ia, mediates platelet binding to collagen, and GPIb mediates binding to von Willebrand's factor (vWf). Platelet GPIIb/IIIa is involved in the binding of fibrinogen. Mutations of these proteins (ie, GPIa and PI^{A2}) have been implicated in increasing the risk for coronary heart disease and cerebral thrombosis.[38,39] A study of a family with premature cardiovascular disease and polymorphisms in both GPIa and GPIIIa demonstrated increased platelet-collagen interaction and procoagulant activity.[40] A "sticky platelet" syndrome has also been described, associated with venous and arterial thrombosis.[41] There are likely many other platelet disorders predisposing to occlusive vascular disease.

Last, it should be emphasized that patients may have more than one risk factor; eg, heterozygosity for both FVL and prothrombin 20210A, or FVL and PS deficiency. Such combinations greatly increase the risk of thrombosis, as does homozygosity for FVL or the prothrombin mutation. In such cases, a history of thrombosis in family members almost always exists. Thrombosis risk is also greatly increased in the presence of other major risk factors such as cancer and diabetes. In these latter situations, thrombotic occlusion of coronary and cerebral arteries may occur in addition to venous thrombosis.

Acquired Thrombophilia

■ Acquired Deficiencies in Antithrombin, Protein C, and Protein S

Deficiencies of AT, PC, and PS may be acquired in the setting of a variety of disorders shown in **Table 11**.3. These three anticoagulant proteins are synthesized by the liver, and therefore levels are decreased when there is immaturity or disease of the liver. In addition, PC and PS require vitamin K for completion of their synthesis; concentrations are reduced when there is vitamin K deficiency or when warfarin is administered. The three anticoagulants are lost in the urine in patients with nephrotic syndrome and in the stool of persons with protein-losing enteropathies. They are consumed when there is disseminated intravascular coagulation or extensive thrombosis. The metabolism of AT is similar to that of albumin; conditions resulting in decreases in albumin, such as major surgery or trauma, also lower AT concentrations, which may be a factor in the pathogenesis of postsurgical thrombosis. Heparin treatment results in a slight decrease in AT levels, while warfarin may cause significant declines in the concentrations of PC and PS, leading, in extreme cases, to thrombosis of cutaneous vessels and skin necrosis. Estrogens, oral contraceptives, and pregnancy are associated with lowering of AT and PS levels. A decrease in PS is a consistent finding in patients with sickle cell disease. Last, about two thirds of PS circulates bound to the C4b-binding protein; increases in this protein occur in endotoxemia and certain other conditions, decreasing the availability of free PS. PC is decreased in patients undergoing marrow transplants who develop veno-occlusive disease, and it is also reduced in those with the antiphospholipid syndrome.

In addition, there are important acquired causes of resistance to aPC. These include pregnancy, oral contraceptives, oral anticoagulants, stroke, increased factor VIII levels, antiphospholipid syndrome, and autoantibodies directed against aPC.[42] Patients with aPC resistance are also susceptible to venous thrombosis; the greater the resistance, the higher the risk.[43]

TABLE 11.3 — ACQUIRED CAUSES OF ANTITHROMBIN, PROTEIN C, AND PROTEIN S DEFICIENCY

Acquired Cause	Antithrombin	Protein C and Protein S
Synthesis	Prematurity, liver disease	Prematurity, liver disease, vitamin K deficiency
Excretion	Nephrotic syndrome, IBD	Nephrotic syndrome, IBD
Consumption	Disseminated intravascular coagulation, postsurgical, posttrauma	Disseminated intravascular coagulation
Medications	Heparin, estrogens, oral contraceptives, L-asparaginase	Warfarin, estrogens, oral contraceptives
Miscellaneous	Pregnancy	Pregnancy,* sickle cell disease,* antiphospholipid antibody syndrome, endotoxemia, * HIV infection*

Abbreviations: HIV, human immunodeficiency virus; IBD, inflammatory bowel disease.

* Protein S deficiency.

■ Antiphospholipid Syndrome

Patients with this syndrome have a positive test for antibodies to phospholipid-protein complexes plus one of the following: venous or arterial thrombosis, livedo reticularis, neuropsychiatric disorder, valvular heart disease, thrombocytopenia, and/or recurrent fetal wastage.[44] The syndrome may be primary, meaning no associated disorders are present, or secondary to systemic lupus erythematosus, other autoimmune disorders, infections, malignancy, or exposure to certain drugs such as chlorpromazine, procainamide, or hydralazine. The diagnosis is based on the clinical findings of thrombosis, either arterial or venous, and a positive test for either anticardiolipin antibodies (ACAs) (titer >40 GPL [IgG Phospholipid units]) or lupus anticoagulant (LA). Antiphospholipid antibodies occur in about a third of patients with systemic lupus erythematosus but are also found in patients with rheumatoid arthritis, sickle cell disease, and in 10% to 15% of apparently healthy elderly individuals.[45]

Antiphospholipid-protein antibodies are a heterogeneous group of antibodies that recognize a variety of phospholipid-binding proteins; these include:

- β_2GP-1
- Prothrombin
- Clotting factors X and XI
- Proteins C and S
- Thrombomodulin
- Annexin V.

These antibodies are detected by ELISA assays that usually include anionic phospholipids such as ACAs or coagulant phospholipids (LA). Goodnight points out that the high-titer (>40 GPL antibodies) are more predictive of disease than low-titer antibodies[46]; antibodies directed against β_2GP-1 are more specific than IgM antibodies, which may be markers for infection rather than thrombosis; LA is more often associated with thrombosis than are ACAs; and last, multiple assays must be performed to assess patient risk for vascular disease.

The term "lupus anticoagulant" arose because the clotting times of phospholipid-based coagulation assays were prolonged by plasma from patients with lupus. This is because the antiphospholipid antibodies in the plasma of these patients interfere with the binding of clotting factors to procoagulant phospholipids. *In vivo*, however, these antibodies interfere with the binding of annexin V and β_2GP-1 to procoagulant phospholipids on cell membranes; this enhances the procoagulant activity of these membranes and is responsible for the thrombophilia.[47,48] In addition, antiphospholipid antibodies indirectly enhance the binding of PS to its plasma inhibitor, the C4b-binding protein, by interfering with the protective effect of β_2GP-1 in maintaining free protein S.[49] Antibodies directed against aPC have also been associated with extensive arterial and venous thrombosis.[50]

Patients have either arterial disease (stroke, digital ischemia, retinal artery occlusion) or recurrent venous thrombosis. The LA is the strongest risk factor for both arterial and venous thrombosis, but ACA >20 units is also an important risk factor for venous thrombosis.[51,52]

■ Diagnosis

An inherited thrombophilia is suspected in persons with thrombosis unexplained by obvious risk factors such as recent orthopedic, neurologic, or other surgery or trauma. The diagnostic approach is shown in **Table 11.4**. A useful algorithm for deciding whether to perform extensive diagnostic studies for inherited thrombophilia is FURY: $\underline{F}$ refers to a positive family history; $\underline{U}$, to clotting at unusual sites; $\underline{R}$, to recurrent episodes of thrombosis; and $\underline{Y}$, to age <45 years. With regard to laboratory investigations, Seligsohn and Lubetsky recommend that a test for resistance to aPC be performed and, if positive, followed by a genetic analysis for FVL and the HR_2 variant.[42] Other causes of aPC resistance include defects in proteins C or S, elevated levels of factor VIII, the use of oral contraceptives, and pregnancy. Further evaluation would include a test for the prothrombin G20210A mutation, screening for the LA and ACAs, and measurement of homocysteine concentration. The second tier of testing includes analysis of protein C, protein S, and AT. Deficiencies or defects in these analytes are much less common and may be acutely affected by the thrombosis itself. Ordinarily, they should be measured at least 2 weeks after oral anticoagu-

TABLE 11.4 — DIAGNOSTIC APPROACH TO THROMBOPHILIA

- History: FURY
  - **F** = positive family history
  - **U** = clotting at unusual sites
  - **R** = recurrent episodes of thrombosis
  - **Y** = age <45 years
- Laboratory studies:
  - aPC by clotting test: if positive, genetic analysis for factor V Leiden and factor V HR_2 mutation
  - Genetic analysis for prothrombin 20210 mutation
  - Lupus anticoagulant; anticardiolipin assay by enzyme-linked immunosorbent assay
  - Homocysteine
  - Antithrombin, proteins C and S (free and total)

Abbreviation: aPC, activated protein C.

lant therapy has been completed, when the effects of treatment and the acute phase of the illness have subsided. Should all of the above tests be unrevealing, further evaluation could include fibrinogen antigen and activity, measures of factors IX, XI, and polymorphisms of plasminogen and factor XIII.

■ Management

Thrombosis usually occurs in patients with more than one risk factor; if an inherited or acquired thrombophilia is present, oral contraceptives should be avoided and prophylaxis against thrombosis should be given after surgery or trauma. The use of antithrombotic drugs is discussed in Chapter 3, *Heparins, Selective Factor Xa Inhibitors, Direct Thrombin Inhibitors, and Warfarin*, but what is unique to the thrombophilic disorders is the duration and intensity of anticoagulant therapy. Venous thrombosis is usually treated with heparin or low molecular weight heparin (LMWH) and warfarin. When the international normalized ratio (INR) obtained by the prothrombin time test is in the range of 2 to 3 for at least 48 hours, the heparins are discontinued. Warfarin is then continued for varying time periods, depending on the perceived risk of recurrence of thrombosis. In patients with inherited thrombophilia, such as that caused by FVL, discontinuing treatment after 3 to 6 months is associated with a recurrence rate of almost 40% after 8 years, as compared with 18% in persons without this mutation.[53] Therefore, continuation of warfarin treatment for >6 months may be considered but must be weighed against the risk of bleeding, which increases with each year of warfarin therapy.[54] In patients with the antiphospholipid syndrome, elevated titers of ACA present 6 months after an episode of venous thromboembolism are predictive of an increased risk of recurrence, and therefore anticoagulants are usually continued indefinitely in such patients.[55]

A problem in the use of warfarin for management of patients with LA is the confounding effect of this pathologic anticoagulant on the INR. Prolongation of the prothrombin time by the LA may be erroneously attributed to the warfarin and result in inadequate dosing of the drug. This may be the reason why some retrospective studies suggested that increasing the intensity of warfarin treatment from an INR of 2 to 3 to an INR of 3 to 4 would be more effective in preventing recurrent episodes of thrombosis.[56,57] However, a recent trial concluded that usual-intensity warfarin (INR 2 to 3) was as effective as high-intensity warfarin (INR 3.1 to 4) for patients with the antiphospholipid syndrome.[58] In pregnant women with antiphospholipid syndrome and a history of thrombosis, low-dose aspirin and heparin or LMWH must be given throughout pregnancy to prevent fetal loss as well as maternal thromboembolism.[59]

REFERENCES

1. Kamphuisen PW, Eikenboom JC, Vas HL, et al. Increased levels of factor VIII and fibrinogen in patients with venous thrombosis are not caused by acute phase reactions. *Thromb Haemost.* 1999;81:680-683.

2. Martinelli I, Mannucci PM, De Stefano V, et al. Different risks of thrombosis in four coagulation defects associated with inherited thrombophilia: a study of 150 families. *Blood.* 1998;92:2353-2358.

3. Ridker PM, Glynn RJ, Miletich JP, Goldhaber SZ, Stampfer MJ, Hennekens CH. Age-specific incidence rates of venous thromboembolism among heterozygous carriers of factor V Leiden mutation. *Ann Intern Med.* 1997:126:528-531.

4. Bucciarelli P, Rosendaal FR, Tripodi A, et al. Risk of venous thromboembolism and clinical manifestations in carriers of antithrombin, protein C, protein S deficiency, or activated protein C resistance. a multicenter collaborative family study. *Arterioscler Thromb Vasc Biol.* 1999;19:1026-1033.

5. Price DT, Ridker PM. Factor V Leiden mutation and the risks for thromboembolic disease: a clinical perspective. *Ann Intern Med.* 1997; 127:895-903.

6. Dang CV, Bell WR, Shuman M. The normal and morbid biology of fibrinogen. *Am J Med.* 1989;87:567.

7. Dahlback B. Procoagulant and anticoagulant properties of coagulation factor V: factor V Leiden (APC resistance) causes hypercoagulability by dual mechanisms. *J Lab Clin Med.* 1999;133:415-422.

8. Tans G, Nicolaes GA, Rosing J. Regulation of thrombin formation by activated protein C: effect of the factor V Leiden mutation. *Semin Hematol.* 1997;34:244-255.

9. Vandenbroucke JP, Koster T, Briet E, Reitsma PH, Bertina RM, Rosendaal FR. Increased risk of venous thrombosis in oral-contraceptive users who are carriers of factor V Leiden mutation. *Lancet.* 1994;344:1453-1457.

10. Lindqvist PG, Svensson PJ, Dahlback B, Marsal K. Factor V Q^{506} mutation (activated protein C resistance) associated with reduced intrapartum blood loss—a possible evolutionary selection mechanism. *Thromb Haemost.* 1998;79:69-73.

11. Grandone E, Margaglione M, Colaizzo D, et al. Factor V Leiden is associated with repeated and recurrent unexplained fetal losses. *Thromb Haemost.* 1997;77:822-824.

12. Ridker PM, Miletich JP, Buring JE, et al. Factor V Leiden mutation as a risk factor for recurrent pregnancy loss. *Ann Intern Med.* 1998; 128:1000-1003.

13. Faioni EM, Franchi F, Bucciarelli P, et al. Coinheritance of the HR2 haplotype in the factor V gene confers an increased risk of venous thromboembolism to carriers of factor V R506Q (factor V Leiden). *Blood.* 1999;94:3062-3066.

14. Makris M, Preston FE, Beauchamp NJ, et al. Co-inheritance of the 20210A allele of the prothrombin gene increases the risk of thrombosis in subjects with familial thrombophilia. *Thromb Haemost.* 1997; 78:1426-1429.

15. van der Meer FJ, Koster T, Vandenbroucke JP, Briet E, Rosendaal FR. The Leiden Thrombophilia Study (LETS). *Thromb Haemost.* 1997;78:631-635.

16. Martinelli I, Sacchi E, Landi G, Taioli E, Duca F, Mannucci PM. High risk of cerebral-vein thrombosis in carriers of a prothrombin gene mutation and in users of oral contraceptives. *N Engl J Med.* 1998;338: 1793-1797.

17. Martinelli I, Taioli E, Bucciarelli P, Akhavan S, Mannucci PM. Interaction between the G20210A mutation of the prothrombin gene and oral contraceptive use in deep vein thrombosis. *Arterioscler Thromb Vasc Biol.* 1999;19:700-703.

18. Hankey GJ, Eikelboom JW. Homocysteine and vascular disease. *Lancet.* 1999;354:407-413.

19. Fermo I, D'Angelo SV, Paroni R, Mazzola G, Calori G, D'Angelo A. Prevalence of moderate hyperhomocysteinemia in patients with early-onset venous and arterial occlusive disease. *Ann Intern Med.* 1995;123: 747-753.

20. Eichinger S, Stumpflen A, Hirschl M, et al. Hyperhomocysteinemia is a risk factor of recurrent venous thromboembolism. *Thromb Haemost.* 1998;80:566-569.

21. Nygard O, Nordrehaug JE, Refsum H, Ueland PM, Farstad M, Vollset SE. Plasma homocysteine levels and mortality in patients with coronary artery disease. *N Engl J Med.* 1997;337:230-236.

22. Harpel PC, Chang VT, Borth W. Homocysteine and other sulfhydryl compounds enhance the binding of lipoprotein (a) to fibrin: a potential biochemical link between thrombosis, atherogenesis, and sulfhydryl compound metabolism. *Proc Natl Acad Sci USA.* 1992; 89:10193-10197.

23. D'Angelo A, Selhub J. Homocysteine and thrombotic disease. *Blood.* 1997:90:1-11.

24. Hajjar KA, Jacovina AT. Modulation of annexin II by homocysteine: implications for atherothrombosis. *J Investig Med.* 1998;46:364-369.

25. Schambeck CM, Hinney K, Haubitz I, Mansouri TB, Wahler D, Keller F. Familial clustering of high factor VIII levels in patients with venous thromboembolism. *Arterioscler Thromb Vasc Biol.* 2001;21:289-292.

26. Mansvelt EP, Laffan M, McVey JH, Tuddenham EG. Analysis of the F8 gene in individuals with high plasma factor VII:C levels and associated venous thrombosis. *Thromb Haemost.* 1998;80:561-565.

27. Koster T, Rosendaal FR, Reitsma PH, van der Velden PA, Briet E, Vandenbroucke JP. Factor VII and fibrinogen levels as risk factors for venous thrombosis: a case-control study of plasma levels and DNA polymorphisms—the Leiden Thrombophilia Study (LETS). *Thromb Haemost.* 1994;71:719-722.

28. van Hylckama Vlieg A, van der Linden IK, Vertina RM, Rosendaal FR. High levels of factor IX increase the risk of venous thrombosis. *Blood.* 2000;95:3678-3682.

29. Meijers JC, Tekelenburg WL, Bouma BN, Bertina RM, Rosendaal FR. High levels of coagulation fator XI as a risk factor for venous thrombosis. *N Engl J Med*. 2000;342:696-701.

30. Morita H, Kurihara H, Tsubaki S, et al. Methylenetetrahydrofolate reductase gene polymorphism and ischemic stroke in Japanese. *Arterioscler Thromb Vasc Biol*. 1998;18:1465-1469.

31. Rosendaal F, Siscovick DS, Schwartz SM, et al. Factor V Leiden (resistance to activated protein C) increases the risk of myocardial infarction in young women. *Blood*. 1997;89:2817-2821.

32. Rosendaal F, Siscovick DS, Schwartz SM, Psaty BM, Raghunathan TE, Vos HL. A common prothrombin variant (20210 G to A) increases the risk of myocardial infarction in young women. *Blood*. 1997;90: 1747-1750.

33. Inbal A, Freimark D, Modan B, et al. Synergistic effects of prothrombotic polymorphisms and atherogenic factors on the risk of myocardial infarction in young males. *Blood*. 1999;93:2186-2190.

34. DeStefano V, Chiusolo P, Paciaroni K, et al. Prothrombin G20210A mutant genotype is a risk factor for cerebrovascular ischemic disease in young patients. *Blood*. 1998;91:3562-3565.

35. Martinelli I, Taioli E, Cetin I, et al. Mutations in coagulation factors in women with unexplained late fetal loss. *N Engl J Med*. 2000;343: 1015-1018.

36. Preston FE, Rosendaal FR, Walker ID, et al. Increased fetal loss in women with heritable thrombophilia. *Lancet*. 1996;348:913-916.

37. Friederich PW, Sanson BJ, Simioni P, et al. Frequency of pregnancy-related venous thromboembolism in anticoagulant factor-deficient women: implications for prophylaxis [published correction appears in *Ann Intern Med*. 1997;126:835 and 1997;127:1138]. *Ann Intern Med*. 1996;125:955-960.

38. Gonzalez-Conejero R, Lozano ML, Rivera J, et al. Polymorphisms of platelet membrane glycoprotein Ib associated with arterial thrombotic disease. *Blood*. 1998;92:2771-2776.

39. Weiss EJ, Bray PF, Tayback M, et al. A polymorphism of a platelet glycoprotein receptor as an inherited risk factor for coronary thrombosis. *N Engl J Med*. 1996;334:1090-1094.

40. Pontiggia L, Lassila R, Pederiva S, Schmid HR, Burger M, Beer JH. Increased platelet-collagen interaction associated with double homozygosity for receptor polymorphism of platelet GPIa and GPIIIa. *Arterioscler Thromb Vasc Biol*. 2002;22:2093-2098.

41. Bick RL, Kaplan H. Syndromes of thrombosis and hypercoagulability. Congenital and acquired causes of thrombosis. *Med Clin North Am*. 1998;82:409-458.

11

42. Seligsohn U, Lubetsky A. Genetic susceptibility to venous thrombosis. *N Engl J Med.* 2001;344:1222-1231.

43. de Visser MC, Rosendaal FR, Bertina RM. A reduced sensitivity for activated protein C in the absence of factor V Leiden increases the risk of venous thrombosis. *Blood.* 1999;93:1271-1276.

44. Love PE, Santoro SA. Antiphospholipid antibodies: anticardiolipin and the lupus anticoagulant in systemic lupus erythematosus and in non-systemic lupus erythematosus disorders. Prevalence and clinical significance. *Ann Intern Med.* 1990;112:682-698.

45. Greaves M. Antiphospholipid antibodies and thrombosis. *Lancet.* 1999;353:1348-1353.

46. Goodnight SH. Antiphospholipid antibodies and thrombosis. In: McArthur JR, Schecter GP, eds. *Hematology 1998.* Washington, DC: American Society of Hematology; 1998:261-265.

47. Rand JH, Wu XX, Andree HA, et al. Antiphospholipid antibodies accelerate plasma coagulation by inhibiting annexin-V binding to phospholipids: a "lupus procoagulant" phenomenon. *Blood.* 1998;92:1652-1660.

48. Rand JH. "Annexinopathies"—a new class of diseases. *N Engl J Med.* 1999;340:1035-1036. Editorial.

49. Merrill JT, Zhang HW, Shen C, et al. Enhancement of protein S anticoagulant function by β_2-glycoprotein-1, a major target antigen of antiphospholipid antibodies. *Thromb Haemost.* 1999;81:748-757.

50. Zivelin A, Gitel S, Griffin JH, et al. Extensive venous and arterial thrombosis associated with an inhibitor to activated protein C. *Blood.* 1999;94:895-901.

51. Horbach DA, van Oort E, Donders RC, Derksen RH, de Groot PG. Lupus anticoagulant is the strongest risk factor for both venous and arterial thrombosis in patients with systemic lupus erythematosus. *Thromb Haemost.* 1996;76:916-924.

52. Ginsburg KS, Liang MH, Newcomer L, et al. Anticardiolipin antibodies and the risk for ischemic stroke and venous thrombosis. *Ann Intern Med.* 1992;117:997-1002.

53. Simioni P, Prandoni P, Lensing AW, et al. The risk of recurrent venous thromboembolism in patients with an arg[506]-gln mutation in the gene for factor V (factor V Leiden). *N Engl J Med.* 1997;336:399-403.

54. Petiti DB, Strom BL, Melmon KL. Duration of warfarin anticoagulant therapy and the probabilities of recurrent thromboembolism and hemorrhage. *Am J Med.* 1986;81:255-259.

55. Schulman S, Svenungsson E, Granqvist S. Anticardiolipin antibodies predict early recurrence of thromboembolism and death among patients with venous thromboembolism following anticoagulant therapy. *Am J Med*. 1998;104:332-338.

56. Rosove MH, Brewer PM. Antiphospholipid thrombosis: clinical course after the first thrombotic event in 70 patients. *Ann Intern Med*. 1992;117:303-308.

57. Khamashta MA, Cuadrado MJ, Mujic F, Taub NA, Hunt BJ, Hughes GR. The management of thrombosis in the antiphospholipid-antibody syndrome. *N Engl J Med*. 1995;332:993-997.

58. Crowther MA, Ginsberg JS, Julian J, et al. A comparison of two intensities of warfarin for the prevention of recurrent thrombosis in patients with the antiphospholipid antibody syndrome. *N Engl J Med*. 2003;349:1133-1138.

59. Danilenko-Dixon DR, Van Winter JT, Homburger HA. Clinical implications of antiphospholipid antibodies in obstetrics. *Mayo Clin Proc*. 1996;71:1118-1120.

11

12 Acute Coronary Syndromes

Patients with unstable angina and non–ST-segment elevation (NSTE) myocardial infarction (MI), collectively referred to as NSTE acute coronary syndrome (ACS), represent a growing population of individuals presenting to the hospital for evaluation. In the United States alone, there are 2.4 million hospitalizations each year for ACS. Accordingly, considerable attention has been given to diagnosis, risk stratification, pharmacologic management, and interventional treatment with the goal of achieving optimal care and establishing "best practice" on a widescale basis.

Pathobiology

The clinical expression of coronary artery disease is driven by a series of pathobiologic events that include plaque disruption and varying degrees of intravascular thromboembolism.[1,2] A majority of patients with unstable angina and NSTEMI have advanced atherosclerotic coronary artery disease with nearly uniform distribution of single-, double-, and triple-vessel involvement; however, it is not the *number* of involved coronary arteries that is unique but the *characteristics* of the underlying atheromatous plaques that are vulnerable to rupture and a dysfunctional endothelium that ineffectively resists thrombosis.[3]

Although plaque disruption is a common theme in ACS, the degree and composition of the associated thrombus burden differ. In contrast to ST-segment elevation MI, the coronary thrombi in patients with unstable angina and NSTEMI are nonocclusive, poorly anchored (ie, prone to embolize), and consist predominantly of platelets with a loose fibrin network[4,5] (**Figure 12.1**). Distal embolization to the microvascular or myocardial perfusion bed is common.

Secondary unstable angina or NSTEMI represents a condition wherein myocardial ischemia is provoked by conditions that increase myocardial oxygen demand such as fever, tachycardia, and hypermetabolic states (eg, thyrotoxi-

FIGURE 12.1 — DISTINCT PATHOBIOLOGIC FEATURES OF STABLE ANGINA AND ACUTE CORONARY SYNDROMES

	Stable Angina	Unstable Angina	Non–ST-Segment Elevation MI	ST-Segment Elevation MI
Inflammation	+	++	++	++
Plaque vulnerability	+	++	++	+++
Thrombosis	—	++	++	+
Embolization	—	++	++	
Thrombus composition	—	Platelets	Platelets	Platelets/fibrin

Abbreviation: MI, myocardial infarction.

cosis) as well as by conditions that reduce coronary blood flow (eg, hypotension) or impair oxygen delivery (eg, anemia, hypoxemia).

Patient Characteristics

Although the signs and symptoms that typify ACS vary considerably, a diagnosis is secured for a majority of patients based on the:

- Presence or absence of traditional atherosclerosis risk factors
- Presenting history
- Physical examination
- Electrocardiogram.

Supporting evidence for myocardial necrosis is secured through serial troponin (T or I) or creatine kinase measurements.

Determining the Probability of Coronary Artery Disease

■ Risk Factors

Individuals who have one or more traditional risk factors for atherosclerotic coronary artery disease or who have previously documented disease (prior MI, coronary angiography with one or more vessels containing a stenosis of ≥70%, revascularization procedure—prior bypass surgery or percutaneous coronary intervention [PCI]) are four to five times more likely to be experiencing myocardial ischemia when they present to the hospital with chest pain than those without existing risk factors or previously documented disease.

■ Electrocardiogram

The surface 12-lead electrocardiogram (ECG) represents an important "first-line" diagnostic test in evaluating patients with suspected myocardial ischemia. It is designed to complement the history and physical examination, providing information that carries considerable predictive value when employed serially in the context of high pretest likelihood of myocardial ischemia (**Table 12.1**). Although a

12

TABLE 12.1 — PATIENT CHARACTERISTICS AND ELECTROCARDIOGRAPHIC FEATURES USEFUL IN DETERMINING THE PROBABILITY OF MYOCARDIAL ISCHEMIA

High probability if:
- Known history of myocardial infarction or angina
- Male ≥60 or female ≥70 years of age
- Variant angina (coronary vasospasm)
- Symmetric T-wave inversion in multiple leads
- ST elevation or depression ≥0.5 mm (in ≥2 leads)
- Hypertension, hypercholesterolemia, smoking, family history of coronary artery disease (any combination of these with diabetes mellitus)
- Hemodynamic change or "dynamic" electrocardiographic changes during chest pain

Intermediate probability if:
- Male <60 or female <70 years of age
- History of peripheral vascular disease
- ST-segment depression <0.5 mm (in ≥2 leads)
- T-wave inversion ≥1 mm in leads with dominant R waves
- At least 2 positive risk factors (excluding diabetes mellitus)

Low probability if:
- Atypical chest pain
- One risk factor (but *not* diabetes mellitus)
- Normal electrocardiogram (during symptoms)
- Normal physical examination
- T-wave flattening or inversion <1 mm in leads with dominant R wave
- Age <35 years for males or <45 years for females

normal ECG does not fully exclude a diagnosis of unstable angina or NSTEMI, the diagnosis should be questioned when serial tracings performed during symptoms remain normal or unchanged. Nevertheless, if the suspicion for myocardial ischemia remains high, observation, biochemical testing, and additional diagnostic testing should be undertaken (**Table 12.2** and **Figures 12.2, 12.3,** and **12.4**).[6]

TABLE 12.2 — EARLY EVALUATION STEPS FOR PATIENTS WITH SUSPECTED MYOCARDIAL ISCHEMIA

- The history, physical examination, 12-lead ECG, and initial serum marker tests should be integrated to assign patients with chest pain to 1 of 4 categories: a noncardiac diagnosis, chronic stable angina, possible ACS, and definite ACS.
- Patients with a noncardiac diagnosis should be managed as dictated by the alternative diagnosis.
- Patients with chronic stable angina should be managed according to existing guidelines for the management of patients with chronic stable angina.
- Patients whose symptoms are suggestive of ACS or are felt to be consistent with a definite ACS but whose initial 12-lead ECG and serum cardiac marker levels are normal, should be observed in a facility with cardiac monitoring (eg, chest pain unit) and a repeat ECG and serum marker measurement should be obtained 4 to 8 hours later.
- If the follow-up 12-lead ECG and serum marker measurements are normal, a stress test to provoke ischemia may be performed. Patients with a negative stress test can be managed as outpatients. Patients with a strongly positive stress test are considered to have myocardial ischemia, and in the presence of the clinical picture of acute ischemia, should be admitted to the hospital for further management.
- Patients who are unable to exercise or who have an abnormal resting ECG should have stress myocardial perfusion imaging.
- Patients believed to have an ACS with an abnormal initial 12-lead ECG should be managed based on the findings of the 12-lead ECG. Patients with ST elevation should be evaluated for immediate reperfusion therapy. Patients with new ST depression and/or T-wave abnormalities should be admitted to the hospital for further management.

Abbreviations: ACS, acute coronary syndrome; ECG, electrocardiogram.

ACC/AHA Guidelines for the management of patients with unstable angina and NSTEMI. *Circulation.* 2000;102:1193-1209.

12

FIGURE 12.2 — ST/T-WAVE CHANGES IN PATIENT WITH MYOCARDIAL ISCHEMIA

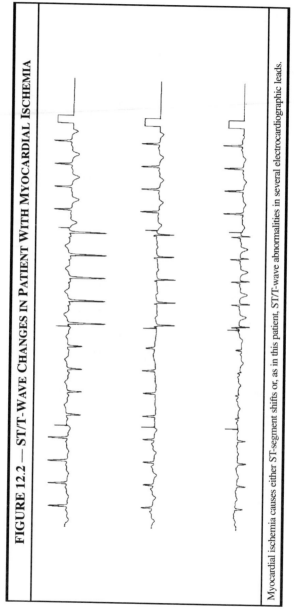

Myocardial ischemia causes either ST-segment shifts or, as in this patient, ST/T-wave abnormalities in several electrocardiographic leads.

FIGURE 12.3 — DEEP SYMMETRIC T-WAVE INVERSIONS IN PATIENT WITH MYOCARDIAL ISCHEMIA

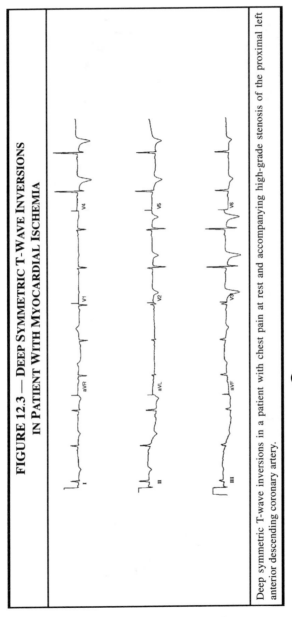

Deep symmetric T-wave inversions in a patient with chest pain at rest and accompanying high-grade stenosis of the proximal left anterior descending coronary artery.

12

207

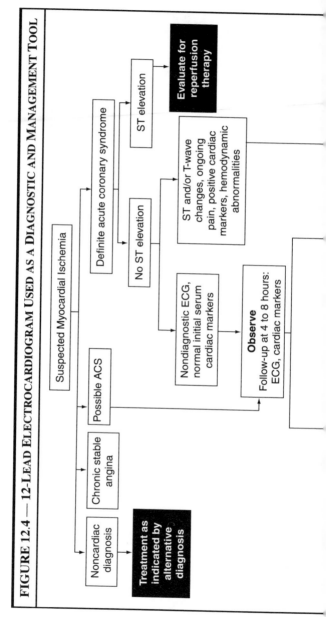

FIGURE 12.4 — 12-LEAD ELECTROCARDIOGRAM USED AS A DIAGNOSTIC AND MANAGEMENT TOOL

Suspected Myocardial Ischemia

- Noncardiac diagnosis
  - **Treatment as indicated by alternative diagnosis**
- Chronic stable angina
- Possible ACS
  - Nondiagnostic ECG, normal initial serum cardiac markers
    - **Observe**
      Follow-up at 4 to 8 hours: ECG, cardiac markers
- Definite acute coronary syndrome
  - No ST elevation
    - ST and/or T-wave changes, ongoing pain, positive cardiac markers, hemodynamic abnormalities
  - ST elevation
    - **Evaluate for reperfusion therapy**

208

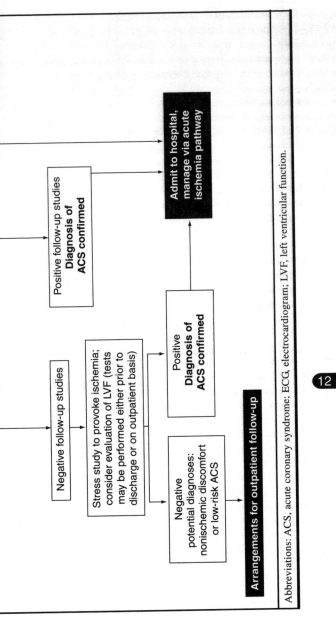

Positive follow-up studies
Diagnosis of ACS confirmed

Negative follow-up studies

Stress study to provoke ischemia; consider evaluation of LVF (tests may be performed either prior to discharge or on outpatient basis)

Positive
Diagnosis of ACS confirmed

Negative potential diagnoses: nonischemic discomfort or low-risk ACS

Admit to hospital, manage via acute ischemia pathway

Arrangements for outpatient follow-up

Abbreviations: ACS, acute coronary syndrome; ECG, electrocardiogram; LVF, left ventricular function.

12

■ **Classification of Unstable Angina**

The Braunwald Classification System is widely used for evaluating patients with unstable angina.[7] It is comprehensive and has been shown to provide both prognostic information and important insights for management.

■ **Risk Stratification**

There are several risk-stratification tools that have been developed over the years; however, the original "high-risk" categorization as defined by the Agency for Health Care Policy and Research provides a clinically useful tool for diagnosis, triage, and management (**Table 12.3**).[8] The importance of ST-segment shifts[9] and biochemical (cardiac enzyme) abnormalities has been emphasized by several experienced groups.

The TIMI Risk Score

Risk stratification is the essential component of patient assessment that can provide both prognostic information and clear direction for management decisions. The Thrombolysis in Myocardial Infarction (TIMI) risk score is an integrated check list that utilizes historical patient information and clinical parameters at hospital presentation to identify

---

TABLE 12.3 — HIGH-RISK FEATURES IN PATIENTS WITH UNSTABLE ANGINA

High-Risk Category (high risk for death or nonfatal myocardial infarction) if *one* or *more* of the following features are present:
- Pulmonary edema with chest pain
- Dynamic mitral insufficiency
- Angina with intermittent S3 gallop or pulmonary rales
- Angina with hypotension
- Prolonged pain (>20 minutes in duration)
- Angina with "dynamic" ST changes
- Persistence of chest pain and electrocardiographic changes despite medical therapy
- Positive troponin T or I assay
- Angina followed by bradyarrhythmias, conduction disturbance, or ventricular tachyarrhythmias

---

individuals at risk for cardiovascular events (**Table 12.4** and **Figure 12.5**).[10]

Hospitalized Patients

■ Monitoring

All patients admitted to the hospital with suspected myocardial ischemia and a diagnosis of unstable angina or NSTEMI should have 12 to 24 hours of continuous ECG monitoring. When available, ST-segment monitoring should be utilized to aid in the identification of high-risk patients.

■ Anti-ischemic Therapy

Optimal management of unstable angina and NSTEMI includes the immediate relief of ischemia and the prevention of serious adverse outcomes (infarction, death). Pharmacologic therapies that specifically address myocardial ischemia include analgesics, nitrates, β-blockers, and calcium channel blockers. Intra-aortic balloon counterpulsation is a mechanical alternative that should be considered

TABLE 12.4 — THE TIMI RISK SCORE FOR UA/NSTEMI	
Characteristics	**Points**
Historical	
Age ≥65 years	1
≥3 Risk factors for CAD	1
Known CAD (stenosis ≥50%)	1
Aspirin use in past 7 days	1
Presentation	
Recent (≤24 hours) severe angina	1
ST-segment deviation ≥0.5 mm	1
↑ Cardiac markers	1
Risk Score = Total Points	(0-7)
Abbreviations: CAD, coronary artery disease; NSTEMI, non–ST-segment elevation myocardial infarction; TIMI, Thrombolysis in Myocardial Infarction; UA, unstable angina.	
Sabatine MS, Antman EM. *J Am Coll Cardiol.* 2003;41(4 Suppl S):89S-95S.	

12

FIGURE 12.5 — RATES OF ALL-CAUSE MORTALITY, MYOCARDIAL INFARCTION, AND SEVERE RECURRENT ISCHEMIA LEADING TO URGENT REVASCULARIZATION

χ^2 trend $P < 0.001$
Hosmer-Lemeshow 3.56_{df8} $P = 0.89$
C Statistic = 0.65

TIMI Risk Score for UA/NSTEMI	0/1	2	3	4	5	6/7
D/MI/UR by 14 Days (%)	4.7	8.3	13.2	19.9	26.2	40.9
Population (%)	4.3	17.3	32.0	29.3	13.0	3.4

Abbreviations: NSTEMI, non–ST-segment elevation myocardial infarction; UA, unstable angina.

Rates of all-cause mortality (D), myocardial infarction (MI), and severe recurrent ischemia leading to urgent revascularization (UR) through 14 days among patients randomized to unfractionated heparin in Thrombolysis In Myocardial Infarction (TIMI) 11B trial, with patients stratified by the TIMI risk score. Population (%): percent of overall trial population with that TIMI risk score.

Adapted from: Antman EM, et al. *JAMA*. 2000;284:835-842.

in patients with refractory angina, hemodynamic compromise, or malignant dysarrhythmias associated with myocardial ischemia. In most instances, intra-aortic balloon pumps serve as a bridge to revascularization (**Table 12.5**).

Antithrombotic Therapy

The pathobiology of ACS dictates a comprehensive antithrombotic regimen that includes one or more platelet antagonists and an anticoagulant (**Table 12.6**).

TABLE 12.5 — MEDICAL THERAPY FOR ACUTE CORONARY SYNDROMES

Agent	Indication	Dose	Duration	Alternatives	Comments
ACE inhibitors	ACS	Variable	Variable	—	Greatest benefit in patients with with reduced LVEF and/or clinical heart failure; have antithrombotic and anti-inflammatory properties as well
β-Blockers	ACS	Titrate to heart rate, symptoms	Indefinite	—	—
Calcium channel blockers	ACS	Titrate to symptoms	Variable	—	Used in patients with refractory angina, AF with rapid ventricular response, particularly when β-blocker contraindicated
Lipid-lowering agents	CHD	Variable	Variable	—	Benefit of high-dose statin therapy in early management of ACS
Nitroglycerin	ACS	Titrate to symptoms (IV preferable for rapid titration)	24-48 hours	—	Benefit beyond 48 hours if recurrent ischemia

Abbreviations: ACE, angiotensin-converting enzyme; ACS, acute coronary syndrome; AF, atrial fibrillation; CHD, coronary heart disease; IV, intravenous; LVEF, left ventricular ejection fraction.

TABLE 12.6 — SUMMARY OF ANTITHROMBOTIC THERAPY IN ACUTE CORONARY SYNDROMES

Class/Agent	Dosing	Clinical Indications	Comment
Oral Antiplatelet Therapy			
Aspirin	162-325 mg (initial) 75-160 mg/d (maintenance)	ACS	True aspirin allergy is rare
Clopidogrel (Plavix)	300 mg (loading) 75 mg/d (maintenance)	ACS, PCI-stenting	Combination therapy with aspirin encouraging
Ticlopidine	500 mg (loading) 250 mg bid (maintenance)	PCI-stenting	Adverse-effect profile concerning
Intravenous Antiplatelet Therapy			
Abciximab (ReoPro)	0.25-μg/kg bolus, 0.125 μg/kg/min (max 10 μg/min) for 12 to 24 hours	ACS/PCI	Greatest benefit with PCI; infusions >12 h not recommended
Eptifibatide (Integrilin)	180 μg/kg × 2 (10 min apart), 2.0 μg/kg/min for 48 to 72 hours*	ACS/PCI	Double-bolus strategy in PCI

			Ideal dosing strategy for PCI being investigated
Tirofiban (Aggrastat)	0.4 mg/kg/min × 30 min, 0.1 mg/kg/min for 48 to 72 hours*	ACS	
Anticoagulants			
Enoxaparin (Lovenox)	1 mg/kg SC bid*	ACS	Combined use with GPIIb/IIIa antagonist and utilization in PCI being investigated
Dalteparin (Fragmin)	120 IU/kg SC bid* (max 10,000 IU bid)	ACS	Experience with GPIIb/IIIa antagonist and PCI limited
Bivalirudin (Angiomax)	1-mg/kg bolus*; 2.5 mg/kg/h 0.75 mg bolus; 1.75 mg/kg/h	PCI PCI	With provisional concomitant GPIIb/IIIa antagonist
Lepirudin (Refludan)	0.4-mg/kg bolus,* 0.15 mg/kg/h	HIT	Target aPTT 60-85 sec
Unfractionated heparin	70-U/kg bolus (max 5000 U), 12-15 U/kg/h (max 1000 U/h)	ACS	Target aPTT 60-85 sec, rebound ischemic events following cessation

Abbreviations: ACS, acute coronary syndrome; aPTT, activated partial thromboplastin time; bid, two times per day; GP, glycoprotein; HIT, heparin-induced thrombocytopenia; PCI, percutaneous coronary intervention; SC, subcutaneous.

* Dose adjustment required for renal insufficiency.

12

■ Platelet Antagonists

The benefits offered by platelet inhibition are well documented and translate to a 60% to 70% reduction in the likelihood of death or MI. Although aspirin has been the agent used in an overwhelming majority of studies, alternative platelet antagonists, like clopidogrel, should be considered in patients with aspirin allergy, intolerance, or resistance. The advantage a clopidogrel/aspirin combination in ACS was recently confirmed in the Clopidogrel in Unstable Angina to Prevent Recurrent Events (CURE) trial.[11-14]

The intravenous (IV) platelet glycoprotein (GP) IIb/IIIa receptor antagonists have added a significant dimension to treatment strategies for ACS. Added benefits (to standard anti-ischemic and antithrombotic therapy) are observed in patients treated medically, as well as in those undergoing PCIs (**Table 12.6**).[15] The greatest overall reduction in adverse events (death, MI, refractory angina) occurs in patients falling within the high-risk category, particularly those with troponin (T or I) positivity.

■ Anticoagulants (Thrombin-Directed Therapy)

Intravenous unfractionated heparin (UFH) given in combination with aspirin is recommended for patients with ACS based on the recognized contribution of platelets and thrombin to arterial thrombosis. Several well-designed studies have documented the benefit of UFH with a 30% reduction in the composite outcome of death or MI and an impressive 50% reduction in recurrent/refractory angina.[16-19]

One of the many recognized challenges of UFH therapy is achieving and maintaining a target level of anticoagulation. Frequent monitoring of the activated partial thromboplastin time (aPTT) is recommended and, when available, point-of-care coagulation instruments for rapid infusion titration (**Table 12.7**).[20] The duration of treatment is determined by the patient's overall clinical status; however, in most instances, a period of 48 to 72 hours is adequate. Intravenous heparin weaning is recommended to minimize "rebound" thrombin generation.[21]

Low molecular weight heparin (LMWH) represents an established treatment and has been shown in several large-scale, randomized trials to be superior to aspirin and, at the very least, equally as efficacious as UFH.[22,23] The findings

216

TABLE 12.7 — PATIENT-SPECIFIC HEPARIN-DOSING NOMOGRAM*

aPTT	Repeat Bolus[†]	Rate Change[†]	Repeat aPTT
<35 sec	60 U/kg	↑ 4 U/kg/h	4 h
35-49 sec	30 U/kg	↑ 3 U/kg/h	6 h
50-70[‡] sec	0	No change	6 h
71-90 sec	0	↓ 2 U/kg/h	6 h
>90 sec	0	↓ 3 U/kg/h	4 h

Abbreviation: aPTT, activated partial thromboplastin time.

* Initial dose: 60-U/kg bolus (not to exceed 5000 U); maintenance infusion: 15-18 U/kg/h. Begin infusion at ≤1200 U/h.

† Patients >65 years of age and those receiving fibrinolytics and/or platelet glycoprotein (GP)IIb/IIIa antagonists have reduced heparin requirements (bolus and infusion).

‡ Target range (for acute coronary syndromes).

of two comparative trials, Efficacy and Safety of Subcutaneous Enoxaparin in Non-Q-Wave Coronary Events (ESSENCE)[24] and Thrombolysis in Myocardial Infarction (TIMI) 11B,[25] support LMWH as the standard of care in high-risk patients with ACS. The recent ACC/AHA Guidelines for ACS[6] provide a level IIa recommendation for enoxaparin over IV UFH as the preferred anticoagulant for ACS patients based upon the clinical trial data described above. A reduced requirement for coagulation monitoring (with the exception of patients with marked renal insufficiency, ie, creatinine clearance <30 mL/min and those of extremes in body weight <50 kg, >120 kg), coupled with the lower incidence of recurrent refractory ischemia requiring coronary angiography/interventions, is responsible for the lower treatment costs for LMWH.

The limitations of UFH during PCI are substantial, not the least of which is its narrow therapeutic index (**Figures 12.6** and **12.7**).[26]

There are several biologic and practical advantages of LMWH compared with UFH in the management of ACS:

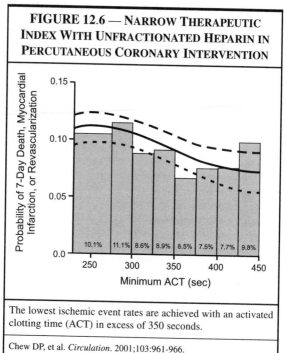

FIGURE 12.6 — NARROW THERAPEUTIC INDEX WITH UNFRACTIONATED HEPARIN IN PERCUTANEOUS CORONARY INTERVENTION

The lowest ischemic event rates are achieved with an activated clotting time (ACT) in excess of 350 seconds.

Chew DP, et al. *Circulation.* 2001;103:961-966.

- Rapid subcutaneous absorption
- Predictable pharmacokinetics and pharmacodynamics
- Reduced platelet activation
- Sustained tissue factor pathway inhibitor (TFPI) release
- Reduced heparin-platelet factor 4–directed antibody production
- Reduced nonspecific binding to plasma proteins.

■ Low Molecular Weight Heparin in Percutaneous Coronary Intervention

There is emerging evidence in support of LMWH as an alternative to UFH in PCI—an important option in the context of maintaining antithrombotic agent consistency when transitioning from medical to mechanical treatment (**Table 12.8**). Although the initial experience with

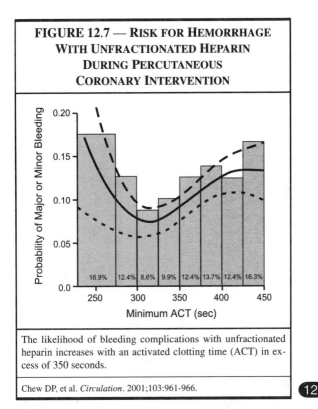

FIGURE 12.7 — RISK FOR HEMORRHAGE WITH UNFRACTIONATED HEPARIN DURING PERCUTANEOUS CORONARY INTERVENTION

The likelihood of bleeding complications with unfractionated heparin increases with an activated clotting time (ACT) in excess of 350 seconds.

Chew DP, et al. *Circulation.* 2001;103:961-966.

12

enoxaparin in the National Investigators Collaborating on Enoxaparin (NICE)-1 registry employed an IV dosing strategy (1.0 mg/kg), there is experience with subcutaneous (SC) administration as well.[27] A single-center study of 451 patients with unstable angina/NSTEMI performed coronary angioplasty and PCI within 8 hours of an SC dose (1 mg/kg enoxaparin) (without additional LMWH or UFH). There were no abrupt closures or urgent revascularizations. Preliminary results from the NICE-3 registry suggest that a small additional dose of enoxaparin 0.3 mg/kg IV could be employed to maintain an adequate level of anticoagulation in cases where the last subcutaneous dose was given ≥8 hours earlier (**Table 12.9**).[28,29]

TABLE 12.8 — CLINICAL EXPERIENCE WITH LMWH ADMINISTERED FOR PCI

Trial/Investigator (No. of Patients)	Route/Dose Administration	GP IIb/IIIa Antagonist	Major Findings
Enoxaparin			
NICE 1 Pilot (60)	IV 1.0 mg/kg	No	Similar safety efficacy and equivalent antifactor Xa to UFH 10,000 U (randomized)
NICE 1 (828)	IV 1.0 mg/kg	No	Favorable bleeding and clinical efficacy; major non-CABG bleeding 0.5% at 30 days
NICE 4 (818)	IV 0.75 mg/kg	Abciximab	Favorable bleeding and clinical efficacy; major non-CABG bleeding 0.2% at 30 days
ESSENCE (142)	SC 1.0 mg/kg	No	Major hemorrhage $\leq 2.0\%$; similar to UFH
Collet (132)	SC 1.0 mg/kg	No	Antifactor Xa levels maintained for 8 hours postdose; favorable clinical outcomes
ACUTE 1 (55)	SC 1.0 mg/kg	Tirofiban	Enhanced platelet inhibition by tirofiban (vs UFH; randomized)
ACUTE 2 (525)	SC 1.0 mg/kg	Tirofiban	No difference in bleeding; slight reduction in recurrent ischemia for enoxaparin (vs UFH; randomized)
POLONIA (100)	IC (local delivery)	No	Reduction in neointimal proliferation and late restenosis

Dalteparin			
Kereiakes (107)	IV 40 vs 60 IU/kg	Abciximab	60 IU/kg provided more consistent antithrombotic effect and fewer clinical thrombotic events
Furman/Kereiakes (40)	IV 60 IU/kg	Abciximab	Similar platelet inhibition with abciximab vs UFH 70 U/kg (randomized)
Marmur/DREAM (110)	IV 60-80 IU/kg	Abciximab	Change in the ACT may be used to monitor therapy
Kotani (30)	IC 5000 IU (local delivery)	No	Reduction in neointimal proliferation and late restenosis
Reviparin			
REDUCE (612)	IV 7000 IU + SC to 28 days	No	Similar major bleeding vs UFH (randomized)

Abbreviations: ACT, activated clotting time; CABG, coronary artery bypass graft; DREAM, Diabetes Reduction Approaches With Ramipril and Rosiglitazone Medications; ESSENCE, Efficacy and Safety of Subcutaneous Enoxaparin in Non–Q-Wave Coronary Events); GP, glycoprotein; IC, intracoronary; IV, intravenous; LMWH, low molecular weight heparin; NICE, National Investigators Collaborating on Enoxaparin; PCI, percutaneous coronary intervention; POLONIA, Polish-American Local Lovenox NIR Assessment Study; REDUCE, Reduction of Restenosis After PTCA, Early Administration of Reviparin in a Double-Blind Unfractionated Heparin and Placebo-Controlled Evaluation; SC, subcutaneous; UFH, unfractionated heparin.

12

TABLE 12.9 — ENOXAPARIN DOSING GUIDELINES AND ALGORITHM FOR NSTE-ACS PATIENTS UNDERGOING PCI

Dosing Guidelines for Initial Enoxaparin-Based Anticoagulation Therapy in Patients With NSTE-ACS:

General Recommendations. Enoxaparin 30-mg IV bolus (optional) followed immediately by 1 mg/kg SC q12h (until diagnostic cardiac catheterization or for 72 to 96 hours). An IV bolus dose should be given when cardiac catheterization is to be performed before therapeutic factor anti-Xa levels are achieved or shortly after presentation.

Enoxaparin Dosing Guidelines and Algorithm for PCI:

Therapeutic Anti-Xa Levels. To ensure that ACS patients promptly achieve therapeutic anti-Xa levels, a 30-mg IV loading dose of enoxaparin is recommended, followed immediately by administration of 1 mg/kg SC q12h. Therapeutic anti-Xa levels also are achieved after ≥2 doses of enoxaparin 1 mg/kg SC q12h have been administered, even in the absence of an initial loading dose.

If an initial 30-mg IV loading dose of enoxaparin has been administered, or ≥2 doses of SC enoxaparin have been administered (with or without IV loading dose):
- If procedure is performed within 8 hours of the last SC dose, no additional enoxaparin needs to be administered.
- If procedure is performed at a point within 8 to 12 hours of the last SC dose, 0.3 mg/kg enoxaparin IV should be administered in the catheterization laboratory.

If an initial 30-mg IV dose of enoxaparin has not been administered and if only one dose of SC enoxaparin has been administered (in a patient without an IV loading dose):
- At time of procedure, patient should receive a booster dose of 0.3 mg/kg prior to catheterization/PCI. The ENOX clotting time may be measured in such patients, and if it is found to be ≥260 seconds, the booster dose may be withheld.

Continued

If no enoxaparin has been previously administered:
- At time of procedure, 1.0 mg/kg enoxaparin IV should be administered in the catheterization laboratory if GP-IIb/IIIa inhibitor is not given; 0.75 mg/kg enoxaparin IV should be administered when a GPIIb/IIIa will be used.

Sheath Removal. Timing of sheath removal depends on a number of factors, among them, whether or not a closure device is employed and time and route of last enoxaparin dose:
- Sheath can be removed 6 to 8 hours after the last SC dose of enoxaparin without a closure device, or immediately if a closure device has been employed.
- Sheath can be removed 4 hours after the 0.3-mg/kg IV supplemental dose for the 8- to 12-hour group, as well as after the 1.0 mg/kg IV (0.75 mg/kg with a GP IIb/IIIa inhibitor) for the group undergoing PCI >12 hours after their last SC dose or who have not received any pretreatment.

Abbreviations: ACS, acute coronary syndrome; ENOX, a rapid, accurate point-of-care test that detects the effect of enoxaparin on coagulation in citrated arterial whole blood; GP, glycoprotein; IV, intravenous; NSTE-ACS, non–ST-segment elevation acute coronary syndrome; PCI, percutaneous coronary intervention; SC, subcutaneous.

Interventional Cardiology Consensus Reports. Consensus Panel Statements for Outcome-Effective and Evidence-Based Patient Management. May 1, 2003.

12

■ **Combination Pharmacotherapy With Low Molecular Weight Heparin and GPIIb/IIIa Receptor Antagonists**

The combined administration of LMWH and GPIIb/IIIa receptor antagonists is particularly attractive in ACS, given its pathobiology that includes both coagulation factors (prothrombinase complex) and activated platelets and their excellent individual track records. The recently completed Integrilin and Enoxaparin Randomized Assessment of Acute Coronary Syndrome Treatment (INTERACT) trial demonstrated superior clinical outcomes and less bleeding when enoxaparin was compared with IV UFH in ACS patients receiving eptifibatide.[30] Superior Yield of the New

Strategy of Enoxaparin, Revascularization and Glycoprotein IIb/IIIa Inhibitors (SYNERGY), a large-scale, randomized, controlled trial evaluating a wide-range of high-risk patients with ACS according to an early invasive treatment strategy, showed convincingly that enoxaparin can be initiated in the emergency department, continued through coronary angiography, and when PCI is indicated. It can be used safely in combination with aspirin, clopidogrel, and a GP IIb/IIIa receptor antagonist. The SYNERGY trial, which included over 10,000 patients worldwide, also shed light on the potential dangers (ischemic/thrombotic and hemorrhagic) associated with transitioning heparin compounds (with differing effects on platelets, endothelial cells, and protective vascular surface proteins) during the course of therapy. The available data from clinical trials (now exceeding 21,000 patients) support the use of enoxaparin in patients with ACS at either low-, moderate-, or high-risk for cardiovascular events.[31,32] The experience to date with combined administration of LMWH and GPIIb/IIIa receptor antagonists is encouraging and suggests that it will likely become a widely employed treatment alternative.[33]

■ Direct Thrombin Inhibitors

The direct thrombin inhibitor hirudin has shown some promise in preventing early ischemic/thrombotic events in patients with ACS.[34] A related molecule, bivalirudin, offers an advantage over UFH in high-risk coronary angioplasty.[35] Preliminary results with pentasaccharide also look promising.

The Randomized Evaluation in PCI Linking Angiomax to Reduced Clinical Events (REPLACE) 2 trial randomized 6010 patients undergoing urgent or elective PCI to either bivalirudin plus provisional platelet GPIIb/IIIa receptor antagonist (abciximab or eptifibatide) administration or UFH plus a GPIIb/IIIa receptor antagonist. Aspirin and clopidogrel pretreatment were recommended. The composite outcome of death, MI, or urgent revascularization at 30 days occurred in 7.1% of UFH-treated patients and 7.6% of bivalirudin-treated patients (odds ratio 0.92, $P = 0.32$). Major bleeding was documented in 4.1% and 2.4% of patients, respectively ($P = 0.001$).[36] The data show that bivalirudin offers an advantage to UFH in urgent and elective coronary angioplasty.

■ Oral Anticoagulant Therapy

Oral anticoagulant therapy with coumarin derivatives (predominantly warfarin) has been studied in patients with ACS. A summary of available information based on data from over 20,000 patients indicates that high-intensity anticoagulation (INR >2.8) reduces cardiovascular complications (relative risk reduction 21%) but increases bleeding risk. Moderate-intensity anticoagulation (INR 2 to 3) also reduces cardiovascular events (relative risk reduction 16%) with less risk for bleeding. The use of moderate-intensity anticoagulation plus aspirin is more effective than aspirin alone (12% relative risk reduction). Last, low-intensity anticoagulation (INR <2) plus aspirin is not more effective than aspirin alone (relative risk reduction 9%) but does increase the risk for bleeding.[37]

■ Fibrinolytic Therapy

Fibrinolytic therapy is not beneficial and, in fact, may be detrimental to patients with unstable angina and NSTEMI.[38]

■ Biochemical Markers

Small elevations in biochemical markers of myocyte injury represent an important indicator of plaque activity, thromboembolic potential, and response to treatment. More specifically, an elevated troponin I (or T) in the first 12 hours of an ACS identifies patients at risk for MI and cardiac death[39] and those most likely to benefit from GPIIb/IIIa antagonists and early invasive management.

■ Management Strategies

Patients with unstable angina and NSTEMI, as previously discussed, represent a spectrum of pathobiology and clinical expression of disease. The available information suggests that risk stratification based on the ECG, hemodynamic profile, biochemical (cardiac markers), and in-hospital course is the key to patient-specific management and optimal outcomes (**Figure 12.8**).

Accumulating data and experience support an early aggressive approach to patient management that includes coronary angiography and revascularization in high-risk individuals (**Tables 12.10, 12.11, and 12.12**).[6,40]

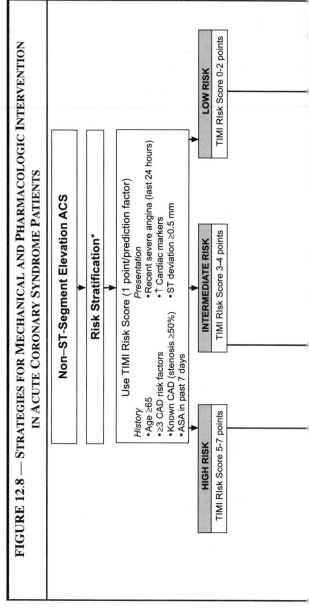

FIGURE 12.8 — STRATEGIES FOR MECHANICAL AND PHARMACOLOGIC INTERVENTION IN ACUTE CORONARY SYNDROME PATIENTS

Non–ST-Segment Elevation ACS

Risk Stratification*

Use TIMI Risk Score (1 point/prediction factor)

History
• Age ≥65
• ≥3 CAD risk factors
• Known CAD (stenosis ≥50%)
• ASA in past 7 days

Presentation
• Recent severe angina (last 24 hours)
• ↑ Cardiac markers
• ST deviation ≥0.5 mm

HIGH RISK
TIMI Risk Score 5-7 points

INTERMEDIATE RISK
TIMI Risk Score 3-4 points

LOW RISK
TIMI Risk Score 0-2 points

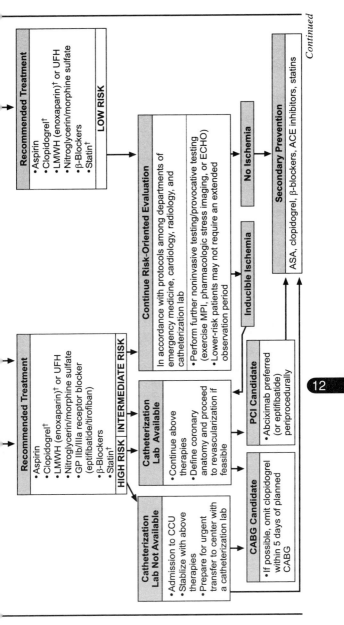

Recommended Treatment
- Aspirin
- Clopidogrel[†]
- LMWH (enoxaparin)[†] or UFH
- Nitroglycerin/morphine sulfate
- β-Blockers
- Statin[†]

LOW RISK

Recommended Treatment
- Aspirin
- Clopidogrel[†]
- LMWH (enoxaparin)[†] or UFH
- Nitroglycerin/morphine sulfate
- GP IIb/IIIa receptor blocker (eptifibatide/tirofiban)
- β-Blockers
- Statin[†]

HIGH RISK | INTERMEDIATE RISK

Continue Risk-Oriented Evaluation

In accordance with protocols among departments of emergency medicine, cardiology, radiology, and catheterization lab

- Perform further noninvasive testing/provocative testing (exercise MPI, pharmacologic stress imaging, or ECHO)
- Lower-risk patients may not require an extended observation period

Catheterization Lab Available
- Continue above therapies
- Define coronary anatomy and proceed to revascularization if feasible

Catheterization Lab Not Available
- Admission to CCU
- Stabilize with above therapies
- Prepare for urgent transfer to center with a catheterization lab

No Ischemia

Inducible Ischemia

PCI Candidate
- Abciximab preferred (or eptifibatide) periprocedurally

CABG Candidate
- If possible, omit clopidogrel within 5 days of planned CABG

Secondary Prevention

ASA, clopidogrel, β-blockers, ACE inhibitors, statins

12

Continued

Abbreviations: ACE, angiotensin-converting enzyme; ACS, acute coronary syndrome; ASA, acetylsalicylic acid; CABG, coronary artery bypass graft; CAD, coronary artery disease; CCU, cardiac care unit; ECHO, echocardiogram; GP, glycoprotein; inflam, inflammatory; LMWH, low molecular-weight heparin; MPI, myocardial perfusion imaging; NTC, nitroglycerin; PCI, percutaneous coronary intervention; TIMI, Thrombolysis in Myocardial Infarction; UFH, unfractionated heparin.

* Consider also inflammatory markers: brain natriuretic peptide (BNP), congestive heart failure (CHF), deep T-wave inversions on electrocardiogram (ECG), etc.

† Based on Class I recommendations from the American College of Cardiology/American Heart Association (ACC/AHA) 2002 Guidelines Update for the Management of Patients With Unstable Angina and Non–ST-Segment Elevation Myocardial Infarction.

Boden WE, Pepine CJ. *J Am Coll Cardiol.* 2003;41(4 Suppl S);1S-6S.

TABLE 12.10 — REVASCULARIZATION IN ACUTE CORONARY SYNDROMES WITHOUT ST-SEGMENT ELEVATION

Coronary Angiography	Mode of Treatment
Left main disease (≥50% stenosis)	
Surgical candidate	CABG
Nonsurgical candidate	PCI
3-Vessel disease, LVEF <50%	CABG
Multivessel disease, LVEF ≥50%, (nondiabetic)	PCI
1- or 2-Vessel disease, large areas of reversible ischemia	CABG or PCI
2-Vessel disease, including proximal LAD, LVEF <50%	CABG
Proximal LAD disease	PCI or CABG

Abbreviations: CABG, coronary artery bypass grafting; LAD, left anterior descending coronary artery; LVEF, left ventricular ejection fraction; PCI, percutaneous coronary intervention.

Summary

12

Unstable angina and NSTEMI represent a spectrum of atherothrombotic disorders. Platelet-rich nonocclusive thrombosis and distal embolization obstructing the microvasculature are the predominant pathobiologic features that develop on a background of advanced atherosclerosis. Anti-ischemic and antithrombotic therapies, including aspirin, clopidogrel, heparin, and IV GPIIb/IIIa receptor antagonists, are the cornerstones of treatment. Direct thrombin inhibitors such as bivalirudin are particularly beneficial in high-risk patients undergoing PCI. An aggressive approach to diagnosis and management based on the TIMI risk score is favored in high-risk patients with hemodynamic instability, recurrent/refractory ischemia, and biochemical markers reflecting myocyte damage.

TABLE 12.11 — ACC/AHA RECOMMENDATIONS FOR ANTIPLATELET THERAPY IN ACS

Class I

1. Antiplatelet therapy should be initiated promptly. ASA should be administered as soon as possible after presentation and continued indefinitely *(Level of Evidence: A)*.

2. Clopidogrel should be administered to hospitalized patients who are unable to take ASA because of hypersensitivity or major gastrointestinal intolerance *(Level of Evidence: A)*.

3. In hospitalized patients in whom an early noninterventional approach is planned, clopidogrel should be added to ASA as soon as possible on admission and administered for at least 1 month *(Level of Evidence: A)*, and for up to 9 months *(Level of Evidence: B)*.*

4. A platelet GPIIb/IIIa antagonist should be administered, in addition to ASA and heparin, to patients in whom catheterization and PCI are planned. The GPIIb/IIIa antagonist may also be administered just prior to PCI *(Level of Evidence: A)*.*

5. In patients for whom a PCI is planned and who are not at high risk for bleeding, clopidogrel should be started and continued for at least 1 month *(Level of Evidence: A)* and for up to 9 months *(Level of Evidence: B)*.*†

6. In patients taking clopidogrel in whom elective CABG is planned, the drug should be withheld for 5 to 7 days *(Level of Evidence: B)*.*

Class IIa

1. Eptifibatide or tirofiban should be administered, in addition to ASA and LMWH or UFH, to patients with continuing ischemia, an elevated troponin, or with other high-risk features in whom an invasive management strategy is *not* planned *(Level of Evidence: A)*.*

2. A platelet GPIIb/IIIa antagonist should be administered to patients already receiving heparin, ASA, and clopidogrel in whom catheterization and PCI are planned. The GPIIb/IIIa antagonist may also be administered just prior to PCI *(Level of Evidence: B)*.*

Continued

Class IIb

1. Eptifibatide or tirofiban, in addition to ASA and LMWH or UFH, to patients without continuing ischemia who have no other high-risk features and in whom PCI is *not* planned *(Level of Evidence: A).**

Class III

1. Intravenous fibrinolytic therapy in patients without acute ST-segment elevation, a true posterior MI, or a presumed new left bundle-branch block *(Level of Evidence: A)*.

2. Abciximab administration in patients in whom PCI is not planned *(Level of Evidence: A).**

Abbreviations: ACC/AHA, American College of Cardiology/American Heart Association; ACS, acute coronary syndrome; ASA, acetylsalicylic acid; CABG, coronary artery bypass grafting; GP, glycoprotein; LMWH, low molecular weight heparin; PCI, percutaneous coronary intervention; UFH, unfractionated heparin.

* New indication; not included in September 2000 guidelines.
† Minor clarification different from full-text version on web site.

Braunwald E, et al. *J Am Coll Cardiol.* 2002;40:1366-1374.

REFERENCES

12

1. Falk E. Unstable angina with fatal outcome: dynamic coronary thrombosis leading to infarction and/or sudden death. Autopsy evidence of recurrent mural thrombosis with peripheral embolization culminating in total vascular occlusion. *Circulation.* 1985;71:699-708.

2. Davies MJ, Thomas A. Thrombosis and acute coronary-artery lesions in sudden cardiac ischemic death. *N Engl J Med.* 1984;310:1137-1140.

3. Furchgott RF, Zawadzki JV. The obligatory role of endothelial cells in the relaxation of arterial smooth muscle by acetylcholine. *Nature.* 1980;288:373-376.

4. Sherman CT, Litvack F, Grundfest W, et al. Coronary angioscopy in patients with unstable angina pectoris. *N Engl J Med.* 1986;315:913-919.

5. Kragel AH, Gertz SD, Roberts WC. Morphologic comparison of frequency and types of acute lesions in the major epicardial coronary arteries in unstable angina pectoris, sudden coronary death and acute myocardial infarction. *J Am Coll Cardiol.* 1991;18:801-808.

TABLE 12.12 — ACC/AHA RECOMMENDATIONS FOR ANTICOAGULANT THERAPY IN ACS

Class I

1. Anticoagulation with subcutaneous LMWH or intravenous UFH should be added to antiplatelet therapy with ASA and/or clopidogrel *(Level of Evidence: A)*.

Class IIa

1. Enoxaparin is preferable to UFH as an anticoagulant in patients with UA/NSTEMI, in the absence of renal failure and unless CABG is planned within 24 hours *(Level of Evidence: A)*.[*][†]

Abbreviations: ACC/AHA, American College of Cardiology/American Heart Association; ACS, acute coronary syndrome; ASA, acetylsalicylic acid; CABG, coronary artery bypass grafting; LMWH, low molecular weight heparin; NSTEMI, non–ST-segment elevation myocardial infarction; UA, unstable angina; UFH, unfractionated heparin.

[*] New indication; not included in the September 2000 guidelines.

[†] Minor clarification different from full-text version on web site.

Braunwald E, et al. *J Am Coll Cardiol*. 2002;40:1366-1374.

6. Braunwald E, Antman EM, Beasley JW, et al. ACC/AHA 2002 guideline update for the management of patients with unstable angina and non–ST-segment elevation myocardial infarction—summary article: a report of the American College of Cardiology/American Heart Association task force on practice guidelines (Committee on the Management of Patients With Unstable Angina). *J Am Coll Cardiol*. 2002;40:1366-1374.

7. Braunwald E. Unstable angina. A classification. *Circulation*. 1989;80:410-414.

8. Braunwald E, Mark DB, Jones RH, et al. Unstable angina: diagnosis and management. Clinical Practice Guideline Number 10. Agency for Health Care Policy and Research and the National Heart, Lung, and Blood Institute, Public Health Service, US Department of Health and Human Services; Rockville, Md; 1994.

9. Kaul P, Fu Y, Chang WC, et al. Prognostic value of ST-segment depression in acute coronary syndromes: insights from PARAGON-A applied to GUSTO-IIb. *J Am Coll Cardiol*. 2001;38:64-71.

10. Sabatine MS, Antman EM. The thrombolysis in myocardial infarction risk score in unstable angina/non–ST-segment elevation myocardial infarction. *J Am Coll Cardiol.* 2003;41(4 Suppl S):89S-95S.

11. Ryan TJ, Anderson JL, Antman EM, et al. ACC/AHA guidelines for the management of patients with acute myocardial infarction: a report of the American College of Cardiology/American Heart Association Task Force on Practice Guidelines (Committee on Management of Acute Myocardial Infarction). *J Am Coll Cardiol.* 1996;28:1328-1428.

12. Ryan TJ, Antman EM, Brooks NH, et al, for the Committee of Management of Acute Myocardial Infarction. 1999 Update: ACC/AHA guidelines for the management of patients with acute myocardial infarction. A report of the American College Cardiology/American Heart Association Task Force on Practice Guidelines. *J Am Coll Cardiol.* 1999;34:890-911.

13. CAPRIE Steering Committee. A randomised, blinded, trial of clopidogrel versus aspirin in patients at risk of ischaemic events (CAPRIE). *Lancet.* 1996;348:1329-1339.

14. The CURE Investigators. Effects of clopidogrel in addition to aspirin in patients with acute coronary syndromes without ST-segment elevation. *N Engl J Med.* 2001;345:494-502.

15. Kong DF, Califf RM, Miller DP, et al. Clinical outcomes of therapeutic agents that block the platelet glycoprotein IIb/IIIa integrin in ischemic heart disease. *Circulation.* 1998;98:2829-2835.

16. Theroux P, Ouimet H, McCans J, et al. Aspirin, heparin, or both to treat acute unstable angina. *N Engl J Med.* 1988;319:1105-1111.

17. Cohen M, Adams PC, Hawkins L, Bach M, Fuster V. Usefulness of antithrombotic therapy in resting angina pectoris or non-Q-wave myocardial infarction in preventing death and myocardial infarction (a pilot study from the Antithrombotic Therapy in Acute Coronary Syndromes Study Group). *Am J Cardiol.* 1990;66:1287-1292.

18. The RISC Group. Risk of myocardial infarction and death during treatment with low dose aspirin and intravenous heparin in men with unstable coronary artery disease. *Lancet.* 1990;336:827-830.

19. Cohen M, Adams PC, Parry G, et al. Combination antithrombotic therapy in unstable rest angina and non-Q-wave infarction in nonprior aspirin users. Primary end points analysis from the ATACS trial. Antithrombotic Therapy in Acute Coronary Syndromes Research Group. *Circulation.* 1994;89:81-88.

20. Becker RC, Ball SP, Eisenberg P, et al. A randomized, multicenter trial of weight-adjusted intravenous heparin dose titration and point-of-care coagulation monitoring in hospitalized patients with active thromboembolic disease. Antithrombotic Therapy Consortium Investigators. *Am Heart J.* 1999;137:59-71.

12

21. Becker RC, Spencer FA, Li Y, et al. Thrombin generation after the abrupt cessation of intravenous unfractionated heparin among patients with acute coronary syndromes: potential mechanisms for heightened prothrombotic potential. *J Am Coll Cardiol.* 1999;34:1020-1027.

22. Gurfinkel EP, Manos EJ, Mejail RI, et al. Low molecular weight heparin versus regular heparin or aspirin in the treatment of unstable angina and silent ischemia. *J Am Coll Cardiol.* 1995;26:313-318.

23. Fragmin and Fast Revascularisation During Instability in Coronary Artery Disease (FRISC II) Investigators. Long-term low-molecular-mass heparin in unstable coronary artery disease: FRISC II prospective randomised multicentre study. *Lancet.* 1999;354:701-707.

24. Cohen M, Demers C, Gurfinkel EP, et al. A comparison of low-molecular-weight heparin with unfractionated heparin for unstable coronary artery disease. Efficacy and Safety of Subcutaneous enoxaparin in Non-Q-Wave Coronary Events Study Group. *N Engl J Med.* 1997;337:447-452.

25. Antman EM, McCabe CH, Gurfinkel EP, et al. Enoxaparin prevents death and cardiac ischaemic events in unstable angina/non-Q-wave myocardial infarction. Results of the Thrombolysis in Myocardial Infarction (TIMI) 11B trial. *Circulation.* 1999;100:1593-1601.

26. Choo JK, Kereiakas DJ. Low molecular weight heparin therapy for percutaneous coronary intervention: a practice in evolution. *J Thromb Thrombolysis.* 2001;11:235-246.

27. Collet JP, Montalescot G, Lison L, et al. Percutaneous coronary intervention after subcutaneous enoxaparin pretreatment in patients with unstable angina pectoris. *Circulation.* 2001;103:658-663.

28. Ferguson JJ. Special report from the 22nd Congress of the European Society of Cardiology. Amsterdam, The Netherlands; August, 2000.

29. Wong GC, Giugliano RP, Antman EM. Use of low-molecular-weight heparins in the management of acute coronary artery syndromes and percutaneous coronary intervention. *JAMA.* 2003;289:331-342.

30. Goodman SG, Fitchett D, Armstrong PW, Tan M, Langer A; Integrilin and Enoxaparin Randomized Assessment of Acute Coronary Syndrome Treatment (INTERACT) Trial Investigators. Randomized evaluation of the safety and efficacy of enoxaparin versus unfractionated heparin in high-risk patients with non-ST segment elevation acute coronary syndromes receiving the glycoprotein IIb/IIIa inhibitor eptifibatide. *Circulation.* 2003;107:238-244.

31. SYNERGY Executive Committee. Superior Yield of the New Strategy of Enoxaparin, Revascularization and Glycoprotein IIb/IIIa inhibitors. The SYNERGY trial: study design and rationale. *Am Heart J.* 2002;143:952-960.

32. Superior Yield of the New Strategy of Enoxaparin, Revascularization and Glycoprotein IIb/IIIa inhibitors (SYNERGY) trial: primary results. Presented at: 53rd Annual Scientific Session of the American College of Cardiology; March 9, 2004; New Orleans, La.

33. Kereiakas DJ, Grines C, Fry E, et al for the NICE-1 and NICE-4 Investigators. Enoxaparin and abciximab adjunctive pharmacotherapy during percutaneous coronary intervention. *J Invasive Cardiol.* 2001; 13:272-278.

34. The Global Use of Strategies to Open Occluded Coronary Arteries (GUSTO) IIB Investigators. A comparison of recombinant hirudin with heparin for the treatment of acute coronary syndromes. *N Engl J Med.* 1996;335:775-782.

35. Bittl JA, Strony J, Brinker JA, et al. Treatment with bivalirudin (hirulog) as compared with heparin during coronary angioplasty for unstable or postinfarction angina. Hirulog Angioplasty Study Investigators. *N Engl J Med.* 1995;333:764-769.

36. Lincoff AM, Bittl JA, Harrington RA, et al. Bivalirudin and provisional glycoprotein IIb/IIIa blockade compared with heparin and planned glycoprotein IIb/IIIa blockade during percutaneous coronary intervention: REPLACE-2 randomized trial. *JAMA.* 2003;289:853-863.

37. Anand SS, Yusuf S. Oral anticoagulants in patients with coronary artery disease. *J Am Coll Cardiol.* 2003;41(4 suppl S):62S-69S.

38. The Thrombolysis in Myocardial Ischemia (TIMI)-IIIB Investigators. Effects of tissue plasminogen activator and a comparison of early invasive and conservative strategies in unstable angina and non-Q-wave myocardial infarction. Results of TIMI IIIB Trial. *Circulation.* 1994;89:1545-1556.

39. Antman EM, Tanasijevic MJ, Thompson B, et al. Cardiac-specific troponin I levels to predict the risk of mortality in patients with acute coronary syndromes. *N Engl J Med.* 1996;335:1342-1349.

40. Smith SC, Dove JT, Jacobs AK, et al. ACC/AHA guidelines of percutaneous coronary intervention (revision of the 1993 PTCA guidelines)—executive summary. A report of the American College of Cardiology/American Heart Association Task Force on Practice Guidelines (committee to revise the 1993 guidelines for percutaneous transluminal coronary angioplasty). *J Am Coll Cardiol.* 2001;37:2215-2238.

12

13

Acute Myocardial Infarction

Rupture of an atherosclerotic plaque with subsequent thrombosis due to platelet aggregation and activation of the intrinsic and extrinsic pathways of coagulation is the initiating event in patients with an acute coronary syndrome (ACS). If there is partial thrombotic occlusion with resultant myocardial necrosis, a non–ST-segment elevation myocardial infarction (STEMI) occurs, as discussed in Chapter 12, *Acute Coronary Syndromes*. When the developing thrombus causes complete occlusion and cessation of blood flow, an acute myocardial infarction (AMI) ensues, heralded by ST-segment elevation on the electrocardiogram (ECG).

The initial goals of antithrombotic and fibrinolytic therapy in patients with STEMI are to achieve rapid and sustained patency of the infarct-related artery and physiologic myocardial perfusion through a combination of pharmacologic agents that:

- Inhibit platelet aggregation
- Inhibit thrombin generation and activity
- Activate endogenous pathways of fibrinolysis, either alone or as an adjunct to mechanical reperfusion modalities.

The long-term goals are to prevent:

- Coronary artery reocclusion
- Thrombotic sequelae of new plaque rupture
- Formation and subsequent embolization of mural thrombi.

Antiplatelet Agents

The most compelling evidence for aspirin's benefit in AMI emerged from the Second International Study of Infarct Survival (ISIS-2)[1] that evaluated outcomes in 17,187 AMI patients treated with intravenous (IV) streptokinase (SK), 160 mg oral aspirin, both, or neither. Aspirin alone was associated with a 35-day mortality reduction of 23%

that increased to 42% when combined with SK (**Figure 13.1**). In addition, aspirin reduced the risk of nonfatal reinfarction by 49% and nonfatal stroke by 46%. Aspirin reduced the rate of early reinfarction due to SK-induced platelet activation (3.8% vs 1.3%).[2] The absolute number of lives saved with aspirin increases dramatically with advancing age: 2.5 per 100 patients treated at <60 years of age, 7 to 8 per 100 treated at >60 years of age.

Thus a dose of 162 mg to 325 mg of nonenteric-coated aspirin represents the cornerstone of initial antiplatelet

FIGURE 13.1 — MORTALITY OUTCOMES FROM ISIS-2

Placebo Infusion and Tablets
568/4300 (13.2%)

Aspirin
461/4295 (10.7%)

Streptokinase
448/4300 (10.4%)

Streptokinase and Aspirin
343/4292 (8.0%)

Cumulative Number of Vascular Deaths

Days From Randomization

Abbreviation: ISIS-2, Second International Studies of Infarct Survival.

ISIS-2. *Lancet*. 1988;11:349-360.

therapy in patients with AMI. Alternatively, aspirin can be administered as a 325-mg suppository in patients with severe nausea or vomiting or a history of peptic ulcer disease. Aspirin is contraindicated in patients with a hypersensitivity to salicylates and should be used with caution in patients with active peptic ulcer disease,[3] although rectal administration may be an appropriate initial option. An alternative approach for patients under age 75 who cannot take aspirin is long-term warfarin therapy, with a goal INR of 2.5.[3]

The benefits of aspirin are seen regardless of patient age or gender and across the broad spectrum of patients with ACS, cerebrovascular disease, and chronic atherosclerotic disease. Lifelong therapy is recommended, at a dose ranging from 75 to 162 mg/day.[2,3]

Given the rapid onset of platelet inhibition derived from a 300-mg loading dose of clopidogrel (four 75-mg tablets) and its benefit compared with aspirin in the Clopidogrel vs Aspirin in Patients at Risk for Ischemic Events (CAPRIE) study, clopidogrel is considered an acceptable alternative for patients unable to take aspirin.[3,4] The favorable results reported in the Clopidogrel in Unstable Angina to Prevent Recurrent Ischemic Events (CURE) trial (in which the combination of clopidogrel and aspirin reduced the cumulative incidence of death, myocardial infarction [MI], and stroke by 20%, at the cost of a slightly higher risk of non–life-threatening bleeding) support combined pharmacotherapy in patients with an ACS.[5]

Fibrinolytic Therapy

The observations of DeWood and other investigators[3,6] that thrombotic occlusion of a coronary artery is the most common cause of acute ST-elevation infarction led to the development of plasminogen activators (summarized in Chapter 4, *Fibrinolytic Agents*). All of the available fibrinolytic agents activate single-chain plasma plasminogen via a direct or indirect enzymatic reaction to the active fibrinolytic agent, double-chain plasmin.[7] Characteristics of the currently available agents, SK, anistreplase, recombinant tissue plasminogen activator (rtPA), reteplase (rPA), and tenecteplase (TNK-tPA) are shown in **Table 4.1**.[3]

■ Benefits of Fibrinolytic Therapy

Observations based on experimental animal models and clinical studies performed in humans demonstrated that prompt recanalization of the infarct artery salvages myocardium, preserves left ventricular performance, and improves outcome in a time-dependent fashion.[8,9] Treatment administered within the initial 2 hours provides the greatest overall benefit.[7] A meta-analysis, including all placebo-controlled trials of fibrinolytic therapy[10] that randomized 1000 or more patients with suspected MI, demonstrated an 18% reduction in 30-day mortality. The largest of these trials, ISIS-2,[1] demonstrated an additive benefit of aspirin, which was associated with a mortality reduction of 53% when given in combination with SK within 4 hours of symptoms. Survival benefit was evident across a broad range of subgroups, including:

- Patients with ST elevation or left bundle branch block (LBBB) within 12 hours of symptom onset
- Diabetics
- Those of advanced age
- Patients with prior MI
- Those with systolic blood pressure considered either low (<100 mm Hg) or high.

Although the magnitude of benefit from fibrinolytic therapy is maximal within the first "golden hour,"[11] the window of opportunity extends to ≥12 hours (in select cases) from symptom onset.[1,12,13]

■ Comparative Trials

Several randomized clinical trials have compared the most widely used fibrinolytic agents, SK and tissue plasminogen activator (tPA): Gruppo Italiano per lo Studio della Sopravvivenza nell'Infarto Miocardico (GISSI)-2[14], ISIS-3[8], and Global Use of Strategies to Open Occluded Coronary Arteries (GUSTO) I[9] (**Table 13.1**). The largest trial, GUSTO I, randomized 41,000 patients with ST-segment elevation to one of four treatment strategies. Accelerated "front-loaded" tPA with IV UFH reduced 30-day mortality by 15% compared with SK with IV or SC UFH (**Figure 13.2**). This benefit was maintained at 1 year (**Figure 13.2**) although hemorrhagic stroke occurred more often with tPA

(0.7%) than with SK (0.4%). A net clinical benefit was still achieved with tPA, as evidenced by nine fewer deaths or disabling strokes per 1000 patients treated.[9] Other complications of MI occurred less frequently as well, including heart failure, cardiogenic shock, allergic reactions, and arrhythmias. The GUSTO angiographic substudy provided strong evidence that rapid achievement of Thrombolysis in Myocardial Infarction (TIMI) 3 (physiologic) flow within the infarct-related coronary artery was a key determinant of favorable outcomes.[11,15] TIMI-3 flow rates at 90 minutes in tPA-treated patients were 55%, compared with an average of 29% in SK-treated patients. Irrespective of the fibrinolytic agent, mortality was lowest (4.2%) in patients with TIMI-3 flow and highest (8.2%) in patients with TIMI-0 or 1 flow at 90 minutes.[15]

In addition to overall survival, TIMI-3 flow status correlated closely with global and infarct region left ventricular function and cavity dilation. These data provided a "proof of concept" platform for fibrinolytic therapy and an evidence-based rationale for establishing early and complete coronary arterial patency and myocardial perfusion as the primary goals of treatment.[3,16-18]

Reteplase, a deletion mutant of tPA, and TNK-tPA, a single-bolus mutant of tPA, were both found to be similar in outcome and efficacy compared with tPA in the GUSTO III[16] and Assessment of the Safety and Efficacy of a New Thrombolytic (ASSENT)-II[17] trials.

13

Complications of Fibrinolytic and Adjunctive Therapy

The major complication associated with fibrinolytic therapy is bleeding, with intracranial hemorrhage representing the most feared and devastating event. The risk of intracranial bleeding ranges from 0.3% in low-risk patients (<65 years of age) to 5% in patients >75 years old with additional risk factors. Nearly two thirds of patients with intracranial hemorrhage will die or sustain significant neurologic disability, particularly in patients >75 years of age, in whom the case fatality rate exceeds 90%.[19] Other sites of serious bleeding, such as genitourinary, gastrointes-

TABLE 13.1 — MORTALITY OUTCOME IN COMPARATIVE TRIALS OF FIBRINOLYTIC THERAPY

Study	No. of Patients	Agents, Dose	Time (h)	Mortality Follow-up	Therapy (%)	Control (%)	RRR (%)/ ARR (%)	P Value
GISSI-2	12,490	SK 1.5 MU, 0.5-1 h vs tPA 100 mg, 3 h; heparin SC vs control	<6	Hospital	SK, 8.6	tPA, 9.0	—	Not significant
International Study Group	20,891	SK 1.5 MU, 0.5-1 h vs tPA 100 mg, 3 h; heparin SC vs control	<6	Hospital	SK, 8.5	tPA, 8.9	—	Not significant
ISIS-3	41,291	SK 1.5 MU, 1 h, APSAC 30 U, 3-5 min, duteplase 0.6 MU/kg; heparin SC vs control	<24	35 d	SK, 10.5	APSAC, 10.6; tPA, 10.3	—	Not significant
INJECT	6,010	SK 1.5 MU, 1 h, rPA 10 U, repeated after 30 min; heparin IV to all	<12	35 d	SK, 9.53	rPA, 9.02	0.51	Not significant

GUSTO I	41,021	SK 1.5 MU, 1 h + heparin SC or IV or SK 1.0 MU 1 h + tPA 1.0 mg/kg 1 h + heparin, or tPA up to 100 mg 1.5 h + heparin	<6	30 d	SK SC heparin, 7.2; SK IV heparin, 7.4	SK, 7.0; tPA, 6.3; rtPA, 6.3	Accelerated tPA vs SK 14/1.0	0.001
GUSTO III	15,059	tPA up to 100 mg, 1.5 h or rPA 10 U, repeated after 30 min; heparin IV to all	<6	30 d	tPA, 7.24	rPA, 7.47	0.23	0.54
COBALT	7,169	tPA up to 100 mg, 1.5 h rtPA 50-mg bolus, repeated (50 or 40 mg) after 30 min; heparin IV to all	<6	30 d	tPA accelerated, 7.53	tPA 2 bolus, 7.98	0.45	Not significant

Abbreviations: APSAC, anisoylated plasminogen-streptokinase activator complex; ARR, absolute risk reduction; COBALT, Continuous Infusion versus Double-Bolus Administration of Alteplase; GISSI, Grupo Italiano per lo Studio della Sopravvivenza neu'Infarcto ous Miocardico; GUSTO, Global Use of Strategies to Open Occluded Coronary Arteries; INJECT, International Joint Efficacy Comparison of Thrombolytics; ISIS, International Study of Infarct Survival; IV, intravenous; MU, megaunit; rPA, reteplase; RRR, relative risk reduction; rtPA, recombinant tissue plasminogen activator; SC, subcutaneous; SK, streptokinase; tPA, tissue plasminogen activator; U, unit.

Cairns JA, et al. Chest. 1998;114(suppl):636S.

13

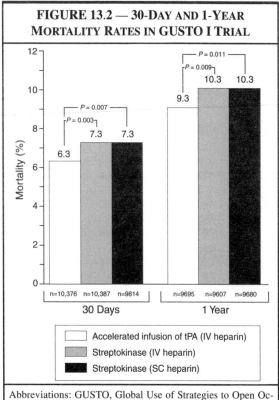

FIGURE 13.2 — 30-DAY AND 1-YEAR MORTALITY RATES IN GUSTO I TRIAL

Abbreviations: GUSTO, Global Use of Strategies to Open Occluded Coronary Arteries; IV, intravenous; SC, subcutaneous; tPA, tissue plasminogen activator.

Superior outcome occurred in the treatment group receiving front-loaded tPA and IV heparin.

tinal, or retroperitoneal, are uncommon (<5%) but can be life-threatening if not quickly recognized and treated. The Fibrinolytic Therapy Trialists reported that for each 1000 patients treated with a fibrinolytic agent, seven major noncerebral hemorrhages and two nonfatal strokes would result, while preventing 18 deaths over 35 days following the MI.[10,20] The incidence of access-site hemorrhage is decreasing with the use of smaller-bore catheters and lower doses of heparin. Allergic reactions occur commonly (1%

to 5%) with SK, but true anaphylactic reactions are rare (<0.5%). Hypotension ranges from 5% to 7% with SK and is less common (2% to 4%) with tPA. Reinfarction rates range from 2% to 4%, depending on the use of conjunctive heparin and aspirin.[20] **Table 4.3** provides a current summary of contraindications and cautions for the administration of fibrinolytic agents.

A novel strategy, employing a reduced 50-mg bolus dose of tPA, followed by immediate angiography and "facilitated" by percutaneous coronary intervention (PCI) for TIMI grade 0, 1, or 2 flow, provided encouraging results.[21] One of the great challenges faced by clinicians is the determination of successful coronary fibrinolysis and physiologic myocardial perfusion. If the patient develops sudden and significant relief of chest pain, full resolution of ST elevation on the ECG, and experiences concomitant salvos of an accelerated idioventricular rhythm, patency and reperfusion are more likely; however, this triad is seen in <10% of patients.[22] Accordingly, mounting interest has focused on rapid resolution of ST elevation determined by continuous (automated) ST-segment analysis as a means to establish a diagnosis.

Recommendations for the Use of Fibrinolytic Agents

The indications for fibrinolytic therapy are summarized in the 2003 American College of Cardiology/American Heart Association (ACC/AHA) consensus guidelines for AMI[3] (**Table 13.2**). Patients <75 years of age with ischemic chest pain and ST elevation >0.1 mV in two or more contiguous leads or bundle branch block presenting within 12 hours of symptom onset are considered optimal candidates.[3] In patients >75 years of age, the absolute benefit of therapy is substantial, although the relative benefit is somewhat less than in patients <75.[10] Benefit also diminishes for treatment given within 12 to 24 hours of symptoms, as well as in patients with blood pressure >180/110 mm Hg, due to the increased risk of intracranial hemorrhage.

Despite the strong clinical trial data supporting these recommendations, a substantial number of patients (≥25%) identified as ideal candidates (based on existing criteria) re-

TABLE 13.2 — DIAGNOSTIC AND TREATMENT MEASURES IN PATIENTS WITH ST ELEVATION OR BUNDLE BRANCH BLOCK

Initial Diagnostic Measures
- Use continuous ECG, automated BP, HR monitoring
- Take targeted history (for AMI inclusions, thrombolysis exclusions), check vital signs, perform focused examination
- Start IVs, draw blood for serum cardiac markers, hematology, chemistry, lipid profile
- Obtain 12-lead ECG
- Obtain chest x-ray (preferably upright)

General Treatment Measures
- Aspirin, 160-325 mg (chew and swallow)
- Nitroglycerin, sublingual: test for Prinzmetal's angina, reversible spasm; anti-ischemic, antihypertensive effects
- Oxygen: sparse data; probably indicated, first 2 to 3 h in all; continue if arterial oxygen saturation is low (<90%)
- Adequate analgesia: small doses of morphine (2 to 4 mg) as needed

Specific Treatment Measures
- Reperfusion therapy: goal—door-to-needle time <30 min; door-to-balloon time <90 min
- Conjunctive antithrombotics: aspirin, heparin (especially with tPA, rPA, or TNKase)
- Adjunctive therapies: β-adrenoceptor blockade if eligible, IV nitroglycerin (for anti-ischemic or antihypertensive effects), ACE inhibitor (especially with large or anterior AMI, heart failure without hypotension [SBP >100 mm Hg], previous MI)
- Early use of statins

Abbreviations: ACE, angiotensin-converting enzyme; AMI, acute myocardial infarction; BP, blood pressure; ECG, electrocardiogram; HR, heart rate; IV, intravenous; rPA, retaplase; SBP, systolic blood pressure; TNKase, tenecteplase; tPA, tissue plasminogen activator.

From: ACC/AHA Joint Guideline Statement.

main untreated, particularly those at highest risk, such as patients with LBBB or heart failure.[23] Thus further efforts are needed to ensure that patients who could benefit from an established and potentially lifesaving means of therapy receive it in a timely manner.

Primary Percutaneous Coronary Intervention

Although fibrinolytic therapy can be administered in virtually any hospital with minimal delay, the rate of TIMI-3 flow plateaus at approximately 50% to 60%. Mechanical reperfusion, using balloon angioplasty or primary coronary stenting, can attain TIMI-3 flow in >85% of patients. A pooled analysis of 10 randomized trials of PCI and fibrinolytic therapy performed by Weaver[24] demonstrated significantly lower rates of the following in favor of mechanical intervention:

- Death (4.4% vs 6.5%)
- Nonfatal reinfarction (7.2% vs 11.9%)
- Hemorrhagic stroke (0.1% vs 1.1%).

A portion of the early benefits had diminished by 1 year.[25,26]

The benefit derived from primary PCI, as with fibrinolytic therapy, is time dependent. Delays beyond 90 minutes from hospital arrival are not uncommon in clinical practice.[27] In addition, only about 20% of US hospitals have onsite capabilities, and of those, one quarter are capable of mobilizing a catheterization team within 60 minutes. Thus for primary PCI to achieve maximal benefit, it must be initiated in a timely manner (door-to-balloon time within 90 minutes of hospital arrival) within 12 hours of symptom onset (or beyond 12 hours if ischemic symptoms persist) by persons skilled in the procedure and supported by an experienced catheterization laboratory team. If the anticipated door-to-balloon time exceeds the door-to-needle time by >60 minutes, fibrinolytic therapy should be administered unless contraindicated. Transfer of an acute MI patient to a hospital capable of performing immediate angioplasty has been shown to be an effective alternate strategy, provided that the initial presentation-to-balloon time in the receiving institution can be lowered to ≤90 minutes.[28] Another strategy is facilitated PCI, where an initial reduced dose of fibrinolytic therapy, a platelet glycoprotein (GP) IIb/IIIa inhibitor, or both are administered, followed by relatively urgent angioplasty. This approach offers the advantages of earlier time to reperfusion, higher TIMI flow in the infarct related coronary artery, greater procedural success rates, and improved survival, but with the limitations of increased cost and bleeding.[3] Several clinical trials are currently assessing this reperfusion strategy. Patients with cardiogenic shock[29] as well as those who are not candidates for fibrinolytic therapy should be considered for immediate coronary angiography and primary PCI.[3]

Overcoming Thrombolytic Resistance

With currently used fibrinolytic strategies, vessel patency (TIMI-2 or -3 flow) is achieved in approximately 60% to 85% of patients, but physiologic reperfusion (TIMI-3 flow), is restored in barely 50%. This "resistance" to optimal reperfusion may be driven by several mechanisms (**Figure 13.3**).[30-32]

The most commonly used antithrombotic strategy, unfractionated heparin (UFH), does not inhibit clot-bound thrombin. The traditional antiplatelet agent, aspirin, has been shown to decrease the risk of reocclusion and reinfarction[1] following coronary thrombolysis but does not inhibit activation of GPIIb/IIIa receptors (and fibrinogen-mediated platelet aggregation).

Several trials have examined the safety and efficacy of combination pharmacotherapy employing fibrinolytic agents and GPIIb/IIIa receptor antagonists. The Integrelin and Reduced Dose of Thrombolytics in Acute Myocardial Infarction (INTRO-AMI) trial evaluated the combination of eptifibatide and reduced-dose tPA, demonstrating a rate of TIMI-3 flow approaching 75% at 90 minutes.[33] The TIMI-14 study tested the combination of abciximab and either reduced dose tPA, rPA, or SK.[34] Abciximab alone produced a TIMI-3 flow rate of 32% at 90 minutes, similar to that obtained with SK alone. The combination of abciximab and SK produced only modest improvement in TIMI flow grade, with a significant increase in hemorrhage. The combination of half-dose tPA (15-mg bolus plus 35 mg over 60 minutes)

FIGURE 13.3 — THROMBOLYTIC RESISTANCE DUE TO ACTIVATION OF THROMBIN AND PLATELETS

Platelets

Fibrin

Thrombin

Thrombus occluding coronary artery

Fibrinolytic therapy

Plasmin cleaves fibrin

Exposes clot-bound thrombin

Activates platelets

Lysed clot
↑ FDPs (antiplatelet and anticoagulant)
↓ Fibrinogen

PAI-1, thromboxane A2, fibrinogen

Reperfusion

New thrombin generation
Platelet activation
Cleaves fibrinogen to fibrin

↑ Platelet activation
↑ Thrombin production
Vasoconstriction
inhibits plasminogen activators

Thrombus formation
Vessel reocclusion

Abbreviations: FDP, fibrin/fibrinogen degradation product; PAI-1, plasminogen activator inhibitor-1.

Moliterno DJ, Topol EJ. *Thromb Haemost*. 1997;78:214-219.

and abciximab produced TIMI-3 flow rates of 77% at 90 minutes, with no significant increase in bleeding (**Figure 13.4**). Myocardial perfusion, as assessed by ST-segment resolution, was also significantly improved.[35]

Although the rPA phase of the TIMI-14 trial as well as the Strategies for Patency Enhancement in the Emergency Department (SPEED) trial demonstrated that the combina-

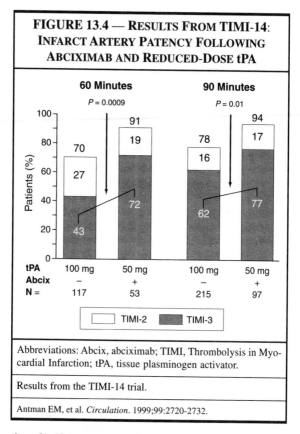

FIGURE 13.4 — RESULTS FROM TIMI-14:
INFARCT ARTERY PATENCY FOLLOWING
ABCIXIMAB AND REDUCED-DOSE tPA

	60 Minutes		90 Minutes	
	P = 0.0009		*P* = 0.01	
TIMI-2	27	19	16	17
TIMI-3	43	72	62	77
Total	70	91	78	94
tPA	100 mg	50 mg	100 mg	50 mg
Abcix	–	+	–	+
N =	117	53	215	97

☐ TIMI-2 ■ TIMI-3

Abbreviations: Abcix, abciximab; TIMI, Thrombolysis in Myocardial Infarction; tPA, tissue plasminogen activator.

Results from the TIMI-14 trial.

Antman EM, et al. *Circulation*. 1999;99:2720-2732.

tion of half-dose rPA (5 + 5 U) and abciximab demonstrated TIMI-3 flow in 63% of patients,[36] the recently completed GUSTO V trial demonstrated equivalent 30-day mortality outcomes between full-dose rPA (5.9%) and half-dose rPA plus abciximab (5.6%). Reinfarction and urgent revascularization did occur less often with combination therapy.[37] The ASSENT-3 trial,[38] using a similar study design, demonstrated similar mortality outcomes in patients receiving full-dose TNK-tPA and reduced-dose UFH (6%) and half-dose TNK-tPA plus abciximab (6.6%), with a trend toward lower mortality when enoxaparin was combined with TNK-tPA (5.4%) (**Figure 13.5**). However, in both trials, patients over the age of 75 receiving the combination of a lytic agent and abciximab experienced a significant increase in intracranial bleeding.

The available data suggest that enhanced rate and extent of thrombolysis is achievable with combined pharmacotherapy; however, the safety and overall benefit can only be established through further investigation.

Heparin Preparations

Heparin is a naturally occurring inhibitor of thrombin, requiring formation of a ternary complex with antithrombin for an inhibitory effect. Several trials performed in the prereperfusion era demonstrated a 17% mortality reduction and a 22% reduction in risk of reinfarction with UFH.[39]

These "historical" data, as well as the reduction in the incidence of venous thromboemboli, provided support for the use of IV UFH or subcutaneous (SC) low molecular weight heparin (LMWH) in patients with MI.[3,40]

Patients with an anterior infarction with anterior akinesis or dyskinesis, significant left ventricular dysfunction, left ventricular aneurysm, congestive heart failure, thrombus in the left ventricle documented by echocardiography, a history of a previous embolic event, and atrial fibrillation are at a high risk for systemic embolization[2] (**Table 13.3**). Although randomized trial data are sparse, there is evidence that the risk of systemic emboli can be reduced by early initiation of heparin therapy.[2] Therefore, independent of the fibrinolytic agent choice, heparin is recommended for patients at high risk for systemic embolism. Unless a contraindication exists, oral anticoagulant therapy with warfarin (target international normalized ratio [INR] 2.5) is continued for several months.

Patients receiving fibrin-selective agents, tPA, rPA, or TNK-tPA should receive weight-adjusted IV UFH (target activated partial thromboplastin time [aPTT] 50-70 seconds) for 48 hours.[3] The dosing strategy is as follows: a 60-U/kg bolus at initiation of fibrinolytic therapy, followed by an initial maintenance dose of 12 U/kg/hr (maximum bolus of 4,000 U) and a 1000 U/hr infusion in patients weighing >70 kg. If non–fibrin-selective fibrinolytics are used, such as SK or anistreplase, patients at low risk for thromboemboli can

13

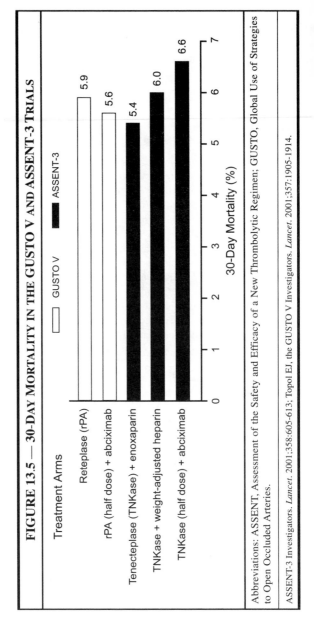

FIGURE 13.5 — 30-DAY MORTALITY IN THE GUSTO V AND ASSENT-3 TRIALS

Abbreviations: ASSENT, Assessment of the Safety and Efficacy of a New Thrombolytic Regimen; GUSTO, Global Use of Strategies to Open Occluded Arteries.

ASSENT-3 Investigators. *Lancet.* 2001;358:605-613; Topol EJ, the GUSTO V Investigators. *Lancet.* 2001;357:1905-1914.

TABLE 13.3 — FACTORS THAT INCREASE THE RISK OF SYSTEMIC EMBOLIZATION FOLLOWING MYOCARDIAL INFARCTION

- Anterior infarction with anterior akinesis or dyskinesis
- Significant left ventricular dysfunction
- Acute left ventricular aneurysm
- Congestive heart failure
- Thrombus in the left ventricle documented by echocardiography
- History of a previous embolic event
- Atrial fibrillation

receive SC heparin 7500 to 10,000 U every 12 hours until ambulatory.

Low Molecular Weight Heparin and Direct-Acting Antithrombins

Low molecular weight heparin provides several potential advantages over conventional UFH, owing to its improved bioavailability, enhanced antithrombotic effects mediated by "upstream" inhibition of the coagulation cascade, and ease of use. Several trials are evaluating the role of LMWH as adjunctive antithrombotic therapy for patients receiving fibrinolytics.[3] As described, ASSENT-3 provided encouraging results for the combination of enoxaparin and TNK-tPA.[38] The National Investigators Collaboration on Enoxaparin (NICE) trials have demonstrated the safety and efficacy of enoxaparin in the catheterization laboratory during PCI, both with and without GPIIb/IIIa receptor antagonists. The EXTRACT (TIMI-25 trial), randomizing 20,000 patients with acute STEMI to either enoxaparin or UFH in conjunction with fibrinolytic therapy and aspirin, will report its findings in 2004.

Warfarin

A meta-analysis of trials performed in the prereperfusion era demonstrated that long-term oral anticoagulation was associated with a modest survival benefit of 20% in men, which was restricted to those with prolonged angina or previous MI.[2] The Warfarin Reinfarction Study (WARIS)[41] included patients with MI (mean 27 days from event) and randomized them to treatment with warfarin (target INR of 2.8 to 4.8) or placebo. There were statistically significant reductions in all-cause mortality (24%), reinfarction (34%), and stroke (55%) in favor of anticoagulant therapy.

The Coumadin Aspirin Reinfarction Study (CARS)[42] tested the efficacy of low-intensity anticoagulation with warfarin 1 mg/day to 3 mg/day plus aspirin 80 mg/day compared with aspirin alone (160 mg/day). Event rates were low and nearly identical in all three study arms of the trial. These results are consistent with a large body of literature that suggests that warfarin is most effective when given in doses capable of increasing the INR to 2 to 3.5 (moderate-to high-intensity anticoagulation).[2]

Several recent trials have compared moderate-intensity (INR 2-3) and high-intensity (INR 2.5-3.5) warfarin therapy with or without aspirin in patients following MI.[42-46] Clinical benefits were found with only a modest increase in bleeding (**Table 13.4**). The AHA/ACC guidelines committee recommend that in the absence of high risk for systemic embolization (**Table 13.3**), warfarin alone (INR 2.5-3.5) or warfarin (INR 2-2.5) plus low-dose aspirin (81 mg) is a reasonable alternative to aspirin in patients <75 years of age. However, the cost and complexity of oral anticoagulation should be weighed against the modest benefit over aspirin alone. New, orally administered direct antithrombins may offer increased safety and ease of administration without monitoring. The ESTEEM trial evaluated clinical outcome and safety of varying doses of ximelagatran, an oral direct-acting thrombin inhibitor, and aspirin 160 mg in 1883 patients with a recent MI. The combination of ximelagatran and aspirin was more effective than aspirin alone in reducing the occurrence of major cardiovascular events at all doses studied; safety and equivalent efficacy was noted with the lowest dose of 24 mg twice daily. Bleeding risk and hepatic transaminase elevation occurred with higher doses. These promising results will require confirmation in a large phase 3 trial.[47]

For patients at high risk for venous or systemic thromboembolism (**Table 13.3**) or reinfarction, a combination of low-dose aspirin plus warfarin (INR 2-3) or warfarin alone (INR 2.5-3.5) is recommended for at least several months following the infarction,[3] reverting to chronic recommendations for anticoagulation after the initial high-risk post-MI period. Treatment is often initiated in the hospital, while the patient is still receiving IV or SC heparin. The availability of LMWH preparations that can be self-administered once or twice per day provide a potential option for earlier hospital discharge with transition to warfarin therapy in the outpatient setting. For patients who have undergone bare metal stenting, clopidogrel can usually be stopped in several weeks; however, longer treatment is recommended with drug-eluting stents and possibly in other patients as well. The benefit of more prolonged therapy is undergoing evaluation. **Figure 13**.6 summarizes these recommendations.

Summary

Acute thrombotic occlusion of an epicardial coronary artery, the most common cause of ST-segment elevation MI, is the end result of platelet activation and aggregation, followed by activation of the extrinsic and intrinsic pathways of coagulation. The clinician's antithrombotic armamentarium includes:

- Fibrinolytics used alone or as part of a facilitated strategy
- Mechanical techniques, such as immediate angioplasty and/or stenting, to restore perfusion and maintain patency
- Antiplatelet agents that inhibit platelet activation as well as aggregation through blockade of the GPIIb/IIIa receptor
- Antithrombotic compounds that prevent propagation of thrombus, particularly after successful reperfusion therapy.

Current research efforts are directed toward defining the safest and most efficacious pharmacologic and mechanical treatments that achieve rapid and sustained patency of the infarct vessel and limit subsequent atherothrombotic events.

13

TABLE 13.4 — ASPIRIN VS WARFARIN THERAPY AFTER STEMI

STUDY DESIGN

Study	Study Design	Drugs Used	ASA	2nd Arm	3rd Arm	Patients
STEMI-Specific Trials						
WARIS-II[1]	Randomized, open label $n = 3630$; FU = mean 4 y	ASA monotherapy vs warfarin monotherapy vs warfarin + ASA	160 mg daily	Dosed to target INR 2.8-4.2	Dosed to target INR 2.0-2.5 + ASA 75 mg daily	Age <75 y; hospitalized for acute MI; % STEMI = 71.8
APRICOT-2[2]	Randomized, open label $n = 308$; FU = 3 mo	ASA monotherapy vs warfarin + ASA	If TIMI 3 post 48 h UFH, 160 mg initially then 80 mg daily	Dosed to target INR 2-3; if TIMI 3 post 48 h UFH, 160 mg initially then 80 mg daily	N/A	Age ≤76 y, acute STEMI ≤6 h prior to thrombolytic therapy; % STEMI = 100
Trials Not Specific to STEMI						
ASPECT-2[3]	Randomized, open label $n = 999$; FU = 26 mo	ASA monotherapy vs warfarin monotherapy vs warfarin + ASA	80 mg daily	Dosed to target INR 3-4	Dosed to target INR 2.0-2.5 + ASA 80 mg daily	Acute MI or UA within preceding 8 wk
CHAMP[4]	Randomized, open label $n = 5059$; FU = median 2.7 y	ASA monotherapy vs Warfarin + ASA	162 mg daily	Dosed to target INR 1.5-2.5 + 81 mg ASA daily	N/A	Acute MI within preceding 14 d prior to enrollment

CARS[5]	Randomized, blinded n = 8803; FU = 33 mo; median = 14 mo	ASA monotherapy vs warfarin 1 mg + ASA	160 mg daily (avg INR at wk 4 = 1.02)	1 mg + 80 mg ASA (avg INR at wk 4 = 1.05)	N/A	Age 21-85 y (82% <70 y); MI 3-21 d (mean 9.6 d) prior to enrollment
			ASA Alone	**Warfarin Alone**		**ASA + Warfarin**
		STUDY RESULTS				
Study	**End Points**		**ASA Alone**	**Warfarin Alone**		**ASA + Warfarin**
STEMI-Specific Trials						
WARIS-II[1]	Death, nonfatal reinfarction, or thromboembolic stroke		20%	16.7% ($P = 0.03$ vs ASA)		15% ($P = 0.001$ vs ASA)
	Major, nonfatal bleeding ($P < 0.001$)		0.17%	0.68%		0.57%
APRICOT-2[2]	Reocclusion (TIMI ≤2) ($P < 0.02$)		28%	N/A		15%
	Total occlusion (TIMI 0-1) ($P < 0.02$)		20%			9%
	Revascularization ($P < 0.01$)		31%			13%
	Reinfarction ($P < 0.05$)		8%			2%
	Event-free survival rate* ($P < 0.01$)		66%			86%
	Bleeding (TIMI major and minor) ($P = $ NS)		3%			5%

13

Continued

Study	End Points	ASA Alone	Warfarin Alone	ASA + Warfarin
Trials Not Specific to STEMI				
ASPECT-2[3]	Death, MI, or stroke (P = 0.0479)	9%	5%	5%
	Major bleeding	1%	1%	2%
	Minor bleeding (P <0.0001)	5%	8%	15%
	Almost 20% of the warfarin and combined group discontinued therapy; 40% in therapeutic range			
CHAMP[4]	Death (P = 0.76)	17.3%	N/A	17.6%
	Recurrent MI (P = 0.78)	13.1%		13.3%
	Stroke (P = 0.52)	3.5%		3.1%
	Major bleeding (P <0.001)	0.72[†]		1.2[†]
CARS[5]	Ischemic stroke (P = 0.0534)	0.6%	N/A	1.1%

Abbreviations: APRICOT-2, Antithrombotics in the Prevention of Reocclusion in Coronary Thrombolysis-2 [trial]; ASA, acetylsalicyclic acid; ASPECT-2, Anticoagulation in the Secondary Prevention of Events in Coronary Thrombosis [study]; CARS, Warfarin (Coumadin) Aspirin Reinfarction Study; CHAMP, Combination Hemotherapy and Mortality Prevention [study]; FU, follow-up; INR, international normalized ratio; MI, myocardial infarction; NA, not applicable; NS, not significant; STEMI, ST-segment elevation myocardial infarction; TIMI, Thrombolysis in Myocardial Infarction; UA, unstable angina; UFH, unfractionated heparin; WARIS-II, Warfarin-Aspirin Reinfarction Study.

* Events are death, revascularization, or reinfarction.
† Reported as number of events per 100 person years of follow-up.

Antman EM, et al. *J Am Coll Cardiol.* 2003. In press.

REFERENCES

1. ISIS-2 (Second International Study of Infarct Survival) Collaborative Group. Randomised trial of intravenous streptokinase, oral aspirin, both, or neither among 17,187 cases of suspected acute myocardial infarction: ISIS-2. *Lancet*. 1988;2:349-360.

2. Cairns JA, Theroux P, Lewis HD Jr, Ezekowitz M, Meade TW. Antithrombotic agents in coronary artery disease. *Chest*. 2001;119(suppl): 228S-252S.

3. Antman EM, Smith SC, Anbe DT, et al. ACC/AHA guidelines for the management of patients with ST-elevation myocardial infarction. A report of the American College of Cardiology/American Heart Association Task Force on Practice Guidelines (Committee on Management of Acute Myocardial Infarction). *J Am Coll Cardiol*. 2003. In press.

4. CAPRIE Steering Committee. A randomised, blinded, trial of clopidogrel versus aspirin in patients at risk of ischaemic events (CAPRIE). *Lancet*. 1996;348:1329-1339.

5. The Clopidogrel in Unstable Angina to Prevent Recurrent Events (CURE) Trial Investigators: Effects of clopidogrel in addition to aspirin in patients with acute coronary syndromes without ST-segment elevation. *N Engl J Med*. 2001;345:494-502.

6. DeWood MA, Spores J, Notske R, et al. Prevalence of total coronary occlusion during the early hours of transmural myocardial infarction. *N Engl J Med*. 1980;303:897-902.

7. Sherry S. *Fibrinolysis, Thrombosis, and Hemostasis: Concepts, Perspectives, and Clinical Applications*. Philadelphia, Pa: Lea and Febiger; 1992:119-160.

8. ISIS-3 (Third International Study of Infarct Survival) Collaborative Group. A randomised comparison of streptokinase vs tissue plasminogen activator vs anistreplase and of aspirin plus heparin vs aspirin alone among 41,299 cases of suspected acute myocardial infarction: ISIS-3. *Lancet*. 1992;339:753-770.

9. The GUSTO Investigators. An international randomized trial comparing four thrombolytic strategies for acute myocardial infarction. *N Engl J Med*. 1993;329:673-682.

10. Fibrinolytic Therapy Trialists' (FTT) Collaborative Group. Indications for fibrinolytic therapy in suspected acute myocardial infarction: collaborative overview of early mortality and major morbidity results from all randomised trials of more than 1000 patients [published correction appears in *Lancet*. 1994;343:742]. *Lancet*. 1994;343:311-322.

13

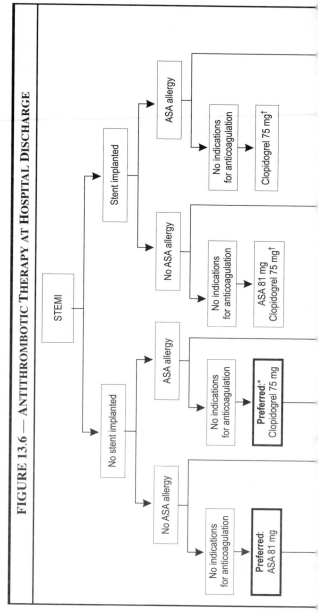

FIGURE 13.6 — ANTITHROMBOTIC THERAPY AT HOSPITAL DISCHARGE

STEMI

No stent implanted

Stent implanted

No ASA allergy

No indications for anticoagulation

Preferred: ASA 81 mg

ASA allergy

No indications for anticoagulation

Preferred:* Clopidogrel 75 mg

No ASA allergy

No indications for anticoagulation

ASA 81 mg
Clopidogrel 75 mg†

ASA allergy

No indications for anticoagulation

Clopidogrel 75 mg†

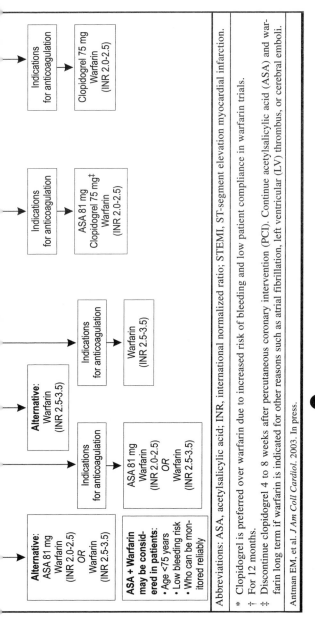

| | | | | | Indications for anticoagulation → Clopidogrel 75 mg Warfarin (INR 2.0-2.5) |

Alternative: ASA 81 mg Warfarin (INR 2.0-2.5) OR Warfarin (INR 2.5-3.5)

Alternative: Warfarin (INR 2.5-3.5)

Indications for anticoagulation → Warfarin (INR 2.5-3.5)

Indications for anticoagulation → ASA 81 mg Warfarin (INR 2.0-2.5) OR Warfarin (INR 2.5-3.5)

Indications for anticoagulation → ASA 81 mg Clopidogrel 75 mg‡ Warfarin (INR 2.0-2.5)

ASA + Warfarin may be considered in patients:
• Age <75 years
• Low bleeding risk
• Who can be monitored reliably

Abbreviations: ASA, acetylsalicylic acid; INR, international normalized ratio; STEMI, ST-segment elevation myocardial infarction.

* Clopidogrel is preferred over warfarin due to increased risk of bleeding and low patient compliance in warfarin trials.

† For 12 months.

‡ Discontinue clopidogrel 4 to 8 weeks after percutaneous coronary intervention (PCI). Continue acetylsalicylic acid (ASA) and warfarin long term if warfarin is indicated for other reasons such as atrial fibrillation, left ventricular (LV) thrombus, or cerebral emboli.

Antman EM, et al. *J Am Coll Cardiol.* 2003. In press.

13

261

11. The GUSTO Angiographic Investigators. The effects of tissue plasminogen activator, streptokinase, or both on coronary-artery patency, ventricular function, and survival after acute myocardial infarction. *N Engl J Med*. 1993;329:1615-1622.

12. Late Assessment of Thrombolytic Efficacy (LATE) study with alteplase 6-24 hours after onset of acute myocardial infarction. *Lancet*. 1993;342:759-766.

13. EMERAS (Estudio Multicentrico Estreptoquinasa Republicas de America del Sur) Collaborative Group. Randomised trial of late thrombolysis in patients with suspected acute myocardial infarction. *Lancet*. 1993;342:767-772.

14. Gruppo Italiano per lo Studio della Sopravvivenza nell'Infarto Miocardico. GISSI-2: a factorial randomised trial of alteplase versus streptokinase and heparin versus no heparin among 12,490 patients with acute myocardial infarction. *Lancet*. 1990;336:65-71.

15. Simes RJ, Topol EJ, Holmes DR Jr, et al for the GUSTO-I Investigators. Link between the angiographic substudy and mortality outcomes in a large randomized trial of myocardial reperfusion. Importance of early and complete infarct artery reperfusion. *Circulation*. 1995;91:1923-1928.

16. The Global Use of Strategies to Open Occluded Coronary Arteries (GUSTO III) Investigators. A comparison of reteplase with alteplase for acute myocardial infarction. *N Engl J Med*. 1997;337:1118-1123.

17. Cannon CP, Gibson CM, McCabe CH, et al. TNK-tissue plasminogen activator compared with front-loaded alteplase in acute myocardial infarction: results of the TIMI 10B trial. Thrombolysis in Myocardial Infarction (TIMI) 10B Investigators. *Circulation*. 1998;98:2805-2814.

18. White HD, Van de Werf FJ. Thrombolysis for acute myocardial infarction. *Circulation*. 1998;97:1632-1646.

19. Gore JM, Granger CB, Simoons ML, et al. Stroke after thrombolysis. Mortality and functional outcomes in the GUSTO-I Trial. *Circulation*. 1995;92:2811-2818.

20. Cairns JA, Kennedy JW, Fuster V. Coronary thrombolysis. *Chest*. 1998;114(suppl):634S-657S.

21. Ross AM, Coyne KS, Reiner JS, et al. Randomized trial comparing angioplasty with a strategy of short acting thrombolysis and immediate planned rescue angioplasty in acute myocardial infarction: the PACT trial. *J Am Coll Cardiol*. 1999;34:1954-1962.

22. Califf RM, O'Neil W, Stack RS, et al. Failure of simple clinical measurements to predict perfusion status after intravenous thrombolysis. *Ann Intern Med*. 1988;108:658-662.

23. Barron HV, Bowlby LJ, Breen T, et al. Use of reperfusion therapy for acute myocardial infarction in the United States: data from the National Registry of Myocardial Infarction 2. *Circulation*. 1998;97: 1150-1156.

24. Weaver WD, Simes RJ, Betriu A, et al. Comparison of primary coronary angioplasty and intravenous thrombolytic therapy for acute myocardial infarction: a quantitative review [published correction appears in *JAMA*. 1998;279:1876]. *JAMA*. 1997;278:2093-2098.

25. Michels KB, Yusuf S. Does PTCA in acute myocardial infarction affect mortality and reinfarction rates? A quantitative overview (meta-analysis) of the randomized clinical trials. *Circulation*. 1995;91: 476-485.

26. The GUSTO IIb Angioplasty Substudy Investigators. A clinical trial comparing primary coronary angioplasty with tissue plasminogen activator for acute myocardial infarction [published correction appears in *N Engl J Med*. 1997;337:287]. *N Engl J Med*. 1997;336:1621-1628.

27. Tiefenbrunn AJ, Chandra NC, French WJ, Gore JM, Rogers WJ. Clinical experience with primary percutaneous transluminal coronary angioplasty compared with alteplase (recombinant tissue-type plasminogen activator) in patients with acute myocardial infarction: a report from the Second National Registry of Myocardial Infarction (NRMI-2). *J Am Coll Cardiol*. 1998;31:1240-1245.

28. Anderson HR, Nielsen TT, Rasmussen K, et al, for the DANAMI-2 Investigators. A comparison of coronary angioplasty with fibrinolytic therapy in acute myocardial infarction. *N Engl J Med*. 2003;349:733-742.

29. Hochman JS, Sleeper LA, Webb JG, et al. Early revascularization in acute myocardial infarction complicated by cardiogenic shock. SHOCK Investigators. Should We Emergently Revascularize Occluded Coronaries for Cardiogenic Shock. *N Engl J Med*. 1999;341:625-634.

30. Moliterno DJ, Topol EJ. Conjunctive use of platelet glycoprotein IIb/IIIa antagonists and thrombolytic therapy for acute myocardial infarction. *Thromb Haemost*. 1997;78:214-219.

31. Cannon CP. Overcoming thrombolytic resistance. *J Am Coll Cardiol*. 1999;34:1395-1402.

32. Ito H, Okamura A, Isakura K, et al. Myocardial perfusion patterns related to immediate thrombolysis in myocardial infarction perfusion grades after coronary angioplasty in patients with acute anterior wall myocardial infarction. *Circulation*. 1996;93:1993-1999.

33. Brener SJ, Zeymer U, Adgey AA, et al. Eptifibatide and low-dose tissue plasminogen activator in acute myocardial infarction: the integrilin and low-dose thrombolysis in acute myocardial infarction (INTRO AMI) trial. *J Am Coll Cardiol*. 2002;39:377-386.

13

34. Antman EM, Giugliano RP, Gibson CM, et al for the TIMI 14 Investigators. Abciximab facilitates the rate and extent of thrombolysis: results of TIMI-14 trial. *Circulation*. 1999;99:2720-2732.

35. de Lemos JA, Antman EM, Gibson CM, et al. Abciximab improves both epicardial flow and myocardial reperfusion in ST-elevation myocardial infarction. Observations from the TIMI 14 trial. *Circulation*. 2000;101:239-243.

36. Herrmann HC, Moliterno DJ, Ohman EM, et al. Facilitation of early percutaneous coronary intervention after reteplase with or without abciximab in acute myocardial infarction: results from the SPEED (GUSTO-4 Pilot) Trial. *J Am Coll Cardiol*. 2000;36:1489-1496.

37. Topol EJ, The GUSTO V Investigators. Reperfusion therapy for acute myocardial infarction with fibrinolytic therapy or combination reduced fibrinolytic therapy and platelet glycoprotein IIb/IIIa inhibition: the GUSTO V randomised trial. *Lancet*. 2001;357:1905-1914.

38. The Assessment of the Safety and Efficacy of a New Thrombolytic Regimen (ASSENT)-3 Investigators. Efficacy and safety of tenecteplase in combination with enoxaparin, abciximab, or unfractionated heparin: the ASSENT-3 randomised trial in acute myocardial infarction. *Lancet*. 2001;358:605-613.

39. MacMahon S, Collins R, Knight C, Yusuf S, Peto R. Reduction in major morbidity and mortality by heparin in acute myocardial infarction. *Circulation*. 1988;78:(suppl 2):II-98. Abstract.

40. Rao AK, Pratt C, Berke A, et al. Thrombolysis in Myocardial Infarction (TIMI) Trial—phase I: hemorrhagic manifestations and changes in plasma fibrinogen and the fibrinolytic system in patients treated with recombinant tissue plasminogen activator and streptokinase. *J Am Coll Cardiol*. 1988;11:1-11.

41. Smith P, Arnesen H, Holme I. The effect of warfarin on mortality and reinfarction after myocardial infarction. *N Engl J Med*. 1990;323:147-152.

42. Coumadin Aspirin Reinfarction Study (CARS) Investigators. Randomized, double-blind trial of fixed low dose warfarin with aspirin after myocardial infarction. *Lancet*. 1997;350:389-396.

43. Fiore LD, Ezekowitz MD, Brophy MT, Lu D, Sacco J, Peduzzi P; the Combination Hemotherapy and Mortality Prevention (CHAMP) Study Group. Department of Veterans Affairs Cooperative Studies Program Clinical Trial comparing combined warfarin and aspirin with aspirin alone in survivors of acute myocardial infarction: primary results of the CHAMP study. *Circulation*. 2002;105:557-563.

44. Anticoagulants in the Secondary Prevention of Events in Coronary Thrombosis (ASPECT) Research Group. Effect of long-term oral anticoagulant treatment on mortality and cardiovascular morbidity after myocardial infarction. *Lancet*. 1994;343:499-503.

45. Brouwer MA, van den Bergh PJ, Aengevaeren WR, et al. Aspirin plus coumarin versus aspirin alone in the prevention of reocclusion after fibrinolysis for acute myocardial infarction: results of the Antithrombotics in the Prevention of Reocclusion in Coronary Thrombolysis (APRICOT)–2 Trial. *Circulation*. 2002;106:659-665.

46. Hurlen M, Abdelnoor M, Smith P, Erikssen J, Arnesen H. Warfarin, aspirin, or both after myocardial infarction. *N Engl J Med*. 2002; 347:969-974.

47. Wallentin L, Wilcox RG, Weaver WD, et al, for the ESTEEM Investigators. Oral ximelagatran for secondary prophylaxis after myocardial infarction: the ESTEEM randomised controlled trial. *Lancet*. 2003;362:789-797.

13

14

Noncardiac Arterial Disease: Peripheral Arterial Vascular Disease and Stroke

Vascular disease of the peripheral arterial circulation, most often caused by atherosclerosis and less commonly by vasculitis (or other nonatherosclerotic arteriopathies), is a chronic process that is responsible for progressive and, at times, incapacitating symptoms, disability, and limb loss. The arterial beds most frequently involved, in order of occurrence, are:

- Femoro-popliteal-tibial
- Aortoiliac
- Carotid and vertebral
- Splanchnic and renal
- Brachiocephalic.

The causes of acute occlusion include:

- Cardioembolism
- Artery-to-artery embolism
- In situ thrombosis
- Trauma
- Vasospasm.

The frequent coexistence of peripheral vascular and coronary artery disease (multibed vascular disease) has been recognized for decades and is clinically important for several reasons. First, it provides a unifying basis for atherosclerosis and its prevention. Second, it offers a biologically plausible explanation for the high cardiovascular mortality (two- to threefold increase) in patients with peripheral vascular disease. Last, the pharmacologic approach to management takes on a more global theme with the objective of preventing atherosclerosis progression and attenuating thrombotic processes, which underlie acute myocardial infarction (MI), stroke, and peripheral arterial occlusion (**Figure 14.1**).

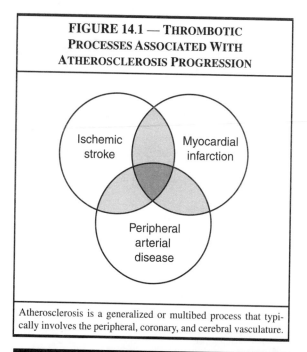

FIGURE 14.1 — THROMBOTIC PROCESSES ASSOCIATED WITH ATHEROSCLEROSIS PROGRESSION

Ischemic stroke

Myocardial infarction

Peripheral arterial disease

Atherosclerosis is a generalized or multibed process that typically involves the peripheral, coronary, and cerebral vasculature.

Vascular Disease

The available data, derived from individual clinical trials and from a frequently cited meta-analysis conducted by the Antiplatelet Trialists' Collaboration, provide strong support for therapies targeting platelet inhibition among patients with vascular disease. In high-risk patients, aspirin therapy 80 mg to 325 mg qd reduced nonfatal MI by one third, nonfatal stroke by one third, and death from all vascular causes by one sixth.[1] The benefit applies to a broad range of individuals, including men and women of all ages and those with hypertension or diabetes mellitus.

Cerebrovascular Disease

Ischemic stroke is a major cause of morbidity and mortality worldwide and, in a large proportion of patients, is caused by atherosclerosis involving the carotid (extracranial) and cerebral (intracranial) vasculature. The benefit of platelet antagonists in patients with prior stroke or transient ischemic attack has been documented by several large-scale clinical trials (**Table 14.1**) and in an overview of all previously conducted trials.[1-11] Ticlopidine or clopidogrel may offer additional benefit (compared with aspirin) in patients with a recent stroke or fixed neurologic defect, reducing the occurrence of fatal or nonfatal stroke by 15% to 20%[5]; however, side effects (including neutropenia) are a concern with long-term administration of ticlopidine. Combined aspirin and dipyridamole preparations (Aggrenox) may offer benefit.

The primary prevention of stroke with pharmacologic therapy (predominantly platelet antagonists) while efficacious has limitations. Patients with advanced carotid disease (stenosis >70%) remain at risk for neurologic events and should be considered for carotid endarterectomy; however, antiplatelet therapy should be continued postoperatively. Anticoagulant therapy with warfarin is preferable following cardioembolic stroke, particularly in the setting of atrial fibrillation.

Peripheral Occlusive Disease

Patients with peripheral vascular (occlusive) disease have specific needs that reflect the disseminated nature of atherosclerosis. Intermittent claudication is a manifestation of ischemic muscle that reflects a fixed obstruction to blood flow and periods of heightened intravascular thrombotic activity.

Because of its dynamic pathobiology and clinical expression, the treatment of patients with peripheral vascular disease has included lifestyle changes (risk-factor modification), vasoactive compounds, muscle-metabolism enhancing drugs, and antithrombotic therapy (aspirin, clopidogrel, or their combination).[12-16]

Critical limb ischemia, as a distinct clinical entity, represents the progression of ischemia to the point of severely compromised nutritive blood flow that threatens tissue viability. The manifestations range from claudication at rest to trophic skin changes and ulceration to overt gangrene and limb loss (**Tables 14.2** and **14.3**). Although revascularization represents the treatment of choice, this is not always fea-

14

269

TABLE 14.1 — RANDOMIZED TRIALS IN PATIENTS WITH EITHER ISCHEMIC STROKE OR TRANSIENT ISCHEMIC ATTACKS RECEIVING PLATELET ANTAGONIST THERAPY

Trial	Patients	Treatment	Comparison(s)	Clinical Outcome(s)	Findings
CAPRIE (1997)	19,185	• Clopidogrel 75 mg qd • Peripheral arterial disease, recent stroke, recent MI	• ASA 325 mg qd	• Ischemic stroke, MI, or vascular death • Stroke • GIH	• PAD patients: RRR 23.8% ($P = 0.0028$) • RRR 7.3% ($P = 0.26$) • 0.52% vs. 0.93% ($P <0.05$)
CAST (1997)	21,106	• ASA 160 mg qd within 48 h	• Placebo	• Mortality • Death or nonfatal stroke	• 3.3% vs 3.9%; OR 14%; $P = 0.004$ • 5.3% vs 5.9%; OR 12%; $P = 0.03$
IST (1997)	19,435	• ASA 300 mg qd within 48 h	• SC heparin • SC heparin + ASA • Neither	• Mortality at 14 days • Recurrent stroke • Death or dependence at 6 mo	• 9.0% vs 9.4%; not significant • 2.8% vs 3.9%; $P <0.001$ • Not significant
ESPS-2 (1996)	6062	• ASA 25 mg bid, dipyridamole 200 mg bid, ASA + dipyridamole* • TIA or completed ischemic stroke within 2 mo	• Placebo	• Mortality • Recurrent stroke	• No difference • ASA RRR 18% ($P = 0.013$) • Dipyridamole RRR 16% ($P = 0.039$) • ASA + dipyridamole RRR 37% ($P <0.001$)
MAST-I (1995)	622	• ASA 300 mg within 6 h	• Untreated • Streptokinase • ASA + streptokinase	• Mortality	• OR 2.7 (1.7-4.3) streptokinase • OR 0.9 (0.6-1.3) ASA + streptokinase

Study	N	Treatment	Comparison	Outcomes	Results
SALT (1991)	1360	• ASA 75 mg qd 1 to 4 mo after cerebrovascular event	—	• Mortality • Stroke • Bleeding event	• 18% RRR • 18% RRR • 7.2% vs 3.2%; $P = 0.001$
UK-TIA 1991	1072	• ASA 300 mg qd, ASA 600 mg bid	• Placebo	• Mortality • GI bleeding	• 15% RRR (−3%–29%) • 3.3% with 300 mg; 6.4% with 1200 mg
CATS (1989)	1072	• Ticlopidine 250 mg bid • Recent thromboembolic stroke	• Placebo	• Stroke, MI, vascular death • As above, but intent-to-treat • Stroke, stroke-related death • Severe side effects	• RRR 30.2% • RRR 23.3%: $P = 0.02$ • RRR 24.1% • 8.2% vs 2.8%
TASS (1989)	3069	• Ticlopidine 250 mg bid • TIA, amaurosis fugax, RIND, minor stroke within 3 mo	• ASA 650 mg bid	• Nonfatal stroke, death • Fatal stroke, nonfatal stroke • Severe neutropenia	• 17% vs 19%; RRR 12%; −2%–26% • 10% vs 13%; RRR 21%; 4%–38% • 13/1529 vs 0/1540

Abbreviations: ASA, aspirin; CAPRIE, Clopidogrel vs Aspirin in Patients at Risk for Ischemic Events; CAST, Chinese Acute Stroke Trial; CATS, Canadian-American Ticlodipine Study; ESPS, European Stroke Prevention Study; GI, gastrointestinal; GIH, gastrointestinal hemorrhage; IST, International Stroke Trial; MAST, Multicenter Acute Stroke Trial; MI, myocardial infarction; OR, odds ratio; PAD, peripheral arterial disease; RIND, reversible ischemic neurologic deficit; RRR, relative risk reduction; SALT, Swedish Aspirin Low-Dose Trial; SC, subcutaneous; TASS, Ticlopidine Aspirin Stroke Study; TIA, transient ischemic attack; UK-TIA, United Kingdom Transient Ischemic Attack.

* Extended-release preparation.

14

TABLE 14.2 — THE PATHOGENESIS OF ACUTE OCCLUSION OF PERIPHERAL ARTERIES

Causes of Acute Occlusion of Peripheral Arteries in Atherosclerotic Patients
- Thrombosis of a native artery with atherosclerotic stenoses
- Thrombosis of an arterial bypass graft
- Embolism from heart, aneurysm, atherosclerotic plaque, or critical stenosis upstream (including cholesterol or atherothrombotic emboli during endovascular procedures)
- Thrombosed aneurysm (with particular regard to popliteal aneurysm)

Causes of Acute Critical Limb Ischemia in Nonatherosclerotic Patients
- Arterial trauma (especially iatrogenic)
- Aortic/arterial dissection
- Arteritis with thrombosis (eg, giant cell arteritis, thromboangiitis obliterans)
- Spontaneous thrombosis associated with hypercoagulable state)
- Popliteal cyst with thrombosis
- Popliteal entrapment with thrombosis
- Vasospasm with thrombosis (eg, ergotism)

Constantini V, Lenti M. *Thromb Res.* 2002;106:V285-V294.

sible, raising the question of pharmacologic alternatives. A majority of clinical trials performed to date have focused on vasodilating compounds such as cilostazol, many of which also possess antithrombotic properties.[17-22]

Acute Arterial Insufficiency

The predominant causes of acute arterial insufficiency are trauma, *in situ* thrombosis, and peripheral embolism. Nontraumatic occlusion can be further classified as thrombotic or embolic. The former is typically associated with advanced atherosclerosis and most often involves the lower extremities. In approximately 85% of cases, arterial embo-

TABLE 14.3 — CLINICAL CLASSIFICATION OF ACUTE LIMB ISCHEMIA

Category	Description/Prognosis	Findings		Doppler Signals	
		Sensory Loss	Muscle Weakness	Arterial	Venous
I. Viable	Not immediately threatened	None	None	Audible	Audible
II. Threatened					
a. Marginally	Salvageable if promptly treated	Minimal (toes) or none	None	(Often) inaudible	Audible
b. Immediately	Salvageable with immediate revascularization	More than toes, associated with rest pain	Mild, moderate	(Usually) inaudible	Audible
III. Irreversible*	Major tissue loss or permanent nerve damage inevitable	Profound, anesthetic	Profound, paralysis (rigor)	Inaudible	Inaudible

* The differentiation between class IIb and III can be difficult at the onset of the leg ischemia.

Rutherford RB, et al. *J Vasc Surg.* 1997;26:517-538. Erratum in: *J Vasc Surg.* 2001;33:805.

14

lism originates within the heart (atrial fibrillation, valvular heart disease, left ventricular mural thrombus). Noncardiac sources include abdominal aortic or femoral aneurysms, ulcerated atherosclerotic plaques, and paradoxic emboli from lower-extremity venous thrombi that cross into the arterial circulation through atrial septal defects, patent foramen ovale, or ventricular septal defects. The most common sites of involvement in descending order of frequency include the iliofemoral, popliteal, and tibial vessels. Diagnostic hallmarks of arterial occlusion are sudden pain with pallor, loss of pulse, and paresthesias. Prolonged ischemia can lead to sensory and motor loss and ultimately tissue necrosis (gangrene).

Acute peripheral emboli are frequently managed with balloon extraction and systemic anticoagulation. The role of anticoagulant therapy (most often with unfractionated heparin [UFH]) is to prevent recurrent cardio- and artery-to-artery embolization. It may also reduce in situ thrombosis in areas of endothelial disruption created by the original thrombus and/or balloon extraction-related trauma. Distal (popliteal artery and below) emboli and acute thrombotic occlusion can be managed with either surgery or selective intra-arterial fibrinolytic therapy. Although a consensus has not been reached, fibrinolytic therapy may be most useful in surgically inaccessible small arteries of the forearm, hand, leg, and foot and in patients who are not considered candidates for surgical intervention.[23] The adjunctive role of platelet glycoprotein (GP) IIb/IIIa antagonists is under investigation, but should be considered with recurring thrombosis despite adequate anticoagulation.

A reduction in cardiovascular events, including MI and vascular death, is a primary goal of antithrombotic therapy in patients with peripheral vascular disease. The Antiplatelet Trialists Collaboration overview documented the benefit of antiplatelet therapy in this subset defined as having either intermittent claudication, peripheral bypass grafts, or peripheral angioplasty.[1] The question that most clinicians ask is "What is the preferred antagonist?" Aspirin or clopidogrel is accepted therapy, with the latter representing a preferable treatment strategy in patients with peripheral vascular disease and known coronary artery disease (dual vascular-bed disease)[2] (**Figure 14.2**). The potential for added benefit with combined strategies of aspirin and clopidogrel has been confirmed in coronary artery disease.

Peripheral Vascular Reconstructive Surgery

Although the available literature suggests that saphenous veins have patency rates that are superior to polytetrafluoroethylene bypass grafts, both are subject to early thrombotic occlusion that stems from in situ thrombogenicity, technical challenges, and in many patients, poor distal runoff. The importance of flow is highlighted by the comparatively low rates of occlusion involving arteries >6 mm in diameter (aortoiliac, femoral) compared with smaller vessels and flow rates >200 mL/minute. Although intermediate and late occlusions may also be thrombotic in origin, neointimal hyperplasia and progressive atherosclerosis dominate the pathobiology.[24,25]

Because the platelets represent the predominant constituent of arterial thrombi, antiplatelet therapy with aspirin or clopidogrel is considered the standard care for patients undergoing reconstructive procedures or angioplasty. Systemic anticoagulation with UFH may be protective at the time of intraoperative vessel cross-clamping. The combination of warfarin and aspirin (or an alternative platelet antagonist) should be reserved for high-risk patients (those with poor vein quality, marginal arterial runoff, and previously failed bypass).[26]

14

Summary

Atherosclerosis is a systemic inflammatory disease that commonly involves a variety of vascular beds. Patients with peripheral vascular disease, in addition to experiencing ischemic symptoms (eg, claudication) are at risk for limb loss, stroke, MI, and cardiovascular death (**Tables 14.4** and **14.5**).[27] Risk-factor modification takes on a global purpose in such patients; antithrombotic therapy, by preventing acute thrombotic events, plays a vital protective role. Aspirin 81 mg/day to 325 mg/day or clopidogrel 75 mg/day should be administered to those with a prior MI or documented multibed vascular disease.

FIGURE 14.2 — CLINICIAN'S APPROACH TO ANTIPLATELET THERAPY IN PATIENTS WITH ATHEROSCLEROTIC VASCULAR DISEASE

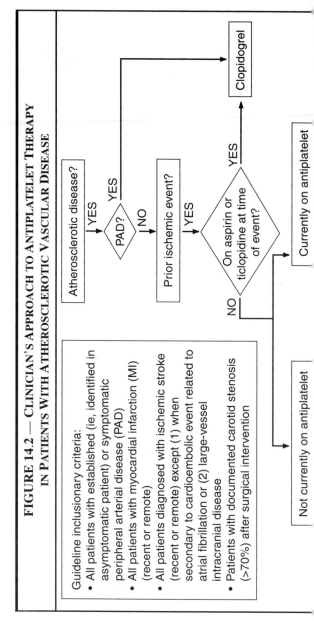

Guideline inclusionary criteria:
- All patients with established (ie, identified in asymptomatic patient) or symptomatic peripheral arterial disease (PAD)
- All patients with myocardial infarction (MI) (recent or remote)
- All patients diagnosed with ischemic stroke (recent or remote) except (1) when secondary to cardioembolic event related to atrial fibrillation or (2) large-vessel intracranial disease
- Patients with documented carotid stenosis (>70%) after surgical intervention

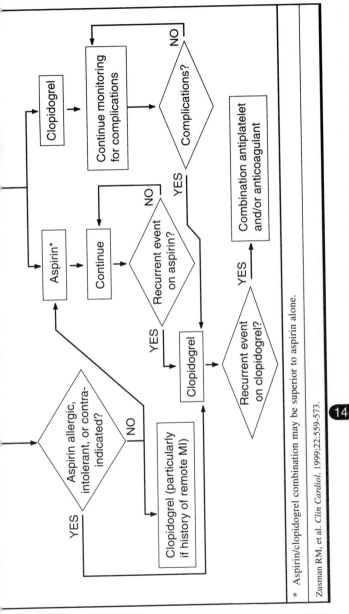

* Aspirin/clopidogrel combination may be superior to aspirin alone.

Zusman RM, et al. *Clin Cardiol.* 1999;22:559-573.

14

277

TABLE 14.4 — CLINICALLY BASED ANTITHROMBOTIC THERAPY IN PERIPHERAL VASCULAR DISEASE		
Clinical Scenario	**Agent**	**Dosing Range/Comments**
Carotid endarterectomy	Aspirin	81-325 mg/d
Prior transient ischemic attack	Aspirin	50-325 mg/d
	Aspirin/persantine	25/200 mg bid
	Clopidogrel	75 mg/d
Acute arterial occlusion/ischemia	Unfractionated heparin*	aPTT 2 × control
	Fibrinolytic therapy	tPA
Chronic lower-extremity ischemia	Aspirin	81-325 mg/d
	Clopidogrel†	75 mg/d
Claudication	Aspirin	81-325 mg/d
	Clopidogrel	75 mg/d
	Cilostazol	50-100 mg bid

Intraoperative anticoagulation during vascular surgery	Unfractionated heparin	aPTT 2-3 × control
Infrainguinal vein bypass	Aspirin	81-325 mg/d
	Clopidogrel	75 mg/d (if aspirin not used)
Infrainguinal prosthetic bypass	Aspirin	81-325 mg/d
Infrainguinal bypass (high thrombotic risk)	Aspirin plus warfarin	81-325 mg/d; INR 2.5 (range 2.0-3.0)
Aortoiliac or renal PCI	Aspirin	325 mg/d
	Clopidogrel	75 mg/d (stenting)

Abbreviations: aPTT, activated partial thromboplastin time; INR, international normalized ratio; PCI, percutaneous coronary intervention; tPA, tissue plasminogen activator.

* Followed by warfarin to INR 2.5 (range 2.0-3.0).
† Clopidogrel may be superior to aspirin for reducing vascular complications.

14

TABLE 14.5 — THE ROLE OF SPECIFIC ANTITHROMBOTIC AGENTS IN PERIPHERAL VASCULAR DISEASE

Condition	ASA	Clopidogrel	Pentoxifylline	Cilostazol	Aggrenox	Heparin
PVD						
Asymptomatic	+++	++	0	–	–	–
With claudication	+++	++	0	++	–	–
Vascular bypass	+++	++	0	0	–	Intraop
Acute occlusion	+++	–	0	0	–	+++
CVD	+++	++	0	0	++	–

Abbreviations: ASA, acetylsalicylic acid; CVD, cerebrovascular disease; PVD, peripheral vascular disease.

REFERENCES

1. Antiplatelet Trialists Collaboration. Secondary prevention of vascular disease by prolonged antiplatelet treatment. *Br Med J.* 1988;296:320-331.

2. CAPRIE Steering Committee. A randomised, blinded trial of clopidogrel versus aspirin in patients at risk of ischaemic events (CAPRIE). *Lancet.* 1996;348:1329-1339.

3. CAST (Chinese Acute Stroke Trial) Collaborative Group. CAST: randomised placebo-controlled trial of early aspirin use in 20,000 patients with acute ischaemic stroke. *Lancet.* 1997;349:1641-1649.

4. International Stroke Trial Collaborative Group. The International Stroke Trial (IST): a randomised trial of aspirin, subcutaneous heparin, both, or neither among 19,435 patients with acute ischaemic stroke. *Lancet.* 1997;349:1569-1581.

5. Hass WK, Easton JD, Adams HP, et al. A randomized trial comparing ticlopidine hydrochloride with aspirin for the prevention of stroke in high-risk patients. Ticlopidine Aspirin Stroke Study Group. *N Engl J Med.* 1989;321:501-507.

6. Gent M, Blakely JA, Easton JD, et al. The Canadian American Ticlopidine Study (CATS) in thromboembolic stroke. *Lancet.* 1989;1:1215-1220.

7. Diener HC, Cunha L, Forbes C, Sivenius J, Smets P, Lowenthal A. European Stroke Prevention Study. 2. Dipyridamole and acetylsalicylic acid in the secondary prevention of stroke. *J Neurol Sci.* 1996;143:1-13.

8. Multicentre Acute Stroke Trial – Italy (MAST-I) Group. Randomised controlled trial of streptokinase, aspirin, and combination of both in treatment of acute ischaemic stroke. *Lancet.* 1995;346:1509-1514.

9. The SALT Collaborative Group. Swedish Aspirin Low-Dose Trial (SALT) of 75 mg aspirin as secondary prophylaxis after cerebrovascular ischaemic events. *Lancet.* 1991;338:1345-1349.

10. Farrell B, Godwin J, Richards S, Warlow C. The United Kingdom transient ischaemic attack (UK-TIA) aspirin trial: final results. *J Neurol Neurosurg Psychiatry.* 1991;54:1044-1054.

11. Lindgarde F, Jelnes R, Bjorkman H, et al for the Scandinavian Study Group. Conservative drug treatment in patients with moderately severe chronic occlusive peripheral arterial disease. *Circulation.* 1989;80:1549-1556.

12. Balsano F, Coccheri S, Libretti A, et al. Ticlopidine in the treatment of intermittent claudication: a 21-month double-blind trial. *J Lab Clin Med.* 1989;114:84-91.

14

13. Ernst E, Kollar L, Matrai A. A double-blind trial of Dextran—haemodilution vs placebo in claudicants. *J Intern Med.* 1990;227:19-24.

14. Brevetti G, Perna S, Sabba C, Martone VD, Condorelli M. Propionyl-L-carnitine in intermittent claudication: double-blind, placebo-controlled, dose titration, multicenter study. *J Am Coll Cardiol.* 1995;26:1411-1416.

15. Belch JJ, Bell PR, Creissen D, et al. Randomized, double-blind, placebo-controlled study evaluating the efficacy and safety of AS-013, a prostaglandin E₁ prodrug, in patients with intermittent claudication. *Circulation.* 1997;95:2298-2302.

16. Liervre M, Azoulay S, Lion L, Morand S, Girre JP, Boissel JP. A dose-effect study of beraprost sodium in intermittent claudication. *J Cardiovasc Pharmacol.* 1996;27:788-793.

17. Ciprostene Study Group. The effect of ciprostene in patients with peripheral vascular disease (PVD) characterized by ischemic ulcers. *J Clin Pharmacol.* 1991;31:81-87.

18. Diehm C, Balzer K, Bisler H, et al. Efficacy of a new prostaglandin E₁ regimen in outpatients with severe, intermittent claudication: results of a multicenter placebo-controlled double-blind trial. *J Vasc Surg.* 1997;256:537-544.

19. Norgren L, Alwmark A, Angqvist KA, et al. A stable prostacyclin analogue (iloprost) in the treatment of ischaemic ulcers of the lower limb. A Scandinavian-Polish placebo controlled, randomised multicenter study. *Eur J Vasc Surg.* 1990;4:463-467.

20. United Kingdom Severe Limb Ischemia Study Group. Treatment of limb threatening ischaemia with intravenous iloprost: a randomised double-blind placebo controlled study. *Eur J Vasc Surg.* 1991;5:511-516.

21. Guilmot JL, Diot E for the French Iloprost Study Group. Treatment of lower limb ischamia due to atherosclerosis in diabetic and nondiabetic patients with iloprost, a stable analogue of prostacyclin: results of a French Multicentre trial. *Drug Invest.* 1991;3:351-359.

22. Rutherford RB, Baker JD, Ernst C, et al. Recommended standards for reports dealing with lower extremity ischemia: revised version. *J Vasc Surg.* 1997;26:517-538.

23. STILE Investigators. Results of a prospective randomized trial evaluating surgery versus thrombolysis for ischemia of the lower extremity. *Ann Surg.* 1994;220:251-268.

24. Eickhoff JH, Buchardt Hansen HJ, Bromme A, et al. A randomized clinical trial of PTFE versus human umbilical vein for femoropopliteal bypass surgery. Preliminary results. *Br J Surg.* 1983;70:85-88.

25. McCollum C, Kenchington G, Alexander C, Franks PJ, Greenhalgh RM. PTFE or HUV for femoro-popliteal bypass: a multi-centre trial. *Eur J Vasc Surg*. 1991;5:435-443.

26. Sarac TP, Huber TS, Back MR, et al. Warfarin improves the outcome of infrainguinal vein bypass grafts at high risk for failure. *J Vasc Surg*. 1998;28:446-457.

27. The sixth (2000) ACCP guidelines for antithrombotic therapy for prevention and treatment of thrombosis. *Chest*. 2001;119(suppl 1):1S-370S.

14

15   Native and Prosthetic Valvular Heart Disease

Scope of the Problem

There are an estimated 250,000 heart valve replacement surgeries performed yearly on a worldwide basis. Mechanical prostheses have an excellent track record of durability (≥25 years) but require lifelong anticoagulation. Improved hemodynamics and reduced thrombogenecity characterize bioprosthetic valves; however, there is the disadvantage of degeneration, particularly in younger individuals. The ideal replacement—a tissue engineered "copy" of a native valve—is decades away in development.

The most feared and devastating complications of native or prosthetic valvular heart disease for patients, clinicians, and surgeons alike are valvular thrombosis and systemic embolism. Although the incidence of thromboembolic events has decreased in North America in parallel with the reduced occurrence of rheumatic heart disease, this has not been the case in other parts of the world. Moreover, despite the improvements in design and surgical technique, thromboembolism remains a serious complication of prosthetic heart valve replacement.

Mechanisms

Clinical, pathologic, and experimental evidence supports two predominant mechanisms for the initiation of thrombosis in patients with native or prosthetic valvular heart disease. The first involves disruption of the vascular endothelial surface and exposure of underlying prothrombotic substrate and/or the introduction of prothrombotic materials into the circulation. The second is mediated by "triggering" of thrombosis in areas of stasis. Early observations established that stasis alone required prolonged periods of time to induce thrombosis; however, the combination of stasis and localized tissue abnormalities and/or a high concentration of coagulation factors is profoundly thrombogenic.[1-3] There is also evidence that prolonged periods of stasis impair tissue perfusion, with resulting endovascular damage and compromised fibrinolytic activity. Extension of thrombus into regions of relative stasis is common and represents an important mechanism for thrombus growth following prosthetic heart valve surgery.[4]

Natural History of Valvular Thrombi

The potential fate of thrombi formed within the cardiovascular system, including those associated with native and prosthetic valvular heart disease, includes:
- Partial or complete lysis
- Organization
- Partial organization with the potential for embolization.

Freshly formed fibrin strands are the most susceptible to lysis. Organization typically begins within 48 hours and is characterized by reduced concentrations of platelets, fibrin, and neutrophils, with a gradual replacement by monocytes, phagocytic cells, and fibroblasts during the first week and smooth muscle cells and connective tissue matrix during the second week. The last step in reducing thrombogenicity, and one of particular importance, is re-endothelialization. As a rule, thrombi formed at sites of inflammation and injury organize more rapidly than stasis-related thrombi.[5,6]

Endothelial cells grow from the point of junction between a prosthetic valve and host tissue. Most believe that endothelium grows to confluence on the prosthetic valve surface, reducing the intermediate and long-term risk of thromboembolism.[7,8] It is clear, however, that despite the important thromboresistant properties of endothelial cells, prosthetic heart valves remain thrombogenic, certainly more so than native valves. This emphasizes the importance of blood flow geometry (high and low shear stress, stasis) as a major contributing factor in thrombogenesis and raises a question of chronic endothelial/neoendothelial cell injury or dysfunction as a lingering risk factor.

Prosthetic Heart Valve Thrombosis

The prerequisite conditions for prosthetic heart valve thrombosis can be defined conceptually in the context of Virchow's triad, with modifications for the introduction of a fourth component, an artificial surface. The traditional and widely cited components—abnormalities of the vascular/endothelial surface, stasis of blood flow, and abnormalities within the circulating blood—are all operational in the setting of prosthetic mechanical heart valve replacement.

The overall "thrombogenic surface" of prosthetic heart valves includes not only the artificial material itself but also the perivalvular excision tissue, sewing ring, and sutures as well. Each element is important, particularly in the early postoperative period when blood flow is reinitiated and the prothrombotic effects of surgery (platelet activation, circulating inflammatory mediators) are at their peak.

Blood flow across the aortic valve is typically rapid and characterized by regions of acceleration and high shear stress. Under these conditions, platelets are activated and erythrocyte membranes are damaged, leading to the release of adenosine diphosphate, further platelet activation, and ultimately, aggregation. The contribution of coagulation factors to overall thrombotic potential is a *secondary phenomenon* (**Figure 15.1**). In contrast, blood flow across the mitral valve is comparatively slow, particularly with coexistent mitral stenosis accompanied by left atrial enlargement or long-standing mitral insufficiency and left ventricular dilatation (**Figure 15.2**). In these settings, coagulation factor activation and interactions with the chamber walls and prosthetic material are the *primary phenomena* favoring thrombus formation, while platelets play a supportive role.

Tissue (bioprosthetic) valves, particularly those placed in the aortic position, often enjoy central unimpeded (laminar) blood flow without regions of either stagnation or acceleration. Although the cloth-covered stent and sewing ring are thrombogenic, the risk of thromboembolism is low, averaging 1% per patient year, and of concern only for the first 3 postoperative months before an organized neointima has developed. In the mitral position, the incidence of arterial thromboembolism is increased two- to threefold, based

FIGURE 15.1 — CHARACTERISTICS OF BLOOD FLOW ACROSS THE AORTIC VALVE

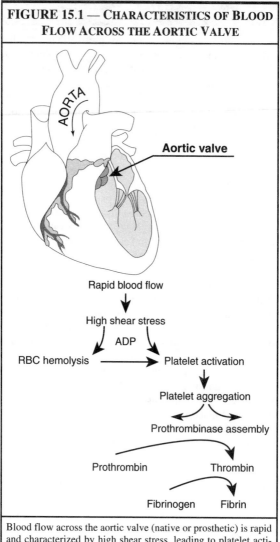

Blood flow across the aortic valve (native or prosthetic) is rapid and characterized by high shear stress, leading to platelet activation (direct and indirect via adenosine diphosphate [ADP] released from hemolyzed red blood cells [RBC]). Thus platelets play a central role in thrombogenicity, while coagulation factors serve in a supportive capacity for thrombus growth.

FIGURE 15.2 — CHARACTERISTICS OF BLOOD FLOW ACROSS THE MITRAL VALVE

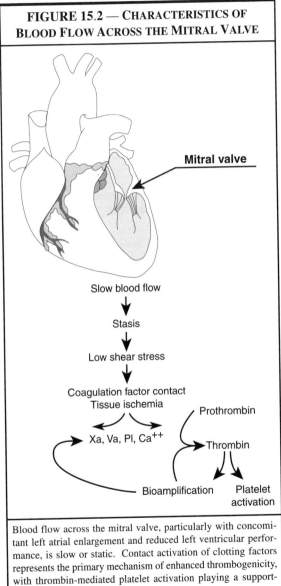

Blood flow across the mitral valve, particularly with concomitant left atrial enlargement and reduced left ventricular performance, is slow or static. Contact activation of clotting factors represents the primary mechanism of enhanced thrombogenicity, with thrombin-mediated platelet activation playing a supporting role.

predominantly on the high incidence of concomitant left atrial enlargement, atrial fibrillation, prior thromboembolism, and reduced left ventricular performance.[9,10]

Mechanical prosthetic heart valves, although more thrombogenic than tissue valves, are also more durable. Technical improvements in prosthesis design and the development of less thrombogenic materials have reduced the risk of thrombotic complications, which, at the present time, occur at an incidence of 3% to 5% per patient year.[11] Similar to tissue valves, mechanical heart valves in the mitral position are associated with a greater risk of thromboembolism than those in the aortic position.[12-14]

Assessing Thromboembolic Risk

■ **Native Valvular Heart Disease**

The risk of thromboembolism in patients with native valvular heart disease is influenced strongly by the site of involvement, chamber dimension, ventricular performance, and the presence of concomitant risk factors such as atrial fibrillation. Prior thromboembolism is considered a strong risk factor for recurrent events regardless of the valvular pathology.

■ **Clinical Experience**

The risk of thromboembolism in patients with prosthetic valvular heart disease is recognized. Despite methodologic limitations, the available information derived from relatively large studies and an ever-expanding clinical experience allows several conclusions to be drawn:

- Thromboprophylaxis for mechanical prostheses is achieved most effectively with oral anticoagulants.
- Antiplatelet therapy *alone* does not offer adequate protection for patients with mechanical prostheses.
- The thrombogenicity of mechanical heart valves, from greatest to least, is as follows: caged ball > tilting disk > bileaflet.
- High-risk patients (increased risk for thromboembolism) benefit from combination (anticoagulant and platelet antagonist) antithrombotic therapy.
- A "threshold" level of anticoagulation is required for benefit.

- High-intensity anticoagulation (international normalized ratio [INR] >3.5) increases the risk for hemorrhagic complications.
- The risk of thromboembolism following bioprosthetic heart valve replacement is greatest during the first 3 postoperative months.[15-20]

Risk Stratification

The management of patients with native and prosthetic valvular heart disease must be approached comprehensively, taking into consideration not only the valve itself but the "company that it keeps" as well. Risk stratification, although focused predominantly on the "thrombotic side" of the equation, must be balanced to include the potential risk of hemorrhage with systemic anticoagulant therapy, particularly in patients with valvular heart disease in whom surgical procedures are being considered[21] (**Tables 15.1** and **15.2**).

Anticoagulant Therapy: Recommendations and Management Guidelines

The recommended approach to patients with native and prosthetic valvular heart disease is based on a composite of clinical trial results and clinical experience.[22] The latter is particularly true of native valvular disease for which few randomized clinical trials have been conducted (**Tables 15.3, 15.4, and 15.5**).

Early Postoperative Anticoagulant Therapy

15

Owing to the paucity of clinical trials, early postoperative anticoagulant therapy has been approached in a variety of ways. Low-dose systemic anticoagulation with either unfractionated heparin or low molecular weight heparin (LMWH) should be instituted once hemostasis has been secured and the risk for thrombosis outweighs the risk of hemorrhage. Unless the clinical conditions dictate otherwise, heparin should be continued until adequate anticoagulation with warfarin has been achieved.

TABLE 15.1 — THROMBOEMBOLIC RISK SCALE

*Low-Risk**
- Atrial fibrillation
- Bioprosthetic heart valve (>3 months postop)
- St. Jude mechanical heart valve (aortic position) (>6 months postop)
- Dilated cardiomyopathy (ejection fraction <35%)

Intermediate-Risk
- Atrial fibrillation and prior thromboembolism (>3 months)
- St. Jude mechanical heart valve (aortic position) plus atrial fibrillation or ejection fraction <35%
- Dilated cardiomyopathy and prior thromboembolism (>3 months)
- Two low-risk factors
- Anterior myocardial infarction <3 months (no other risk factors)
- St. Jude mechanical heart valve ≤6 months postop or in mitral position
- Bjork-Shiley (tilting-disk) mechanical heart valve (aortic position)

High-Risk
- Atrial fibrillation and prior thromboembolism (<3 months)
- Dilated cardiomyopathy and prior thromboembolism (<3 months)
- Bjork-Shiley mechanical heart valve (mitral position) and any other risk factor
- St. Jude mechanical heart valve (aortic position) and ≥1 intermediate-risk factor
- Caged-ball mechanical heart valve (mitral position)

Very High-Risk
- Antiphospholipid antibody syndrome plus prior event or additional risk factors
- Cardioversion ≤2 weeks
- Arterial thromboembolic event ≤1 month
- Caged-ball mechanical heart valve (any position) plus additional risk factors
- Any combination of ≥2 risk factors

* Any of the low-risk factors plus *no* prior thromboembolism.

UMASS-Memorial Medical Center; 2003.

TABLE 15.2 — HEMORRHAGIC RISK SCALE

Low-Risk
- Dental procedures*
- Cataract surgery
- Angiography (diagnostic)
- Cystoscopy
- Breast biopsy
- Arthroscopic surgery

Intermediate-Risk
- Total hip replacement
- Total knee replacement
- Laparoscopic surgery
- Maxillofacial surgery
- Transurethral prostate removal
- Hysterectomy
- Colonoscopy with biopsy
- Prostate biopsy
- Skin graft

High-Risk
- Major abdominal surgery
- Major thoracic surgery
- Brain/central nervous system surgery
- Radical prostatectomy
- Skin graft
- Liver biopsy
- Kidney biopsy

* Exception: multiple extractions.

UMASS-Memorial Medical Center; 2003.

The institution of oral anticoagulant therapy requires careful monitoring because of the wide variability in postoperative warfarin response and potential danger of excessive anticoagulation. Higher initial doses, ≥5 mg, frequently cause INR values above the target range. Accordingly, 2.5 mg may be preferable in this particular setting.[23] Following hospital discharge, a structured means for close patient follow-up (coordinated anticoagulation clinic) is recommended.

TABLE 15.3 — ANTITHROMBOTIC THERAPY FOR PATIENTS WITH NATIVE VALVULAR HEART DISEASE

Native Valvular Heart Disease	Recommendations
Rheumatic Mitral Valvular Disease	
Prior thromboembolism	Oral anticoagulant, INR 2.5
Paroxysmal or chronic AF	Oral anticoagulant, INR 2.5
LA diameter >5.5 cm	Oral anticoagulant, INR 2.5
MVA <1.0 cm², LA enlargement >5.5 cm	Oral anticoagulant, INR 2.5
Recurrent embolism (despite oral anticoagulant)	Add aspirin 80 to 100 mg qd or clopidogrel 75 mg qd
Mitral Annular Calcification	
Uncomplicated	No antithrombotic therapy
AF or systemic embolism	Oral anticoagulant, INR 2.5

Mitral Valve Prolapse	
Uncomplicated	No antithrombotic therapy
TIA	Aspirin 325 mg qd
Recurrent TIAs	Oral anticoagulant, INR 2.5 or clopidogrel 75 mg qd
Systemic embolism	Oral anticoagulant, INR 2.5
Aortic Valvular Disease	
Sinus rhythm	No antithrombotic therapy
Chronic AF or systemic embolism	Oral anticoagulant, INR 2.5

Abbreviations: AF, atrial fibrillation; INR, international normalized ratio; LA, left atrium; MVA, mitral valve area; TIA, transient ischemic attack.

15

TABLE 15.4 — ANTITHROMBOTIC THERAPY FOR PATIENTS WITH BIOPROSTHETIC HEART VALVES OR VALVE REPAIR

Valve Type/Position	INR	Duration of Treatment
Mitral position	2.5	3 months
Aortic position	2.5	3 months
Atrial fibrillation	2.5	Long-term
LA thrombosis	2.5	3 to 6 months
Systemic embolism	2.5	3 to 12 months
Systemic embolism despite anticoagulant therapy	2.5*	Minimum 12 months
Valve repair†	2.5	3 months

Abbreviations: INR, international normalized ratio; LA, left atrium (includes left atrial appendage).

* Add aspirin 80 to 100 mg qd or clopidogrel 75 mg qd.
† With or without annuloplasty ring.

Bridging Therapy

Decisions regarding periprocedural or "bridging" anticoagulant therapy in patients with mechanical heart valves (and other forms of valvular heart disease requiring long-term anticoagulation) have been complicated by the virtual absence of randomized trials. Cohort studies and institutional data sets support the safety of LMWH (when anticoagulant therapy is required) for relatively brief periods of time (up to 7 days).[24] Upon review of an increasing body of clinical data, the FDA recently removed the "Black Box" warning against the use of enoxaparin in patients with mechanical prosthetic heart valves. However, there are insufficient data to confirm the safety and efficacy of LMWH (or other anticoagulants) in pregnant patients with mechanical heart valves.[25]

TABLE 15.5 — SUMMARY OF RECOMMENDATIONS FOR PATIENTS WITH MECHANICAL HEART VALVES

Valve Type/Position	INR Target
Bileaflet, aortic	2.5 (3.0 if AF, LA >5.5 cm, or LVEF <35%)
Tilting-disk, aortic	3.0
Bileaflet, mitral	3.0 or 2.5 plus aspirin 80 to 100 mg qd
Tilting-disk, mitral	3.0 or 3.0* plus aspirin 80 to 100 mg qd
Caged-ball/disk	3.0 plus aspirin 80 to 100 mg qd
Systemic embolism despite anticoagulant therapy	3.0 plus aspirin 80 to 100 mg qd

Abbreviations: AF, atrial fibrillation; INR, international normalized ratio; LA, left atrium; LVEF, left ventricular ejection fraction.

* With additional risk factors.

Summary

Antithrombotic therapy in the form of oral anticoagulation with or without concomitant platelet antagonists is an important consideration for patients with prosthetic as well as those with native valvular heart disease. Each patient should be assessed carefully to determine the inherent risk of thromboembolism, the expected benefit from antithrombotic treatment, and the potential hemorrhagic risk. The development of patient management guidelines and coordinated anticoagulation clinics has streamlined the decision-making process substantially and elevated the standard of care. Strategies for bridging therapy are being developed; however, the safety of thromboprophylaxis during pregnancy requires further investigation to establish "best practice."

15

REFERENCES

1. Hewson W. Experimental inquiries. I. An inquiry into the properties of the blood, with some remarks on some of its morbid appearances; and an appendix relating to the discovery of the lymphatic system in birds, fish, and the animals called amphibians. London, T Cadell, 1771. Quoted by Wessler S: Thrombosis in the presence of vascular stasis. *Am J Med.* 1962;33:648.

2. Wessler S. Thrombosis in the presence of vascular stasis. *Am J Med.* 1962;33:648.

3. Malone PC, Morris CJ. The sequestration and margination of platelets and leukocytes in veins during conditions of hypokinetic and anaemic hypoxia: potential significance in clinical postoperative venous thrombosis. *J Pathol.* 1978;125:119-129.

4. Sevitt S. The structure and growth of valve-pocket thrombi in femoral veins. *J Clin Pathol.* 1974;27:517-528.

5. Wessler S, Freiman DG, Balloon JD, et al. Experimental pulmonary embolism with serum induced thrombi. *Am J Pathol.* 1961;38:89.

6. Scott GB. A quantitative study of the fate of occlusive red venous thrombi. *Br J Exp Pathol.* 1968;49:544-550.

7. Harker LA, Slichter SJ, Sauvage LR. Platelet consumption by arterial prostheses: the effects of endothelialization and pharmacologic inhibition of platelet function. *Ann Surg.* 1977;186;594-601.

8. Clagett GP, Robinowitz M, Maddox Y, Langloss JM, Ramwell PW. The antithrombotic nature of vascular prosthetic pseudointima. *Surgery.* 1982;91:87-94.

9. Cohn LH, Mudge GH, Pratter F, Collins JJ. Five to eight-year follow-up of patients undergoing porcine heart-valve replacement. *N Engl J Med.* 1981;304:258-262.

10. Geha AS, Hammond GL, Laks H, Stansel HC, Glenn WW. Factors affecting performance and thromboembolism after porcine xenograft cardiac valve replacement. *J Thorac Cardiovasc Surg.* 1982;83:377-384.

11. Edmunds LH Jr. Thromboembolic complications of current cardiac valvular prostheses. *Ann Thorac Surg.* 1982;34:96-106.

12. Starr A, Grunkemeier GL. Selection of a prosthetic heart valve. *JAMA.* 1984;251:1739-1742.

13. Yoganathan AP, Corcoran WH, Harrison EC, Carl JR. The Björk-Shiley aortic prosthesis: flow characteristics, thrombus formation and tissue overgrowth. *Circulation.* 1978;58:70-76.

14. Daenen W, Nevelsteen A, van Cauwelaert P, de Maesschalk E, Willems J, Stalpaert G. Nine years' experience with the Björk-Shiley prosthetic valve: early and late results of 932 valve replacements. *Ann Thorac Surg*. 1983;35:651-663.

15. Horstkotte D, Schulte HD, Bircks W, Strauer BE. Lower intensity anticoagulation therapy results in lower complication rates with the St. Jude medical prosthesis. *J Thorac Cardiovasc Surg*. 1994;107:1136-1145.

16. Vogt S, Hoffmann A, Roth J, et al. Heart valve replacement with the Björk-Shiley and St. Jude medical prostheses: a randomized comparison in 178 patients. *Eur Heart J*. 1990;11:583-591.

17. Acar J, Iung B, Boissel JP, et al. AREVA: multicenter randomized comparison of low-dose versus standard dose anticoagulation in patients with mechanical prosthetic heart valves. *Circulation*. 1996; 94:2107-2112.

18. Sethia B, Turner MA, Lewis S, Rodger RA, Bain WH. Fourteen years' experience with the Björk-Shiley tilting disc prosthesis. *J Thorac Cardiovasc Surg*. 1986;91:350-361.

19. Heras M, Chesebro JH, Fuster V, et al. High risk of thromboemboli early after bioprosthetic cardiac valve replacement. *J Am Coll Cardiol*. 1995;25:1111-1119.

20. Bloomfield P, Kitchin AH, Wheatley DJ, Walbaum PR, Lutz W, Miller HC. A prospective evaluation of the Björk-Shiley, Hancock, and Carpentier-Edwards heart valve prostheses. *Circulation*. 1986;73: 1213-1222.

21. Horstkotte D, Piper C, Wiemer M. Optimal frequency of patient monitoring and intensity of oral anticoagulation therapy in valvular heart disease. *J Thromb Thrombolysis*. 1998;5(suppl 1):S19-S24.

22. Hirsch J, Dalen JE, Guyatt G. The Sixth (2000) ACCP Guidelines for Antithrombotic Therapy for Prevention and Treatment of Thrombosis. *Chest*. 2001;119(suppl 1):1S-2S.

23. Ageno W, Turpie AG, Steidl L, et al. Comparison of a daily fixed 2.5-mg warfarin dose with a 5-mg, international normalized ratio adjusted, warfarin dose initially following heart valve replacement. *Am J Cardiol*. 2001;88:40-44.

24. Montalescot G, Polle V, Collet JP, et al. Low molecular weight heparin after mechanical heart valve replacement. *Circulation*. 2000;101: 1083-1086.

25. Clinical Cardiology Consensus Reports. Anticoagulation and enoxaparin use in patients with prosthetic heart valves and/or pregnancy. An evidence-based review and focused analysis of current controversies and clinical strategies. *American Health Consultants*. 2002;3:1-20.

16 Atrial Fibrillation

Prevalence and Classification

Atrial fibrillation (AF) is a common arrhythmia encountered in routine clinical practice and is an important and independent risk factor for stroke. More than 2 million adults in the United States are afflicted with AF, and its prevalence increases markedly with advancing age. AF affects 4% of the population over age 60 and more than 10% of those over 80. AF is more common in men than in women, but since women outnumber men in the older age groups, the total number of men and women with AF is essentially equal.[1]

Patients with AF fall into three categories:

- Valvular or rheumatic
- Nonvalvular
- "Lone."

The prevalence of rheumatic heart disease has decreased dramatically in the past century. Nonvalvular AF is the most common form encountered in clinical practice in North America, often in association with other cardiac conditions such as hypertensive heart disease, heart failure due to systolic or diastolic abnormalities of the left ventricle, and chronic ischemic heart disease. In the absence of organic heart disease, AF is considered lone.[2]

Risk of Cerebral Thromboembolism

When the left atrium fibrillates, there is stasis of blood flow and increasing likelihood of thrombus formation. Upon release or embolization into the circulation, stroke and its attendant disability can occur.

Atrial fibrillation accompanying rheumatic valvular heart disease or a prosthetic valve is associated with a particularly high rate of cerebral thromboembolism. While nonvalvular AF was once considered a harmless disorder, it is now recognized as the most common cause of cardio-embolic stroke (**Figures 16.1** and **16.2**).[3,4]

Although patients with nonvalvular AF are at significant risk for stroke, there are several well-recognized risk factors that increase occurrence rates further. These include prior transient ischemic attacks (TIAs) or stroke, history of hypertension, diabetes mellitus, congestive heart failure, angina, and increasing age[1,5] (**Table 16.1**).

Echocardiography, a diagnostic test that can detect chamber enlargement, valvular regurgitation, and other cardiac abnormalities, can provide important information that guides assessment of stroke risk (**Table 16.2**).[6,7]

Left atrial enlargement has been suggested as a risk factor for stroke, although its positive predictive value remains unproven.[6] Complex aortic plaque, as well as the left atrium and its appendage, are well visualized by transesophageal echocardiography (TEE) because of the close proximity of the left atrium to the esophagus. The appearance of spontaneous echocardiography contrast "or smoke" in the left atrium suggests stasis of blood flow and, with it, a greater risk for thrombosis in the left atrium or its appendage. The presence of left atrial thrombus substantially increases the risk for thromboembolism.[6-8]

Effectiveness of Antithrombotic Therapy

The goals for the clinical management of AF are to 1) determine, and whenever possible, correct the underlying proarrhythmic substrate, and 2) reduce the adverse hemodynamic and thromboembolic consequences of the arrhythmia through control of ventricular rate and/or maintenance of sinus rhythm. Because normal sinus rhythm may not be achieved or sustained easily, the focus of attention often shifts to stroke prevention by means of antithrombotic therapy. Two important recent clinical trials, Atrial Fibrillation Follow-up Investigation of Rhythm Management (AFFIRM)[9] and Rate Control vs Electrical Cardioversion for Persistent Atrial Fibrillation (RACE)[10] compared a strategy of control of ventricular rate with maintenance of sinus rhythm in the setting of continued oral anticoagulation.

FIGURE 16.1 — STROKE: EMBOLI OF CARDIAC ORIGIN

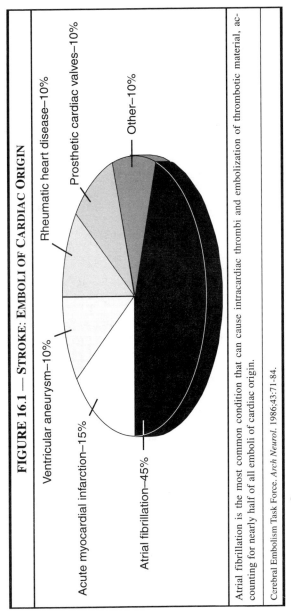

Rheumatic heart disease—10%

Prosthetic cardiac valves—10%

Other—10%

Ventricular aneurysm—10%

Acute myocardial infarction—15%

Atrial fibrillation—45%

Atrial fibrillation is the most common condition that can cause intracardiac thrombi and embolization of thrombotic material, accounting for nearly half of all emboli of cardiac origin.

Cerebral Embolism Task Force. *Arch Neurol.* 1986;43:71-84.

16

303

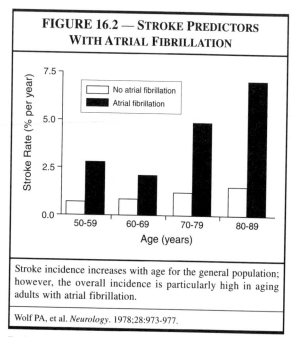

FIGURE 16.2 — STROKE PREDICTORS WITH ATRIAL FIBRILLATION

Stroke incidence increases with age for the general population; however, the overall incidence is particularly high in aging adults with atrial fibrillation.

Wolf PA, et al. *Neurology.* 1978;28:973-977.

Both approaches were associated with a similar frequency of embolic events. When strokes occurred with either strategy, most often there was a subtherapeutic international normalized ratio (INR) or unplanned stopping of warfarin. Both studies demonstrated a nonsignificant trend toward increased mortality in the rhythm-control arm, despite the use of warfarin with each strategy. Although a majority of patients with AF are candidates for anticoagulation therapy, only a relatively small proportion actually receive it.[11] In both community and academic settings, <60% of patients with strong indications for anticoagulation therapy are actually prescribed warfarin.[12-14]

Five large-scale randomized clinical trials performed in Denmark, the United States, and Canada[15-19] have shown definitively that oral anticoagulation therapy with warfarin, titrated to an INR of 2.0 to 4.5 prevents stroke with a very low risk for major hemorrhage (**Table 16.3**).

A meta-analysis of randomized trials demonstrated that anticoagulation therapy reduced the risk of stroke by 68%,

TABLE 16.1 — STROKE PREDICTORS WITH ATRIAL FIBRILLATION: RISK-STRATIFICATION SCHEME

Stratification	Clinical Features	Stroke Rate (%/y)
High risk	Prior stroke or TIA or systemic embolism; age >75 years, hypertension, poor LV systolic function; rheumatic mitral valve disease or prosthetic heart valve	4 to 12
Moderate risk	Age 65 to 75 years; CAD with preserved LV function, thyrotoxicosis	2 to 4
Low risk	No high- or moderate-risk features, eg <65 years old, and no cardiovascular disease	1

Abbreviations: CAD, coronary artery disease; LV, left ventricular; TIA, transient ischemic attack.

Fintel D, Hofmann C. *The American Family Physicians Guide to Preventing Strokes and Lowering Health Risks in Patients With Atrial Fibrillation.* Lisle, Ill: Illinois Academy of Family Physicians; 2000; and Albers G, et al. *Chest.* 2001;119(suppl 1):194S-206S.

with almost no increase in the frequency of intracranial or major bleeding.[5] Women experienced an even greater reduction in stroke risk (84%) compared with men (60%).[5] Based on the existence of strong and compelling data, an expert panel of the American College of Chest Physicians issued a directive for the use of anticoagulation therapy with warfarin in appropriately chosen patients with AF.[1] According to their consensus recommendations, oral warfarin therapy titrated to a goal INR of 2.5, range 2 to 3, should be strongly considered for all eligible patients who are at high risk for stroke.[1]

Ximelagatran is a new orally administered direct-acting thrombin inhibitor not yet approved by the Food and

16

TABLE 16.2 — STROKE PREDICTORS WITH ATRIAL FIBRILLATION: ECHOCARDIOGRAPHIC FINDINGS

Transthoracic Echocardiography (TTE)
- Left ventricular ejection fraction <50%
- Large left atrium (>2.5 cm/M^2 body surface area)

Transesophageal Echocardiography (TEE)
- Echocardiography "smoke" in left atrium
- Left atrial appendage thrombus

Fintel D, Hofmann C. *The American Family Physicians Guide to Preventing Strokes and Lowering Health Risks in Patients With Atrial Fibrillation.* Lisle, Ill: Illinois Academy of Family Physicians; 2000.

TABLE 16.3 — STROKE REDUCTION BY WARFARIN THERAPY

Warfarin reduced the risk of stroke by:
- 68% overall
- 60% in men
- 84% in women

Atrial Fibrillation Investigators. *Arch Intern Med.* 1994;154:1449-1457.

Drug Administration. This agent has short half-life with a quick onset and offset of antithrombotic activity and requires no anticoagulation monitoring. The Stroke Prevention Using Oral Thrombin Inhibitor in Atrial Fibrillation (SPORTIF III) trial[20] compared the 36-mg twice-daily dose of ximelagatran to warfarin in 3407 patients with chronic or paroxysmal atrial fibrillation. The primary end point of stroke and systemic embolic events occurred at a rate of 2.3% in the warfarin group and 1.6% in the ximelagatran group, leading to a 29% reduction in risk with the newer agent, fulfilling the goal of noninferiority. Major and minor bleeding was reduced from 29.5% with warfarin to 25.5% with ximelagatran ($P = 0.007$). These promising results of less bleeding with at least equivalent efficacy were confirmed in the SPORTIF V trial. Elevated liver enzymes in 6% to 8% of patients will require further evaluation.

Risk Stratification and Risk Reduction With Warfarin Therapy

Risk stratification can be used to reliably identify patients who are at high risk for stroke and those who will benefit most from anticoagulation therapy. Treatment reduces absolute stroke rates by 3.2%, 4.0%, and 6.9% for patients with AF and concomitant risk factors who are <65, 65 to 75, and >75 years of age, respectively.[5] Thus warfarin therapy in older patients with AF can result in a substantial reduction (70% to 85% relative risk) for life-threatening and crippling consequences of stroke. Even in the uncommon circumstance of elderly patients (>75 years) with no other risk factors, treatment with warfarin can reduce the risk of stroke considerably.[1]

The epidemiology-based concept of "number needed to treat to show benefit" is useful in understanding the impact of anticoagulation therapy, combining the absolute rate of stroke with the relative reduction in stroke risk provided by warfarin therapy (**Table 16.4**).[2,21] The data demonstrate that only 15 patients with prior stroke or TIA would require warfarin treatment for 1 year to prevent a life-threatening or disabling stroke. The higher the clinical risk of stroke, the greater the protection afforded by anticoagulation. When more than one risk factor is present, increased age strikingly decreases the "number needed to treat," clearly demonstrating the elevated stroke risk in older patients with additional risk factors.

Risks Versus Benefits of Warfarin Therapy

The major risk of anticoagulation therapy is bleeding, particularly in the presence of gastrointestinal or genitourinary disease, or in a setting in which trauma is more likely (alcoholism, Parkinson's disease, or previous stroke with significant neurologic impairment). However, despite the potential for increased bleeding risk, pooled data from the five largest randomized trials of anticoagulation therapy demonstrate only a small increase in risk for major hemorrhage in patients treated with warfarin compared with con-

16

TABLE 16.4 — NUMBER OF ATRIAL FIBRILLATION PATIENTS TREATED WITH WARFARIN TO PREVENT A STROKE

Category	Actual Risk Reduction Rate (%/y)	Number Needed to Treat
Age <65 years and one or more risk factors	3.2	31
Age 65 to 75 years, and one or more risk factors	4.0	25
Age >75 years, and one or more risk factors	6.9	14
Hypertension	3.7	27
Diabetes	5.8	17
Prior stroke or transient ischemic attack	6.6	15
Congestive heart failure	5.2	19
Angina pectoris	5.8	17
Myocardial infarction	4.9	20

Fintel D, Hofmann C. *The American Family Physicians Guide to Preventing Strokes and Lowering Health Risks in Patients With Atrial Fibrillation.* Lisle, Ill: Illinois Academy of Family Physicians; 2000.

trol groups—1% vs 1.3% annually (**Table 16.5** and **Figure 16.3**).[5]

TABLE 16.5 — RISK OF BLEEDING: ANNUAL OCCURRENCE OF MAJOR BLEEDING EVENTS	
Event	**Frequency** (%)
Major Bleeding	
Patients receiving placebo	1.0
Warfarin-treated patients	1.3
Intracranial Bleeding	
Patients receiving placebo	0.1
Warfarin-treated patients	0.3
Atrial Fibrillation Investigators. *Arch Intern Med* 1994;154:1449-1457.	

The Role of Antiplatelet Agents

Thrombus developing within the left atrium or left atrial appendage in atrial fibrillation is dependent upon stasis of blood flow and activation of soluble coagulation factors; however, several studies have evaluated the reduction of stroke risk by aspirin therapy, administered in doses of 75 mg to 325 mg.[15,16,22] In two randomized trials, Danish Atrial Fibrillation Aspirin Coagulation (AFASAK)[15] and European Atrial Fibrillation Trial (EAFT),[22] risk reduction with aspirin failed to achieve statistical significance (16% and 17%, respectively). In contrast, the American Stroke Prevention in Atrial Fibrillation (SPAF)-1 trial[16] showed a significant reduction (42%) with aspirin treatment at a daily dose of 325 mg. A pooled analysis of these three trials demonstrated a 21% reduction in the risk of ischemic stroke (8.1% in control patients and 6.3% in aspirin-treated patients; $P = 0.05$; number needed to treat = 50),[1,23] suggesting that aspirin therapy is associated with a clinically important decrease in stroke risk among patients with AF. Several studies directly compared the efficacy of aspirin with warfarin. In the AFASAK[15] and EAFT[22] trials, warfarin therapy significantly decreased the risk of primary events

16

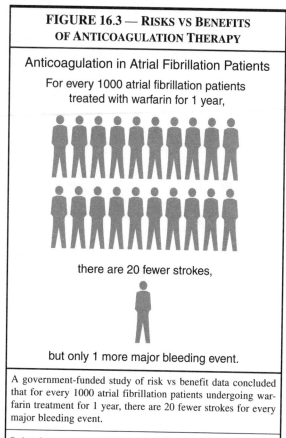

FIGURE 16.3 — RISKS VS BENEFITS OF ANTICOAGULATION THERAPY

Anticoagulation in Atrial Fibrillation Patients

For every 1000 atrial fibrillation patients treated with warfarin for 1 year,

there are 20 fewer strokes,

but only 1 more major bleeding event.

A government-funded study of risk vs benefit data concluded that for every 1000 atrial fibrillation patients undergoing warfarin treatment for 1 year, there are 20 fewer strokes for every major bleeding event.

Patient Outcomes Research Team. Agency for Health Care Policy and Research (AHCPR); 1995. Pub No. 95-0091.

by 48% and 40%, respectively, as compared with aspirin. The SPAF-3 study evaluated the efficacy of fixed-dose, low-intensity warfarin therapy (INR 1.2 to 1.5; maximum daily dose, 3 mg) plus aspirin.[24] This arm was prematurely terminated because of a substantially increased rate of primary outcome events (7.9% per year) compared with patients receiving standard adjusted-dose warfarin, target INR 2 to 3 (1.9% per year). All patients participating in this trial had at least one clinical risk factor for stroke. Thus low-intensity anticoagulation plus aspirin is ineffective in high-risk patients.[24] In addition, there is a considerably greater risk reduction associated with warfarin therapy (68%) than with aspirin therapy (21%) in high-risk patients when compared with control patients.[5] Considered collectively, the data support aspirin treatment solely for patients at low risk for stroke (<65 years old and no other risk factors) or those who have contraindications for warfarin therapy.[2]

Clopidogrel and ticlopidine are effective for stroke prevention; however, there are as yet no clinical trial data supporting their primary use in patients with AF.

Alternative, Nonpharmacologic Approaches

For patients with a definite contraindication for oral anticoagulation (ie, significant fall risk, intracranial or systemic bleeding, or noncompliance) there are several nonpharmacologic modalities available. These include surgical exclusion or amputation of the left atrial appendage, percutaneous implantation of an occlusion device (experimental), surgical Maze procedure, or radiofrequency ablation of AF triggers in the pulmonary veins. At the current time, the efficacy of these new approaches is still under evaluation.

Initiating and Monitoring Antithrombotic Therapy

The initial evaluation of a patient with AF should include a careful history, physical examination, selected laboratory studies, and diagnostic tests as indicated[2] (**Table 16.6**). **Table 16.7** displays recommendations for warfarin or aspirin therapy, dependent on age and the presence or absence of other risk factors.[1, 2]

When initiating warfarin therapy in the outpatient setting, clinicians must be mindful of differing dose requirements and potential interactions (**Figure 16.4**). Initial starting doses are typically 5 mg in patients <65 years of age, decreasing to 3 mg in patients >75 years of age. Since warfarin exerts its action by preventing hepatic carboxylation of vitamin K–dependent clotting factors, 3 to 5 days

16

TABLE 16.6 — RECOMMENDED STRATEGY FOR MANAGING PATIENTS WITH ATRIAL FIBRILLATION

- Slow ventricular response
- Identify and correct the underlying triggers/causes of AF
- Assess risks vs benefits of electrical or pharmacologic cardioversion. Before and after cardioversion, use anticoagulant therapy according to ACCP guidelines
- For a patient who remains in chronic or paroxysmal AF, anticoagulate with warfarin (target INR 2.5, range 2 to 3). Aspirin therapy is recommended for patients age <65 years with "lone AF"

Abbreviations: AF, atrial fibrillation; ACCP, American College of Chest Physicians; INR, international normalized ratio.

TABLE 16.7 — CHEST 2001 SUMMARY OF RECOMMENDATIONS

Age (y)	Risk Factors*	Recommendation
<65	Absent	Aspirin
	Present	Warfarin (target INR 2.5, range 2 to 3)
65-75	Absent	Aspirin or warfarin
	Present	Warfarin (target INR 2.5, range 2 to 3)
>75	All patients	Warfarin (target INR 2.5, range 2 to 3)

Abbreviation: INR, international normalized ratio.

* Prior transient ischemic attack, systemic embolus or stroke, hypertension, poor left ventricular function, rheumatic mitral valve disease, prosthetic heart valve.

Albers G, et al. *Chest.* 2001;119(suppl 1):194S-206S.

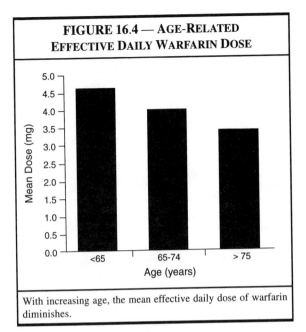

FIGURE 16.4 — AGE-RELATED EFFECTIVE DAILY WARFARIN DOSE

With increasing age, the mean effective daily dose of warfarin diminishes.

are generally required to achieve a full anticoagulation effect. Given delayed expression of drug effect, along with the increased sensitivity of older individuals to warfarin, it is appropriate to "go low and slow" when initiating therapy and to change weekly dose by only 1 to 2 mg at a time when INR values fall out of the therapeutic range of 2 to 3. When initiating therapy, anticoagulation status should be monitored every 1 to 3 days until the INR is stable, followed by weekly monitoring. Routine monthly testing is appropriate once patients have stabilized. An INR should be checked within 3 days of starting or stopping medications known to interact with warfarin and at any time the patient experiences signs or symptoms of bleeding or thrombosis.[2]

The therapeutic window is the level of therapy that achieves an optimal balance between patient benefit and risk. When administering anticoagulation therapy for AF, this window is the range of anticoagulation intensity, measured by the INR, that reliably prevents thromboembolic events with a minimum risk of hemorrhagic events. Hylek

16

and colleagues, based on a large anticoagulation clinic population, reported that the risk of thromboembolic events in patients with AF rises dramatically with an INR <2, doubling at an INR of 1.7, and tripling at an INR of 1.5 (**Figure 16.5**).[25] Conversely, the risk of hemorrhage increases dramatically as the INR increases to levels >3 (**Figure 16.6**).[26] The therapeutic window (**Figure 16.7**) therefore represents the optimum INR range of 2 to 3, at which the risks of both hemorrhage and thromboemboli are minimized.

Improving the Paradigm for Outpatient Anticoagulation

The traditional approach to outpatient anticoagulation therapy management involves phlebotomy, a delay period (to receive test results from an outside laboratory), retrieval of the patient's records, attempts by the office staff (nurse or physician) to reach the patient and discuss changes in dose, and documentation of these changes in the medical

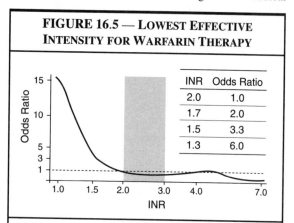

FIGURE 16.5 — LOWEST EFFECTIVE INTENSITY FOR WARFARIN THERAPY

INR	Odds Ratio
2.0	1.0
1.7	2.0
1.5	3.3
1.3	6.0

Hylek and colleagues studied the lowest effective intensity for anticoagulant therapy with warfarin. They determined that an intensity of anticoagulation expressed as international normalized ratio (INR) values <2.0 resulted in a substantially higher risk of stroke.

Hylek EM, et al. *N Engl J Med*. 1996;335:540-546.

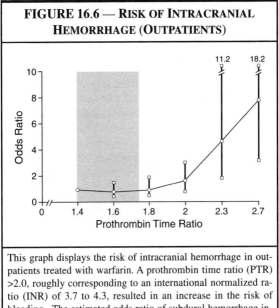

FIGURE 16.6 — RISK OF INTRACRANIAL HEMORRHAGE (OUTPATIENTS)

This graph displays the risk of intracranial hemorrhage in outpatients treated with warfarin. A prothrombin time ratio (PTR) >2.0, roughly corresponding to an international normalized ratio (INR) of 3.7 to 4.3, resulted in an increase in the risk of bleeding. The estimated odds ratio of subdural hemorrhage increased 7.6-fold as the PTR increased from 2.0 to 2.5. Note: Shade to PTR = 1.75.

Hylek EM, Singer DE. *Ann Intern Med.* 1994;120:897-902.

record. The development of rapid and reliable point-of-care coagulation monitors, such as the CoaguChek and ProTime devices, offers an attractive alternative. This technology, coupled with computerized data bases and experienced anticoagulation clinic providers represents an emerging coordinated strategy to achieve optimal care. Anticoagulation clinics, whether based in the hospital or in an outpatient-practice setting, have demonstrated clear benefits over a traditional office-based approach, including reduced episodes of under- or over-anticoagulation, clinical events, hospitalizations, and emergency room (ER) visits (**Table 16.8**).[27]

16

FIGURE 16.7 — THERAPEUTIC WINDOW

Thromboembolic events may occur at an international normalized ratio (INR) value of <2.0. Conversely, clinical events associated with hemorrhage increase with increasing intensity of anticoagulation. The Chest 2001 Guidelines recommend a target INR of 2.5 (range 2.0 to 3.0) for atrial fibrillation.

Challenges for the Future: Improving the Delivery of Antithrombotic Therapy for Atrial Fibrillation

The utilization of warfarin and aspirin therapy for stroke prevention in AF has increased substantially in the past decade,[28] due in part to the publication of landmark trials demonstrating the benefit of treatment and the promulgation of guidelines by the Consensus Committee of the American College of Chest Physicians. Recent trends suggest, however, that treatment rates have plateaued — a concerning trend that mandates national education efforts for physicians and health care systems regarding treatment choices in patients with AF (**Figure 16.8**). The implementation of anticoagulation therapy with warfarin could prevent 40,000 strokes per year, at a cost saving of more than $600 million annually.[11]

TABLE 16.8 — MONITORING ANTICOAGULATION OUTCOMES: ANTICOAGULATION CLINICS VS USUAL MEDICAL CARE

Anticoagulation Outcome	Clinics (%)	Usual (%)
Rates of bleeding	8.1	35.3
Rates of thromboembolic events	3.3	11.8
Incidence of warfarin-related		
Hospitalizations	5.0	19.0
Emergency-room visits	6.0	22.0

Chiquette E, et al. *Arch Intern Med.* 1998;158:1641-1647.

FIGURE 16.8 — WARFARIN UTILIZATION

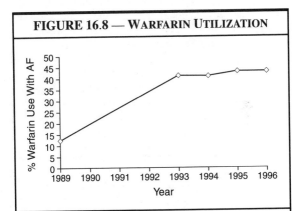

When evaluating warfarin use in 2.8 million patient visits over an 8-year period, it is obvious that warfarin use increased after the publication of results of several randomized clinical trials that evaluated stroke prevention in atrial fibrillation (AF). Subsequent utilization has remained constant (flat) despite additional publications on the efficacy of warfarin in stroke prevention and the underutilization of antithrombotic therapy in patients with AF.

Stafford RS, Singer DE. *Circulation.* 1998;97:1231-1233.

16

Summary

Atrial fibrillation is a common arrhythmia with a prevalence that increases with age. Patients with AF have an increased risk for thromboembolic complications, most importantly, stroke. The results of several international large-scale, randomized trials have provided convincing evidence that coexisting demographic and clinical characteristics determine the overall likelihood of stroke. Furthermore, these studies demonstrate conclusively that antithrombotic therapy with warfarin in patients at moderate or high risk and with aspirin in patients at low risk or those unable or unwilling to take warfarin, can significantly reduce thromboembolic complications, with enormous potential savings in human suffering and economic cost. Comprehensive approaches to management that include point-of-care coagulation monitoring and coordinating anticoagulation clinics offer great promise in elevating the standard of care. Promising new treatments, such as ximelagatran, may offer the benefit of efficacy similar to warfarin with a lower bleeding risk and no need for coagulation monitoring, increasing the likelihood that a greater number of patients will receive anticoagulant therapy. Further evaluation of the data will be required.

REFERENCES

1. Albers G, Dalen J, Laupacis A, et al. Antithrombotic therapy in atrial fibrillation. *Chest*. 2001;199(suppl 1):194S-206S.

2. Fintel D, Hofmann C. *The American Family Physicians Guide to Preventing Strokes and Lowering Health Risks in Patients With Atrial Fibrillation*. Lisle, Ill: Illinois Academy of Family Physicians; 2000.

3. Cerebral Embolism Task Force. Cardiogenic brain embolism. *Arch Neurol*. 1986;43:71-84.

4. Wolf PA, Dawber TR, Thomas HE Jr, Kannel WB. Epidemiologic assessment of chronic atrial fibrillation and risk of stroke: the Framingham Study. *Neurology*. 1978;28:973-977.

5. Atrial Fibrillation Investigators. Risk factors for stroke and efficacy of antithrombotic therapy in atrial fibrillation. Analysis of pooled data from five randomized controlled trials. *Arch Intern Med*. 1994; 154:1449-1457.

6. Atrial Fibrillation Investigators. Echocardiographic predictors of stroke in patients with atrial fibrillation: a prospective study of 1066 patients from 3 clinical trials. *Arch Intern Med.* 1998;158:1316-1320.

7. Ezekowitz MD, Levine JA. Preventing stroke in patients with atrial fibrillation. *JAMA.* 1999;281:1830-1835.

8. Stroke Prevention in Atrial Fibrillation Investigators Committee on Echocardiography. Transesophageal echocardiographic correlates of thromboembolism in high-risk patients with nonvalvular atrial fibrillation. *Ann Intern Med.* 1987;147:1561-1564.

9. Wyse DG, Waldo AL, DiMarco JP, et al. A comparison of rate control and rhythm control in patients with atrial fibrillation. The atrial fibrillation follow-up investigation of rhythm management (AFFIRM) investigators. *N Engl J Med.* 2002;347:1825-1833.

10. Van Gelder IC, Hagens VE, Bosker HA, et al. A comparison of rate control and rhythm control in patients with recurrent persistent atrial fibrillation. *N Engl J Med.* 2002;347:1834-1840.

11. Patient Outcomes Research Team. Secondary and tertiary prevention of stroke. Agency for Health Care Policy and Research (AHCPR); 1995. Publication 95-0091.

12. Stafford RS, Singer DE. Recent national patterns of warfarin use in atrial fibrillation. *Circulation.* 1998;97:1231-1233.

13. Brass LM, Krumholz HM, Scinto JD, Mathur D, Radford M. Warfarin use following ischemic stroke among Medicare patients with atrial fibrillation. *Arch Intern Med.* 1998;158:2093-2100.

14. Go AS, Hylek EM, Borowsky LH, et al. Warfarin use among ambulatory patients with nonvalvular atrial fibrillation: The Anticoagulation and Risk Factors in Atrial Fibrillation (ATRIA) study. *Ann Intern Med.* 1999;131:927-934.

15. Peterson P, Boysen G, Godtfredsen J, Anderson ED, Anderson B. Placebo controlled randomised trial of warfarin and aspirin for prevention of thromboembolic complications in chronic atrial fibrillation. The Copenhagen AFASAK study. *Lancet.* 1989;1:175-179.

16. Stroke Prevention in Atrial Fibrillation Investigators. Stroke Prevention in Atrial Fibrillation Study. Final results. *Circulation.* 1991;84:527-539.

17. Boston Area Anticoagulation Trial for Atrial Fibrillation Investigators. The effect of low-dose warfarin on the risk of stroke in patients with nonrheumatic atrial fibrillation. *N Engl J Med.* 1990;323:1505-1511.

18. Connolly SJ, Laupacis A, Gent M, Roberts RS, Cairns JA, Joyner C. Canadian Atrial Fibrillation Anticoagulation (CAFA) Study. *J Am Coll Cardiol.* 1991;18:349-355.

16

19. Ezekowitz MD, Bridgers SL, James KE, et al for the Veterans Affairs Stroke Prevention in Nonrheumatic Atrial Fibrillation Investigators. Warfarin in the prevention of stroke associated with nonrheumatic atrial fibrillation. *N Engl J Med*. 1992;327:1406-1412.

20. Halperin JL. SPORTIF III. A long-term randomized trial comparing ximelagatran with warfarin for prevention of stroke and systemic embolism in patients with nonvalvular atrial fibrillation. Presented at the 52nd Annual Scientific Sessions of the American College of Cardiology; Chicago, Ill: March 20-April 2, 2003.

21. Akhtar W, Reeves WE, Movahed A. Indications for anticoagulation in atrial fibrillation [published correction appears in *Am Fam Physician*. 1999;59:1122]. *Am Fam Physician*. 1998;58:130-136.

22. European Atrial Fibrillation Trial Study Group. Optimal oral anticoagulation therapy in patients with nonrheumatic atrial fibrillation and recent cerebral ischemia. *N Engl J Med*. 1995;333:5-10.

23. Fihn S, Callahan CM, Martin DC, McDonnell MB, Henikoff JG, White RH. The risk for and severity of bleeding complications in elderly patients treated with warfarin. The National Consortium of Anticoagulation Clinics. *Ann Intern Med*. 1996;124:970-979.

24. Stroke Prevention in Atrial Fibrillation Investigators. Adjusted-dose warfarin versus low-intensity, fixed-dose warfarin plus aspirin for high-risk patients with atrial fibrillation: stroke prevention in atrial fibrillation III randomized clinical trial. *Lancet*. 1996;348:633-638.

25. Hylek EM, Skates SJ, Sheehan MA, Singer DE. An analysis of the lowest effective intensity of prophylactic anticoagulation for patients with nonrheumatic atrial fibrillation. *N Engl J Med*. 1996;335:540-545.

26. Hylek EM, Singer DE. Risk factors for intracranial hemorrhage in outpatients taking warfarin. *Ann Intern Med*. 1994;120:897-902.

27. Chiquette E, Amato MG, Bussey HI, et al. Comparison of an anticoagulation clinic with usual medical care: anticoagulation control, patient outcomes, and health care costs. *Arch Intern Med*. 1998;158:1641-1647.

28. Stafford RS, Singer DE. Recent national patterns of warfarin use in atrial fibrillation. *Circulation*. 1998;97:1231-1233.

17 Venous Thromboembolic Disease and Pulmonary Embolism

Incidence

Venous thromboembolism is common and leads to disability, economic loss, and even death. The true incidence is uncertain, but a report from Minnesota provides some revealing statistics.[1] The health records of 2218 persons residing in Olmstead County over a 25-year period and having a deep vein thrombosis (DVT) or pulmonary embolism (PE) were reviewed. The rate of DVT was 48 per 100,000, and PE, 69 per 100,000. Projected to the entire US population, this would be 201,000 new cases of venous thromboembolism per year (107,000 DVT and 94,000 PE).

Anatomy and Pathophysiology

The venous anatomy of the lower extremities is complex and varies from person to person.[2] Constant features are the proximal veins: the iliacs, common femoral, superficial and deep femoral, and popliteals (**Figure 17.1**). The iliac veins are in the pelvis, and the common femoral is a very short segment extending under the inguinal ligament. The superficial femoral vein is the major, long conduit down the thigh to the knee. The deep femoral vein is rarely the site of disease. The popliteal vein branches into the anterior and posterior tibial veins and the peroneal vein in highly variable fashion. These veins distal to the popliteal vein are the major calf veins; there are also soleal and gastrocnemius veins. The greater and lesser saphenous veins are the superficial veins of the leg and connect to the deep system via perforating veins. Patients may have a superficial thrombophlebitis (reported to occur frequently in patients with factor V Leiden [FVL]), calf-vein thrombosis, proximal vein thrombosis, or various combinations of proximal and distal vein clots.

17

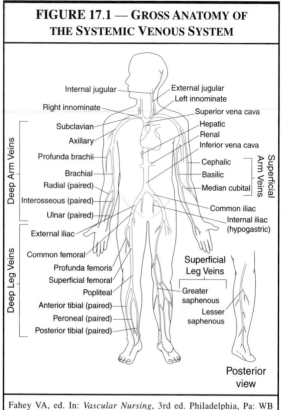

FIGURE 17.1 — GROSS ANATOMY OF THE SYSTEMIC VENOUS SYSTEM

Fahey VA, ed. In: *Vascular Nursing*, 3rd ed. Philadelphia, Pa: WB Saunders Co; 1999:23.

More than 100 years ago, Virchow established that thrombi forming in the veins of the lower extremities or pelvis can embolize to the lungs.[3] He described his famous triad of risk factors for venous thromboembolism:

- Blood hypercoagulability
- Stasis of flow
- Vessel-wall injury.

The factors that have been associated with hypercoagulability may be congenital, acquired, or both, and are discussed in Chapter 11, *Inherited/Acquired Coagulation and Platelet Disorders (Thrombophilia)*. However, it must be emphasized that it is a combination of risk factors that most often is associated with venous thrombosis. It is unlikely that only two or three risk factors are involved in the actual development of a thrombus; for example, a study that recorded simply whether patients were heterozygous for FVL preoperatively did not find an association with the postoperative development of thromboembolism after joint arthroplasty.[4] As more reliable associations are made between risk factors and venous thrombosis, screening for multiple risk factors prior to surgery or pharmacotherapy may become an accepted procedure.

Stewart,[5] in an experimental model of venous thrombosis, describes four stages in the pathogenesis of venous thrombi:

- *Stage 1*: Initiation, characterized by the development of small tears in the endothelium of thin-walled veins.
- *Stage 2*: Adherence of neutrophils and platelets, with release of cathepsin, neutrophil activation peptide-2, β-thromboglobulin, and adenosine diphosphate.
- *Stage 3*: Coagulation, associated with platelet activation and fibrin deposition.
- *Stage 4*: Layering, characterized by trapping of erythrocytes and activation of neutrophils and platelets by fibrin.

Thrombi form within the cusps of venous valves and gradually accrete fibrin (stage 4) until they either obstruct the lumen or embolize. The factors determining which path is followed are obscure. Large thrombi may be found occluding major veins with no evidence of embolization, or massive pulmonary embolization may occur with no apparent residual thrombi in the major veins. In animal studies, Wessler and associates observed that 5 days were required for experimentally formed emboli to become adherent to the subendothelium of the pulmonary arteries.[6] Whether a similar period is necessary for pathologic thrombi to attach to human veins is unknown but might have an important bearing on when activity should be permitted after a DVT is diagnosed.[7]

One reason for difficulty in determining the duration of thrombosis is that there may be no symptoms as long as the thrombi do not completely occlude the vein lumen. However, such thrombi may embolize at any time; this accounts for the presence of pulmonary emboli in patients who have never had leg symptoms. Furthermore, most noninvasive tests for DVT rely on detection of venous occlusion as a surrogate marker for venous thrombosis. Nonobstructing thrombi are frequently not recognized by these techniques but become apparent on radiocontrast venography (see below).

Diagnosis

The diagnosis of DVT and PE is difficult and requires a mixture of clinical suspicion and objective testing.[8] A complete history, with attention to specific symptoms and signs, should be recorded; a thorough family history is also invaluable. The laboratory evaluation is critical in establishing an unequivocal diagnosis, but most of the tests currently used are not of uniformly high sensitivity and specificity. Thus an accurate diagnosis requires experience and attention to detail.

Signs and Symptoms of Deep Vein Thrombosis

The cardinal symptoms of DVT are pain and swelling in the lower extremity. The pain may be sharp and sudden in onset or come on more gradually and be reported as drawing in character. There may be little or no swelling, or the entire lower extremity may be enormous. On examination, there is frequently a reddish-purple discoloration of the leg in comparison with the noninvolved side. One may also see a prominent venous pattern on the affected limb. If there is associated superficial phlebitis, there may be tenderness over the saphenous vein itself and a cord may be palpable; otherwise, diffuse calf tenderness and warmth of the leg may be present. The Homans' sign (pain in the calf with dorsiflexion of the foot) is present in only about half the cases and is neither sensitive nor specific for DVT.

Deep vein thrombosis may be simulated by a ruptured Baker's cyst. These cysts are often located in the popliteal fossa; when they rupture, they produce sudden, severe pain, redness, swelling, and leg tenderness mimicking the signs and symptoms of DVT. Another "look-alike" is a simple cellulitis, which is usually associated with redness of the skin, warmth, swelling, and pain. Heterotopic ossification occurs in the thigh and pelvic girdle muscles of persons with spinal cord injury and motor paralysis. The deposition of calcium salts in the muscles results in redness and warmth of the overlying skin and swelling of the involved muscle groups, simulating proximal vein thrombosis. Large hematomas of the thigh may produce warmth, leg swelling, tenderness, and skin discoloration. Leg pains may be due to muscle cramps, and leg swelling occurs in heart failure and pregnancy, though usually bilaterally. Because there are so many entities that may be confused with DVT, laboratory studies are required to confirm the diagnosis.

Signs and Symptoms of Pulmonary Embolism

Patients with PE may be entirely asymptomatic or complain only of vague fatigue or breathlessness on exertion. Chest pain may be absent or described as a lancinating pain with every breath, making any activity impossible. Occasionally, patients note only a dull ache, a feeling of chest heaviness, or palpitations. Cough and hemoptysis are relatively infrequent. Often, PE is associated with otherwise unexplained fever (with temperature as high as 39°C). Tachycardia is the rule, tachypnea is often present, and if the embolus is large, syncope may occur. Chest examination may be entirely unremarkable, or there may be dullness and decreased breath sounds at one lung base, indicating the presence of a pleural effusion. Infrequently, a pleural rub is present. Sometimes, there is rib tenderness, leading to the mistaken impression that symptoms are due to chest trauma rather than to PE.

The differential diagnosis is broad and includes pneumonia, pleurisy, pneumothorax, atelectasis, pulmonary edema, congestive heart failure, bronchitis, lung malignancy, septicemia, orthostasis, and musculoskeletal pain. Even experienced clinicians may mistake one of these dis-

17

orders for PE. Therefore, objective testing is essential whenever the diagnosis is suspected.

Laboratory Testing for Deep Vein Thrombosis

A diagnostic algorithm has been proposed by Perrier and Bounameaux (**Figure 17.2**).[9] The first step is the performance of a rapid and sensitive test for D-dimer; several such tests, such as SimpliRed (AGEN® Biomedical, Ltd. Brisbane, Australia) and Vidas DD® (bioMerieux, Marcy l'Etoile, France), have been studied extensively.[10,11] D-Dimer is a proteolytic product of the degradation of fibrin, and is released into the circulation when fibrin thrombi undergo lysis. A negative test reliably excludes thrombosis unless there is a moderate or high pretest probability of thrombosis.[10] Factors that affect pretest probability are the presence of active cancer, paralysis or lower-extremity cast, major surgery within the previous 4 weeks or bedridden for more than 3 days, tenderness along the deep veins, thigh, and/or calf swelling, or a strong family history of venous thromboembolism.[12] If these are present, or if the physician considers that thromboembolism is the most likely explanation for the patient's symptoms based on other findings,[13] then further testing must be performed. Additional testing is also required if the D-dimer is positive, since false-positive results may occur in patients with liver or kidney disease, as well as after trauma or surgery. The next step is to perform duplex ultrasound.[14] This noninvasive technique provides a clear diagnosis in the majority of patients with symptomatic thrombi. The veins of greatest interest (common femoral, superficial femoral, popliteal) are readily located; they should be easily compressible by the ultrasound transducer. Lack of compressibility is characteristic of venous thrombosis and indicates venous hypertension due to outflow obstruction by thrombus. Thrombi may occasionally be visualized and collateral circulation recognized. A review of nine published studies noted that the sensitivity and specificity of compression ultrasound in the diagnosis of symptomatic proximal vein thrombosis were 96% and 98%, respectively.[15] In asymptomatic patients, complete

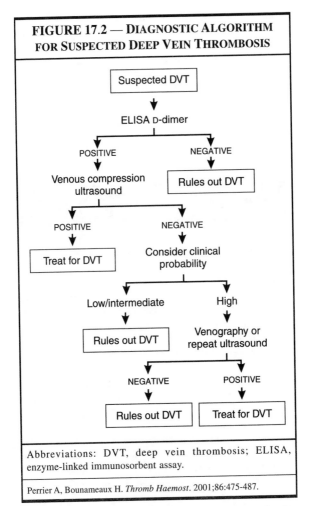

FIGURE 17.2 — DIAGNOSTIC ALGORITHM FOR SUSPECTED DEEP VEIN THROMBOSIS

Suspected DVT

↓

ELISA D-dimer

POSITIVE → Venous compression ultrasound

NEGATIVE → Rules out DVT

Venous compression ultrasound:

POSITIVE → Treat for DVT

NEGATIVE → Consider clinical probability

Low/intermediate → Rules out DVT

High → Venography or repeat ultrasound

NEGATIVE → Rules out DVT

POSITIVE → Treat for DVT

Abbreviations: DVT, deep vein thrombosis; ELISA, enzyme-linked immunosorbent assay.

Perrier A, Bounameaux H. *Thromb Haemost.* 2001;86:475-487.

obstruction of the veins is usually not present, and veins may remain compressible. Under these circumstances, the sensitivity of ultrasound declines to 62%, although the test remains very specific (97%). Sensitivity is also lost in patients with calf-vein thrombosis, where the vagaries of the venous anatomy in the calf may mislead the ultrasonographer, and up to 60% of thrombi may be missed. Other limitations of ultrasound include having only a short segment of vein involved and attempting to recognize fresh thrombus in a patient with old DVT.[14]

When there is strong clinical suspicion of DVT but the ultrasound is negative or equivocal, contrast venography is the test of choice. This is an invasive procedure which entails injecting contrast material into a vein on the dorsum of the foot and using fluoroscopy to follow the course of the dye as it makes its way to the pelvis. If an appropriate amount of contrast is injected, all veins with the exception of the deep femoral vein are visualized.

Diagnostic Testing for Pulmonary Embolism

A diagnostic algorithm for PE is shown in **Figure 17.3**. Again, one begins with the rapid D-dimer test, which is usually very sensitive to the presence of pulmonary emboli. In a patient with low clinical probability, a negative test rules out PE[13]; if the test is positive, compression ultrasound will indicate whether DVT is present. Identification of a thrombus is an indication for anticoagulant therapy. The ventilation/perfusion lung scan has traditionally been selected as the initial method for the objective diagnosis of PE. Interpretation of the test requires a concomitant chest x-ray, which most often is either normal or shows an effusion. Other signs, such as Hampton's hump or prominent pulmonary vasculature, are far less frequent. The lung scan is performed by doing a ventilation scan using xenon and a perfusion scan with iodinated albumin microspheres. A ventilated area that is not perfused is prima facie evidence of a PE, especially if the chest x-ray is normal in the area of interest. Unfortunately, such positive scans are found in only 15% of cases, and normal scans occur in only 8%; the majority of scans are of intermediate (44%) or low (33%) probability.[16] Thus lung scanning alone is not helpful in a majority of patients. Efforts have been made to improve the diagnostic value of lung scans by combining the scan results with the clinical assessment of disease likelihood.[12] For example, if there is a high clinical probability of a PE and the scan is positive, then a PE can be confirmed by pulmonary angiography 96% of the time. On the other hand, if there is a low clinical probability and the scan is a low-probability scan, PE is present in only 4%. For intermediate scans, the probabilities improve from 50% to 66% with high clinical probability and to 16% with low clinical probability.

Ventilation/perfusion scans are clearly not optimal studies for PE and are being supplanted as first-line tests by helical computed tomography (CT). This technique displays thrombi located in the main pulmonary arteries. In institutions with the appropriate equipment, helical CT has the advantage that it is available at all times, whereas lung scans are usually obtainable only during regular hours. A disadvantage is lack of sensitivity to smaller emboli. Two critical analyses of the literature concluded that CT has not yet been evaluated by high quality studies.[17,18] One algorithm suggests that CT be performed in all patients in whom there is an intermediate or high clinical suspicion of PE. If no PE is demonstrated, ultrasound of the legs could be done to ensure that thrombi are not present,[15] and anticoagulants would be withheld. This approach needs to be examined in a controlled, randomized clinical trial. When the diagnosis of PE is equivocal, pulmonary angiography is the definitive study. However, it is invasive, carries a dye load, requires expertise, and is expensive.

Management

The properties of the various anticoagulants in clinical use or under development are discussed in Chapter 3, *Heparins, Selective Factor Xa Inhibitors, Direct Thrombin Inhibitors, and Warfarin*. In this section, the prevention of thromboembolism in medical and surgical patients will be briefly reviewed, and the management of patients presenting with DVT or PE will be described, the feasibility of outpatient management explored, and the indications for fibrinolytic agents examined.

■ Thromboprophylaxis

Medical patients hospitalized for acute illness are at risk for venous thromboembolism (VTE). In a clinical trial that enrolled patients with congestive heart failure (New York Heart Association class III and IV) and those with acute respiratory failure, infections, and rheumatic diseases,

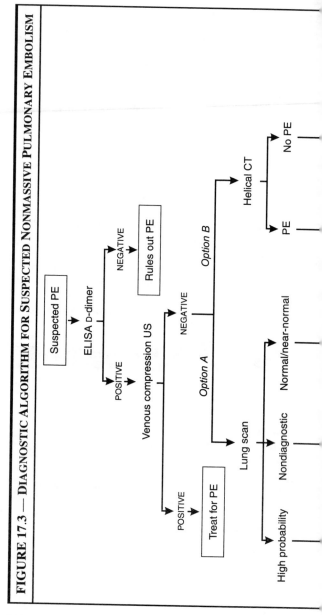

FIGURE 17.3 — DIAGNOSTIC ALGORITHM FOR SUSPECTED NONMASSIVE PULMONARY EMBOLISM

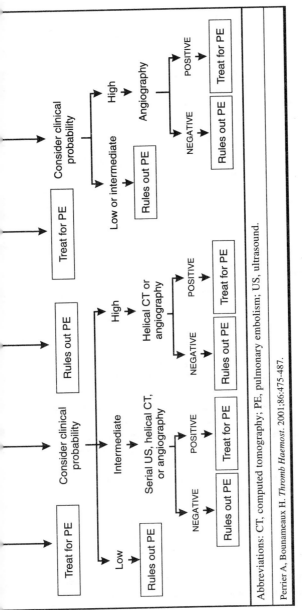

Abbreviations: CT, computed tomography; PE, pulmonary embolism; US, ultrasound.

Perrier A, Bounameaux H. *Thromb Haemost*. 2001;86:475-487.

17

the frequency of VTE in the placebo group was 14.9%.[19] A second study that included less severely ill patients (30% had chronic obstructive pulmonary disease, not intubated, as well as the aforementioned groups) found a 5% frequency of VTE in the placebo group (the PREVENT trial).[20] In the first study, enoxaparin in a subcutaneous (SC) dose of 40 mg once daily decreased the frequency of VTE to 5.5% (P <0.001), and in the second study, dalteparin in a SC dose of 5000 U once daily also resulted in a statistically significant decline in VTE (to 2.8%, P <0.0015). In neither study was bleeding significantly increased. Therefore, SC low molecular weight heparin (LMWH) is strongly recommended for the prevention of VTE in high-risk medical patients. The benefit of thromboprophylaxis with anticoagulants has also been demonstrated in patients with stroke, cancer, and other medical conditions.[21]

Persons undergoing surgical procedures are also at risk for VTE, and may be stratified according to risk.[21] The lowest risk group is comprised of patients <40 years of age having minor surgery with no additional risk factors; at moderate risk are those aged 40 to 60 having nonmajor surgery. At high risk are patients >60 years of age and those >40 years of age having major surgery; and at highest risk are patients with previous VTE, cancer, or other hypercoagulable conditions, and those undergoing most orthopedic and trauma surgery. Thromboprophylaxis ranges from the use of elastic stockings or compression devices for those at low risk to LMWH, fondaparinux, warfarin, or combinations of anticoagulants with mechanical devices for those at highest risk. **Table 3.1** shows the indications for surgical prophylaxis using LMWH approved by the Food and Drug Administration (FDA). In high-risk patients, anticoagulant prophylaxis should be continued for 4 to 5 weeks after the procedure.[22]

■ Deep Vein Thrombosis

Once the diagnosis of DVT has been established, the patient should be assessed as to whether the thrombosis is idiopathic or secondary to a defined risk factor such as surgery, trauma, cancer, antiphospholipid antibody syndrome, or inherited thrombophilia. If the latter are suspected, blood samples should be obtained for measurements of proteins

C and S, antithrombin, lupus anticoagulant, anticardiolipin antibody, homocysteine, and genetic testing for FVL and the prothrombin 20210A mutation. Abnormalities noted in these tests may affect the duration of the anticoagulant treatment, but it should be noted that proteins C and S may be low during the acute phase of an illness but subsequently will return to normal. Low values of these proteins should always be confirmed by repeat testing 3 to 6 months later.

Treatment for acute DVT is usually initiated with LMWH. In the past 10 years, more than a dozen controlled, double-blind, clinical trials have compared various LMWHs with unfractionated heparin (UFH) in the management of acute DVT. Lensing and associates performed a meta-analysis of 10 studies and noted that there was a statistically significant risk reduction in symptomatic thromboembolic complications, clinically important bleeding, and mortality with the use of LMWH.[23]

In the early 1990s, a relatively large study of venous thrombosis treatment compared tinzaparin with UFH.[24] Over 400 patients were randomized to receive either SC tinzaparin 175 U/kg once daily or UFH infused intravenously according to the Hull protocol shown in **Table 9.2**. To maintain blinding of the study, patients randomized to tinzaparin received an intravenous (IV) placebo, and patients treated with UFH received an SC placebo. The activated partial thromboplastin time (aPTT) was used to monitor the heparin treatment, but the results of the test and the adjustments of heparin dose were performed by third parties not involved in the clinical management of the patients. This rigorous study design permitted an unbiased assessment of treatment outcomes. Warfarin was started on day 2 and the heparin discontinued on day 6; patients were followed for 3 months. Despite the use of IV UFH, new thromboembolic events occurred in 6.9% of patients assigned to UFH; the figure for tinzaparin was lower (2.8%; $P = 0.07$). While major bleeding was recorded in 5% of those receiving UFH, this complication occurred in only 0.5% of those on tinzaparin ($P = 0.006$). Finally, 21 UFH-treated patients died as compared with 10 treated with tinzaparin ($P = 0.049$). Thus, by every measure, tinzaparin was superior to UFH.

Low molecular weight heparins available in the United States are shown in **Table 17.1**. Two of these, enoxaparin and tinzaparin, are currently approved by the FDA for the treatment of venous thrombosis. Tinzaparin is given in a once-daily dose of 175 U/kg. Enoxaparin may be given either twice daily in a dose of 1 mg/kg or once daily in a dose of 1.5 mg/kg.[25] Coincidentally with the dose of LMWH, warfarin may be started in a dose of 5 mg. This particular dose of warfarin is selected because studies by Harrison and colleagues have shown that this dose is most likely to result in prothrombin time being in the therapeutic range by days 3 to 5.[26] However, prothrombin time must be assessed frequently and the doses of warfarin adjusted accordingly. For example, if the international normalized ratio (INR) is still only ≤1.2 on day 3 of warfarin dosing, the dose should be escalated by 2.5 mg daily until the INR is above 2.0, and then the dose can be adjusted downward. In the patient who is very sensitive to warfarin, the INR will be >1.5 by day 2 of therapy and the dose should be reduced by 2.5 mg. A great many factors affect sensitivity to warfarin; these include patient's diet, concomitant drugs, and mutations in the P-450 cytochrome system that is responsible for warfarin metabolism.[27] While some of these factors can be anticipated (for example, meager food intake in the postoperative patient or concurrent antibiotic therapy), other factors affecting warfarin responsiveness may only become apparent during administration of the drug.

Low molecular weight heparin should be continued until the INR has been >2.0 for 48 hours. This ensures that the levels of coagulation factors (prothrombin, factors VII, IX and X) have declined to sufficiently low levels that re-

TABLE 17.1 — LOW MOLECULAR WEIGHT HEPARINS USED FOR THE TREATMENT OF THROMBOEMBOLISM	
Drug (Trade)	**Dose**
Dalteparin (Fragmin)	100 U/kg q 12 h; 200 U/kg daily
Enoxaparin (Lovenox)	1 mg/kg q 12 h; 1.5 mg/kg daily
Tinzaparin (Innohep)	175 U/kg daily

current thrombosis is considered unlikely. In the majority of patients, a maintenance dose of 5 mg warfarin is satisfactory, but in young patients higher doses are usually necessary, and in elderly patients or those on restricted diets, lower doses suffice. Prothrombin times are usually obtained twice weekly until the INR consistently is in the 2 to 3 range and then biweekly or even monthly in stable patients. In those patients whose prothrombin times are quite labile, home testing of the INR may be recommended. A drop of blood, obtained from a fingerstick puncture, is presented to a machine that displays the prothrombin time and INR. This permits the patient to self-monitor the INR and in consultation with medical personnel determine the best dosing regimen compatible with the patient's lifestyle. In one study, patients performing self-testing had more INRs within the therapeutic range than patients who were on standard management.[28]

■ Outpatient Therapy

Patients with acute DVT may be treated at home if several criteria are met:

- The thrombus should be distal to the iliac vein. Iliac vein thrombi usually cause considerable leg swelling and discomfort and frequently embolize to the lungs. Patients with such thrombi need to be managed under physician supervision until leg swelling has decreased and fear of embolization has abated; a 2- to 3-day period is appropriate.

- The presence of pulmonary emboli warrants close supervision for at least 72 hours, until the patient is hemodynamically stable and further risk of embolization has subsided.

- Patients with risk factors for bleeding, such as liver disease, peptic ulcer, and thrombocytopenia, should be given anticoagulants with great caution and only in the hospital setting.

- The patient or caregiver must be instructed on the technique for administering the LMWH and must be considered reliable.

- There must be provision for obtaining prothrombin times in the outpatient setting, since warfarin is being given concurrently with LMWH.

17

- The patient should be geographically accessible in the event of thrombus recurrence or an untoward reaction to the medication.
- Third-party payers must be educated about the cost-benefits of home therapy and willing to provide financial coverage for treatment.

■ Duration of Treatment

Following the transition from LMWH to warfarin, a decision must be made about the duration of oral anticoagulation. The British Thoracic Society conducted a study comparing 4 weeks of anticoagulation with 3 months of therapy.[29] Approximately 350 patients were randomized to each treatment. Of those treated for 4 weeks, 7.8% had recurrent thrombosis vs 4% of those receiving anticoagulants for 3 months ($P = 0.04$), prompting a recommendation that at least 3 months of treatment be given. Prandoni and associates noted that the recurrence rate of DVT in patients treated for 3 months was 10% at 1 year and 20% at 2 years, suggesting that a longer treatment period might be beneficial.[30] Six weeks of anticoagulation were compared with 6 months by Schulman and colleagues; the 6-month group had about half the recurrence rate as the 6-week group.[31] Kearon and associates randomized patients to receive either 3 months or at least 6 months of anticoagulation.[32] The study was stopped when it was observed that 17 of 83 patients whose anticoagulation was discontinued after 3 months had recurrent thromboembolism as compared with only one of 79 patients who continued on anticoagulation ($P < 0.001$). Finally, a second study by Schulman and colleagues compared 6 months' treatment with treatment that was continued indefinitely in patients with a second episode of venous thromboembolism and showed a cumulative probability of recurrence of 24% vs 4% at 4 years.[33] However, when anticoagulation is discontinued, recurrence rates are high; in the study by Agnelli and colleagues, the rate of recurrence was 5% per patient year in patients discontinuing anticoagulants after 1 year of treatment.[34]

Does this mean that anticoagulation should be continued indefinitely in all patients with DVT? The risk of bleeding must also be considered. In the Kearon study, only one patient randomized to 3 months of anticoagulation had any bleeding, as compared with nine patients in the >6-month group ($P = 0.03$). Patients receiving anticoagulation for an indefinite period in the second Schulman study had an 8.6% risk of major hemorrhage, as compared with 2.7% in the 6-month group. Thus bleeding becomes an important factor when anticoagulation is continued beyond 6 months.

Can the risk of recurrent thromboembolism be estimated more precisely and the duration of treatment modified accordingly? The British Thoracic Society study referred to earlier found that the subset of patients who developed thrombosis in association with a defined risk factor, such as surgery or trauma, did not have an increased rate of recurrence when treatment was stopped at 4 weeks. This important observation needs to be confirmed by a prospective randomized trial of treatment duration in persons with this particular risk factor. Residual thrombus may also be predictive of recurrent thrombosis. Prandoni and associates reported that 41 of 58 episodes of recurrent thromboembolism occurred in patients with residual thrombosis whose anticoagulation was discontinued. No recurrences were observed in those who remained on oral anticoagulants.[35]

Are persons with inherited thrombophilia at greater risk for recurrence? In a study of patients with the prothrombin 20210A mutation, Eichinger and colleagues found no increase in recurrence rates as compared with those without the mutation.[36] Whether heterozygosity for FVL increases recurrence rates is controversial. After 3 to 6 months of anticoagulation, Simioni and associates noted that the recurrence rate in those with FVL was almost 40% at 8 years, as compared with 18% in those without the mutation.[37] However, Eichinger and associates found a recurrence rate at 2 years of only 8.9% in those with FVL and 9.7% in those without,[38] and Rintelen and colleagues, in a retrospective review, could detect no increase in rate, which was 4.8% per year for those with FVL and 5% per year in controls.[39] Patients with hyperhomocysteinemia appear to have a high recurrence rate when anticoagulation is stopped after 6 months.[40] Whether this high recurrence rate can be lowered by decreasing serum homocysteine with folic acid treatment needs to be examined.

The following guidelines for the duration of anticoagulant therapy have been proposed by the Consensus Conference of the American College of Chest Physicians:[41]

- First event with reversible or time-limited risk factors: 3 months
- First event with idiopathic thromboembolism: 6+ months
- For patients with recurrent idiopathic thromboembolism or a continuing risk factor such as cancer, antiphospholipid antibody syndrome, or deficiency of antithrombin: 12+ months
- The duration of therapy needs to be individualized in patients with deficiency of protein C or S, multiple thrombophilic conditions, homocysteinemia, and homozygous factor V Leiden.
- Isolated symptomatic calf vein thrombosis should be treated for at least 6 to 12 weeks. If anticoagulants are not given, serial noninvasive studies should be performed for 10 to 14 days to assess for proximal extension of the thrombus.

Because of risk of recurrence of venous thrombosis persists even with 6 months of warfarin therapy, switching to a lower dose rather than stopping the drug may be considered. The PREVENT investigators reported that less-intense warfarin therapy (INR 1.5-2.0) was effective in preventing thrombosis recurrence.[42] Monitoring was limited to every 8 weeks, and adverse events were infrequent. Only 14 of 225 patients had recurrences. However, another recent study compared full-dose warfarin (INR 2-3) with lower-dose warfarin (INR 1.5-1.9) started 3-plus months after a DVT.[43] In this trial, the recurrence rate with full-dose warfarin was only six of 369 and was significantly lower than with lower-dose therapy (16 of 369). Surprisingly, the rate of bleeding was no higher in the full-dose warfarin group, including major bleeding and overall bleeding. Based on these results, continuing full-dose anticoagulation for 6 months to 1 year is reasonable for most patients, and for patients whose INR is more difficult to control, switching to lower-intensity treatment after 6 months is an option.

■ Management of Venous Thromboembolism in Pregnancy

Pregnancy may occur in a woman with a history of VTE or a thrombotic event may occur in a pregnant patient. In the woman with a previous thrombosis, it is important to ascertain whether the thrombosis was related to a transient risk factor, such as surgery or trauma, or whether there is an ongoing risk factor, such as a congenital thrombophilia. Examples of the latter would be FVL, prothrombin 20210 mutation, deficiencies of antithrombin or protein C or S, and hyperhomocysteinemia. If not previously recorded, these factors should be studied (recognizing that protein S often declines during pregnancy).

In a study of 44 women who had no evidence of thrombophilia and only transient risk factors, there were no recurrences of VTE during pregnancy if anticoagulants were withheld antepartum and given 4 to 6 weeks postpartum.[44] However, three of 51 women (5.9%) with abnormal laboratory results or idiopathic thrombosis had recurrent thrombi during pregnancy; these women should receive prophylactic doses of heparin or LMWH during their pregnancy. Women who experience VTE during pregnancy are treated with full therapeutic doses of heparin (see Chapter 18, *Complications of Antithrombotic Therapy*, under section entitled *Heparin During Pregnancy*) or LMWH throughout the remaining months of their pregnancies, and anticoagulants are continued for at least 4 weeks postpartum.[45] If LMWH is given, anti-Xa levels are obtained during the first trimester and early in the third trimester to confirm that levels are in the 0.5 to 1.2 U/mL range; more frequent monitoring may be performed if there is a marked weight gain during the pregnancy.

To avoid excessive postpartum bleeding, many patients will be scheduled for induction of labor so that anticoagulant can be held 24 to 36 hours prior to delivery. This may also permit the use of epidural anesthesia, which otherwise would be contraindicated. The LMWH is resumed the day after the delivery if bleeding is not abnormal, and warfarin may be introduced at the same time. After 5 days of warfarin therapy, the INR should be >2.0 and the LMWH may be discontinued. As noted in Chapter 18, warfarin does not appear in the breast milk in sufficient quantities to adversely

17

affect the neonate. Warfarin is continued for at least 6 weeks postpartum or longer if there are ongoing risk factors for recurrent VTE.

Complications of Deep Vein Thrombosis and Management of Pulmonary Embolism

■ Postphlebitic Syndrome

Failure of recanalization of thrombosed veins leads to the postphlebitic syndrome, which is characterized by pain and swelling of the leg and induration, discoloration, and eventually ulceration of the skin of the involved extremity. Prandoni and colleagues recorded a cumulative incidence of the post-thrombotic syndrome of 22.8% after 2 years, 28% after 5 years, and 29.1% after 8 years.[30] Franzeck and colleagues also observed post-thrombotic changes in 28% of patients in their series.[46] The most common cause of these changes was found to be a combination of reflux and vein obstruction. This results in venous hypertension and increased flow through the superficial venous system. Chronic congestion of the skin is accompanied by thickening, pruritus, pigmentation, and ulceration.

There are several possible reasons for the development of the postphlebitic syndrome. First, thrombi located proximally in the common femoral vein or ileofemoral vein may completely obstruct venous outflow. If these thrombi do not undergo early recanalization, postphlebitic syndrome is a likely outcome. Second, recurrent episodes of DVT may eventually occlude the majority of venous outflow vessels. Finally, inadequate anticoagulation therapy during the acute episode may allow thrombus to extend to the collateral veins, further impairing venous outflow and resulting in a greater frequency of recurrent DVT.[47]

Prevention of postphlebitic syndrome requires early, intensive anticoagulation, which is continued long enough to prevent recurrent DVT (see *Duration of Treatment*, this chapter). Also, the use of compression stockings is beneficial. In a randomized trial, Brandjes and associates observed that wearing a sized-to-fit compression hose decreased the occurrence of all postphlebitic syndrome from 47% to 20%, and the severe syndrome from 23% to 11% (both *P* <0.001).[48] The stocking was worn on the involved leg beginning 2 to 3 weeks after the acute DVT and was worn during the daylight hours for up to 2 years. This is a safe and inexpensive measure that should be offered to all patients. In addition, there may be a role for fibrinolytic therapy to recanalize ileofemoral or common femoral thrombi. Three agents are currently available: streptokinase (SK), urokinase (UK), and tissue plasminogen activator (tPA).

The systemic administration of SK or UK results in the lysis of thrombi in less than half of all patients[49]; this is because venous thrombi may be quite long and prolonged exposure to the lytic agent is required. Furthermore, major bleeding occurs in 8% to 38% with SK, much higher than the 10% with heparin therapy. With prolonged infusion of tPA (35 hours), 40% clot lysis was achieved in four of seven patients, but 22% of all patients treated had major bleeding.[50] Even if the majority of the thrombus undergoes lysis, there may be no benefit unless the patency of the vessel is fully restored. Therefore, there have been attempts to combine lytic therapy with physical destruction of the thrombus, using catheter-directed thrombolysis. The catheter is introduced into the popliteal vein and advanced into the thrombus; the lytic agent is then sprayed into the clot. The catheter is gradually advanced and the clot lysed until flow is restored. Stents may be placed to maintain vessel patency. In a series of 312 infusions, complete lysis was achieved in 31%, and major bleeding occurred in 11%. Pulmonary emboli occurred in 1% and there were two deaths.[51] The vein was still patent in 60% of patients at the 1-year follow-up visit. This approach is appropriate for patients with iliac or ileofemoral vein thrombosis who live near centers with the expertise to perform this sophisticated treatment. Contraindications to fibrinolytic therapy include a history of stroke, major surgery, or head injury within the past 2 weeks or any potential bleeding lesions in noncompressible areas: ie, gastrointestinal or genitourinary tract. Arterial blood gas determinations and intramuscular **17** injections are avoided in patients receiving fibrinolytic agents.

■ **Pulmonary Embolism**

Patients with moderate PE are treated with UFH or LMWH, but those with submassive or massive PE may require fibrinolytic therapy. The decision to give a fibrinolytic agent is based on the presence of the following: hemodynamic instability with hypotension, symptomatic hypoxemia, and elevated right-heart pressure with signs of right-heart overload. When clinical suspicion of massive PE is high, one should not wait for diagnostic laboratory tests but rather immediately institute thrombolysis. In patients who are more stable, obtaining a spiral CT examination, a ventilation/perfusion scan, or a pulmonary angiogram is warranted to unequivocally establish the diagnosis of PE. An echocardiogram will confirm the presence of right-heart strain.

FDA-approved regimens for the treatment of PE are shown in **Table 17.2**.[52] Tissue plasminogen activator may be administered in a bolus dose of 15 mg (especially if the patient is in shock), and then 50 mg is infused over the first hour and 35 mg over the second hour for a total dose of 100 mg over 2 hours. Heparin is not given concomitantly with any fibrinolytic agent but rather is started as a continuous infusion of 500 U/hr immediately at the conclusion of fibrinolytic therapy. An aPTT is obtained and the dose of heparin adjusted to prolong the aPTT to 1.5 to 2.5 times

TABLE 17.2 — REGIMENS APPROVED BY THE FOOD AND DRUG ADMINISTRATION FOR THE TREATMENT OF PULMONARY EMBOLISM

Drug	Dose
Streptokinase	250,000 U as a loading dose over 30 min, followed by 100,000 U/hr for 24 hrs
Urokinase	4,400 U/kg as a loading dose over 10 min, followed by 4,400 U/kg/hr for 12 to 24 hrs
tPA	100 mg as a continuous intravenous infusion over 2 hrs

Abbreviation: tPA, tissue plasminogen activator.

Goldhaber SZ. *Disorders of Thrombosis.* Philadelphia, Pa: WB Saunders Company; 1996:321-328.

the control value. Alternatively, LMWH may be given in full therapeutic SC doses at the conclusion of the thrombolytic treatment.

The contraindications to fibrinolytic therapy are as noted, but are all relative, depending on the severity of the PE. For example, the occurrence of a large PE in a patient with a history of stroke would not contraindicate the use of a fibrinolytic agent, as the drug may be lifesaving in this circumstance. However, it must be recognized that the risk of intracranial hemorrhage with tPA approaches 1%, which must be taken into consideration when recommending thrombolysis. It is always advisable to discuss the risks and benefits of therapy with the patient prior to embarking on a potentially dangerous course of management.

■ Vena Caval Filters

Insertion of a vena caval filter is an option for the prevention of venous thromboembolism. The usual indication for filter placement is the presence of a fresh thrombus in the veins of the lower extremity or pelvis in a patient unable to receive treatment doses of anticoagulants. Such patients generally have experienced major bleeding or have a strong contraindication for systemic anticoagulation. Another indication is impaired pulmonary reserve such that even a small PE could be fatal. Other, more controversial indications, are recurrent PEs despite "adequate" anticoagulation, and contraindications for other methods of prophylaxis in a patient at high risk for thromboembolism. Filters are moderately effective; the frequency of PE in patients with filters is 2.6% to 3.8%.[53] However, the frequency of DVT is 6% to 32%, and inferior vena caval thrombosis, 3.6% to 11.2%. In the only published randomized trial of filters, 400 high-risk patients received conventional anticoagulant therapy, and half the group was randomized to also have a filter placed.[54] Although the filter group had fewer PEs, at a 2-year follow-up, the frequency of DVT was almost twice as high in the filter group as in those without filters (20.8% vs 11.6%), and there was no difference in survival.

17

REFERENCES

1. Silverstein MD, Heit JA, Mohr DN, Petterson TM, O'Fallon WM, Melton LJ 3rd. Trends in the incidence of deep vein thrombosis and pulmonary embolism: a 25-year population-based study. *Arch Intern Med.* 1998;158:585-593.

2. Rohrer MJ. The systemic venous system: basic considerations. In: Fahey VA, ed. *Vascular Nursing.* 3rd ed. Philadelphia, Pa: WB Saunders Company; 1999:23.

3. Virchow RLK. *Thrombosis and Emboli.* Matzdorff AC, Bell WR, trans. Canton, Oh: Science History Publications; 1998:234.

4. Ryan DH, Crowther MA, Ginsberg JS, Francis CW. Relation of factor V Leiden genotype to risk for acute deep venous thrombosis after joint replacement surgery. *Ann Intern Med.* 1998;128:270-276.

5. Stewart GJ. Neutrophils and deep vein thrombosis. *Haemostasis.* 1993;23(suppl 1):127-140.

6. Wessler S, Freiman DG, Ballon JD, Katz JH, Wolff R, Wolf E. Experimental pulmonary embolism with serum-induced thrombi. *Am J Path.* 1961;38:89-101.

7. Aschwanden M, Labs KH, Engel H, et al. Acute deep vein thrombosis: early mobilization does not increase the frequency of pulmonary embolism. *Thromb Haemost.* 2001;85:42-46.

8. Anand SS, Wells PS, Hunt D, Brill-Edwards P, Cook D, Ginsberg JS. Does the patient have deep vein thrombosis [published correction appears in *JAMA.* 1998;279:1614 and 1998;280:328]? *JAMA.* 1998; 279:1094-1099.

9. Perrier A, Bounameaux H. Cost-effective diagnosis of deep vein thrombosis and pulmonary embolism. *Thromb Haemost.* 2001;86:475-487.

10. Kearon C, Ginsberg JS, Douketis J, et al. Management of suspected deep venous thrombosis in outpatients by using clinical assessment and d-dimer testing. *Ann Intern Med.* 2001;135:108-111.

11. Perrier A, Howarth N, Didier D, et al. Performance of helical computed tomography in unselected outpatients with suspected pulmonary embolism. *Ann Intern Med.* 2001;135:88-97.

12. Wells PS, Ginsberg JS, Anderson DR, et al. Use of a clinical model for safe management of patients with suspected pulmonary embolism. *Ann Intern Med.* 1998;129:997-1005.

13. Wells PS, Anderson DR, Rodger M, et al. Excluding pulmonary embolism at the bedside without diagnostic imaging: management of patients with suspected pulmonary embolism presenting to the emergency department by using a simple clinical model and d-dimer. *Ann Intern Med.* 2001;135:98-107.

14. Kearon C, Ginsberg JS, Hirsh J. The role of venous ultrasonography in the diagnosis of suspected deep venous thrombosis and pulmonary embolism. *Ann Intern Med.* 1998;129:1044-1049.

15. Lensing AWA, Buller HR. Objective tests for the diagnosis of venous thrombosis. In: Hull R, Pineo GF, eds. *Disorders of Thrombosis.* Philadelphia, Pa: WB Saunders Company; 1995:239-257.

16. The Pioped Investigators. Value of the ventilation/perfusion scan in acute pulmonary embolism. Results of the prospective investigation of pulmonary embolism diagnosis (PIOPED). *JAMA.* 1990;263: 2753-2759.

17. Rathbun SW, Raskob GE, Whitsett TL. Sensitivity and specificity of helical computed tomography in the diagnosis of pulmonary embolism: a systematic review. *Ann Intern Med.* 2000;132:227-232.

18. Mullins MD, Becker DM, Hagspiel KD, Philbrick JT. The role of spiral volumetric computed tomography in the diagnosis of pulmonary embolism. *Arch Intern Med.* 2000;160:293-298.

19. Samama MM, Cohen AT, Darmon JY, et al. A comparison of enoxaparin with placebo for the prevention of venous thromboembolism in acutely ill medical patients. Prophylaxis in Medical patients with Enoxaparin Study Group. *N Engl J Med.* 1999;341:793-800.

20. Leizorovicz A, Cohen AT, Turpie AGG, et al. A randomized placebo controlled trial of dalteparin for the prevention of venous thromboembolism in 3706 acutely ill medical patients: the PREVENT Medical Thromboprophylaxis Study. *J Thromb Haemost.* 2003;1(suppl 1). Abstract OC396.

21. Geerts WH, Heit JA, Clagett GP, et al. Prevention of venous thromboembolism. *Chest.* 2001;119(suppl 1):132S-175S.

22. Hull RD, Pineo GF, Stein PD, et al. Extended out-of-hospital low-molecular-weight heparin prophylaxis against deep venous thrombosis in patients after elective hip arthroplasty: a systematic review. A*nn Intern Med.* 2001;135:858-869.

23. Lensing AW, Prins MH, Davidson BL, Hirsh J. Treatment of deep venous thrombosis with low-molecular-weight heparins. A meta-analysis. *Arch Intern Med.* 1995;155:601-607.

24. Hull RD, Raskob GE, Pineo GF, et al. Subcutaneous low-molecular-weight heparin compared with continuous intravenous heparin in the treatment of proximal-vein thrombosis. *N Engl J Med.* 1992;326:975-982.

25. Merli G, Spiro TE, Olsson CG, et al. Subcutaneous enoxaparin once or twice daily compared with intravenous unfractionated heparin for treatment of venous thromboembolic disease. *Ann Intern Med.* 2001;134:191-202.

17

26. Harrison L, Johnston M, Massicotte MP, Crowther M, Moffat K, Hirsh J. Comparison of 5-mg and 10-mg loading doses in initiation of warfarin therapy. *Ann Intern Med*. 1997;126:133-136.

27. Aithal GP, Day CP, Kesteven PKL, Daly AK. Association of polymorphisms in the cytochrome P450 CYP2C9 with warfarin dose requirement and risk of bleeding complications. *Lancet*. 1999;353: 717-719.

28. Watzke HH, Forberg E, Svolba G, Jimenez-Boj E, Krinninger B. A prospective controlled trial comparing weekly self-testing and self-dosing with the standard management of patients on stable oral anticoagulation. *Thromb Haemost*. 2000;83:661-665.

29. Research Committee of the British Thoracic Society. Optimum duration of anticoagulation for deep-vein thrombosis and pulmonary embolism. *Lancet*. 1992;340:873-876.

30. Prandoni P, Lensing AW, Cogo A, et al. The long-term clinical course of acute deep venous thrombosis. *Ann Intern Med*. 1996;125:1-7.

31. Schulman S, Rhedin AS, Lindmarker P, et al. A comparison of six weeks with six months of oral anticoagulant therapy after a first episode of venous thromboembolism. Duration of Anticoagulation Trial Study Group. *N Engl J Med*. 1995;332:1661-1665.

32. Kearon C, Gent M, Hirsh J, et al. A comparison of three months of anticoagulation with extended anticoagulation for a first episode of idiopathic venous thromboembolism [published correction appears in *N Engl J Med*. 1999;341:298]. *N Engl J Med*. 1999;340:901-907.

33. Schulman S, Granqvist S, Holmstrom M, et al. The duration of oral anticoagulant therapy after a second episode of venous thromboembolism. Duration of Anticoagulation Trial Study Group. *N Engl J Med*. 1997;336:393-398.

34. Agnelli G, Prandoni P, Santamaria MB, et al. Three months versus one year of oral anticoagulant therapy for idiopathic deep venous thrombosis. *N Engl J Med*. 2001;345:165-169.

35. Prandoni P, Lensing AW, Prins MH, et al. Residual venous thrombosis as a predictive factor of recurrent venous thromboembolism. *Ann Intern Med*. 2002;137:955-960.

36. Eichinger S, Minar E, Hirschl M, et al. The risk of early recurrent venous thrombembolism after oral anticoagulant therapy in patients with the G20210A transition in the prothrombin gene. *Thromb Haemost*. 1999;81:14-17.

37. Simioni P, Prandoni P, Lensing AW, et al. The risk of recurrent venous thromboembolism in patients with an Arg[506] to Gln mutation in the gene for factor V (factor V Leiden). *N Engl J Med*. 1997;336:399-403.

38. Eichinger S, Pabinger I, Stumpflen A, et al. The risk of recurrent venous thromboembolism in patients with and without factor V Leiden. *Thromb Haemost.* 1997;77:624-628.

39. Rintelen C, Pabinger I, Knobl P, Lechner K, Mannhalter C. Probability of recurrence of thrombosis in patients with and without factor V Leiden. *Thromb Haemost.* 1996;75:229-232.

40. Eichinger S, Stumpflen A, Hirschl M, et al. Hyperhomocysteinemia is a risk factor of recurrent venous thromboembolism. *Thromb Haemost.* 1998;80:566-569.

41. Hyers TM, Agnelli G, Hull RD, et al. Antithrombotic therapy for venous thromboembolic disease. *Chest.* 2001;119(suppl 1):176S-209S.

42. Ridker PM, Goldhaber SZ, Danielson E, et al. Long-term, low-intensity warfarin therapy for the prevention of recurrent venous thromboembolism. *N Engl J Med.* 2003;348:1425-1434.

43. Kearon C, Ginsberg JS, Kovacs MJ, et al. Comparison of low-intensity warfarin therapy with conventional-intensity warfarin therapy for long-term prevention of recurrent venous thromboembolism. *N Engl J Med.* 2003;349:631-639.

44. Brill-Edwards P, Ginsberg JS, Gent M, et al, for the Recurrence of Clot in This Pregnancy Study Group. Safety of withholding heparin in pregnant women with a history of venous thromboembolism. Recurrence of Clot in This Pregnancy Study Group. *N Engl J Med.* 2000;343:1439-1444.

45. Bates SM, Ginsberg JS. How we manage venous thromboembolism during pregnancy. *Blood.* 2002;100:3470-3478.

46. Franzeck UK, Schalch I, Bollinger A. On the relationship between changes in the deep veins evaluated by duplex sonography and the postthrombotic syndrome 12 years after deep vein thrombosis. *Thromb Haemost.* 1997;77:1109-1112.

47. Hull RD, Raskob GE, Brant RF, Pineo GF, Valentine KA. Relation between the time to achieve the lower limit of the APTT therapeutic range and recurrent venous thromboembolism during heparin treatment for deep vein thrombosis. *Arch Intern Med.* 1997;157:2562-2568.

48. Brandjes DPM, Buller HR, Heijboer H, et al. Randomised trial of effect of compression stockings in patients with symptomatic proximal-vein thrombosis. *Lancet.* 1997;349:759-762.

49. Kwaan HC. Thrombolytic therapy for deep vein thrombosis. *J Lab Clin Med.* 1992;119:450-451. Editorial.

50. Marder VJ, Brenner B, Totterman S, et al. Comparison of dosage schedules of rt-PA in the treatment of proximal deep vein thrombosis. *J Lab Clin Med.* 1992;119:485-495.

17

51. Mewissen MW, Seabrook GR, Meissner MH, Cynamon J, Labropoulos N, Haughton SH. Catheter-directed thrombolysis for lower extremity deep venous thrombosis: report of a national multicenter registry. *Radiology*. 1999;211:39-49.

52. Goldhaber SZ. Thrombolytic therapy for venous thromboembolism. In: Hull R, Pineo GF, eds. *Disorders of Thrombosis*. Philadelphia, Pa: WB Saunders Company; 1995:321-328.

53. Streiff MB. Vena caval filters: a comprehensive review. *Blood*. 2000;95:3669-3677.

54. Decousus H, Leizorovicz A, Parent F, et al. A clinical trial of vena caval filters in the prevention of pulmonary embolism in patients with proximal deep-vein thrombosis. *N Engl J Med*. 1998;338:409-415.

18 Complications of Antithrombotic Therapy

Introduction

The major complication of antithrombotic therapy is bleeding. Most of the agents in current clinical use have a narrow therapeutic index, ie, the ratio of the toxic dose to the effective dose for a therapeutic effect is small. Therefore, patients receiving these agents must be closely supervised and many of the drugs require laboratory monitoring. Because of these considerations, there has been a great impetus to develop safer agents that do not need laboratory control. Many of these drugs are currently in clinical trials. **Table 18.1** lists the adverse reactions associated with antithrombotic agents.

Warfarin

Hemorrhage is the most common adverse effect associated with warfarin administration. To predict the risk of bleeding, Beyth and colleagues[1] developed a five-point scoring system, with one point given for each of the following:

- Age >65 years
- History of stroke
- History of gastrointestinal bleeding
- Specific comorbid conditions (recent myocardial infarction [MI], elevated serum creatinine, hematocrit <30%, or diabetes).

Low-risk patients had a score of 0; intermediate-risk patients, 1 or 2; and high-risk, 3 or 4. The risk of bleeding in these three groupings at 12 months was 3%, 8%, and 30%, respectively. A Mayo Clinic study observed that malignancy was also a risk factor for bleeding, but that age, sex, history of gastrointestinal hemorrhage, peptic ulcer, alcohol abuse, hypertension, and stroke were not associated with major bleeding.[2] This discrepancy in study outcomes reflects

18

TABLE 18.1 — ADVERSE REACTIONS ASSOCIATED WITH ANTITHROMBOTIC AGENTS

Adverse Effect	Warfarin	Heparin	LMWH	Fibrinolytics	Antiplatelet
Bleeding	Yes	Yes	Yes	Yes	Yes
Thrombocytopenia	No	1% to 3%	<1%	No	Abciximab, 1%; Ticlopidine, 1%
Skin/muscle necrosis	Yes	Yes	Rare	No	No
Osteoporosis	?No	Yes	Rare	No	No
Alopecia	Yes	Yes	Rare	No	No
Other	No	Eosinophilia; hypoaldosteronism; elevated transaminases	No	No	No

Abbreviation: LMWH, low molecular weight heparin.

the fact that the risk of bleeding with warfarin treatment is multifactorial (**Table 18.2**). In addition, and perhaps most important, outcomes are related to the experience and expertise of those giving this anticoagulant. Several studies have noted that complications are far less frequent in patients managed by coordinated anticoagulation clinics.[3]

TABLE 18.2 — FACTORS INFLUENCING THE RISK OF WARFARIN-INDUCED BLEEDING

- Age
- Diet
- Medications
- Changes in therapy
- Duration of therapy
- Concurrent diseases
- Genetic polymorphisms

■ Genetic Factors

Warfarin (S-component) is metabolized by the P-450 cytochrome (CYP) 2C9 of the liver. There are two allelic variants of CYP 2C9, and these are much less efficient in metabolizing warfarin than the wild-type cytochrome. Patients with these alleles require lower doses of warfarin to achieve an anticoagulant effect and because of their increased sensitivity to the drug, are more likely to experience bleeding complications.[4] Since most patients requiring warfarin are unlikely to be tested for the presence of these cytochrome alleles, it would seem prudent to initiate warfarin therapy with a relatively low dose of 5 mg. Harrison and colleagues showed that when 10 mg was used as the starting dose, patients were significantly more likely to be overanticoagulated than when they were given 5 mg.[5] At 60 hours after the initiation of warfarin therapy, nine of 25 patients in the 10-mg group, but none of the 24 patients in the 5-mg group, had international normalized ratios (INRs) >3.0. Four of the patients in the 10-mg group eventually required vitamin K because of excessive anticoagulation.

■ Diet

The antagonist of warfarin, vitamin K, is found in fresh vegetables, butter, oils, meat products, and avocado.[6] There-

18

fore, the composition of the diet will have an important influence on the intensity of treatment. In one study of patients who had been poorly controlled on oral anticoagulants, administration of a diet of known vitamin K composition resulted in more stable anticoagulation.[7] Diet is especially important in patients with concurrent illnesses, whose nutrition may be marginal. Such patients have heightened sensitivity to warfarin and an increased risk of anticoagulant-associated bleeding. On the other hand, the use of enteral supplements containing vitamin K promotes resistance to warfarin. Prior to initiating warfarin therapy, the nutritional status of the patient should be assessed and the doses of warfarin correspondingly adjusted.

■ **Drugs**

Many commonly used medications have significant interactions with warfarin. In 1994, Wells and associates reviewed all reports of warfarin-drug interactions and found original reports of 186 such interactions.[8] Potentiation of warfarin effect was observed with six antibiotics, five cardiac drugs, two anti-inflammatory agents, two histamine$_2$-blockers, and alcohol in persons with concomitant liver disease (**Table 18.3**). Inhibition of warfarin effect was noted with three antibiotics, three central nervous system (CNS) drugs, cholestyramine, and sucralfate. Since that time, an important interaction between acetaminophen and warfarin was recognized,[9] and it has also been suggested that certain herbal remedies, such as ginkgo biloba, ginseng, and garlic, may enhance the effects of warfarin. In general, patients should be alerted to the possibility of warfarin-drug interactions. They should notify their caregivers whenever there is a change in their diet or medications. INR measurements should be performed during the period of potential drug interaction and the dosage of warfarin adjusted to assure that prothrombin times remain within the therapeutic range.

■ **Changes and Duration of Warfarin Treatment**

A study of 96 patients followed for up to 23 years showed that thromboembolism occurred most often during periods of high variability in the prothrombin time ratios.[10] A decline in the INR to <1.5 increases the frequency of

TABLE 18.3 — DRUG-WARFARIN INTERACTIONS

Drug	Potentiate	Inhibit
Antibiotics	Co-trimoxazole Erythromycin Fluconazole Isoniazid Metronidazole Miconazole Ciprofloxacin	Griseofulvin Rifampin Nafcillin
Cardiac drugs	Clofibrate Amiodarone Propranolol Sulfinpyrazone	—
Antipyretics, Anti-inflammatories	Acetaminophen Phenylbutazone Piroxicam	—
Histamine$_2$-blockers	Cimetidine Omeprazole	—
Central nervous system agents	Fluoxetine	Barbiturates Carbamazepine Chlordiazepoxide
Other	Lovastatin Tamoxifen Androgens	Cholestyramine Antithyroid drugs Sucralfate

thrombotic events to as high as 17.5%, as compared with 2.3% for INRs within the 2 to 3 range.[11] Instability of the prothrombin time may occur because of changes in diet or medications, poor compliance, or interruption of anticoagulation for any reason. The latter is usually engendered by the need for an invasive procedure. However, it should be recognized that certain types of surgery, such as cataract extraction and dental procedures, do not require cessation of anticoagulation. The main risk in these operations is related to the method of administration of the anesthetic agent; retrobulbar injections or lingual nerve blocks may be associated with hematoma formation. If such injections are re-

18

quired or if more extensive procedures are undertaken, warfarin should be withheld for approximately 4 days to allow the INR to decline to below 1.5[12,13]; this level does not increase bleeding. The warfarin may be resumed in the evening after surgery. Heparin needs to be given preoperatively only if venous or arterial thrombosis has occurred within the past month, and it need not be started until the INR is <2. Postoperatively, patients will need anticoagulant prophylaxis, given either intravenously or subcutaneously, depending on thrombosis risk, and continued until an INR of ≥2 is sustained for at least 48 hours.

Several recent studies have emphasized that warfarin therapy for conditions such as atrial fibrillation and recurrent venous thromboembolism should be continued for many months, if not indefinitely. This long duration of oral anticoagulation increases the risk for bleeding. Using the prediction rule described previously, Beyth and colleagues observed that patients prospectively classified into low-, medium-, and high-risk categories had cumulative incidences of bleeding at 48 months of 3%, 12%, and 53%, respectively.[14]

■ Management of Warfarin-Induced Bleeding

The first step in the management of bleeding in patients taking warfarin is to stop the drug. However, recovery of clotting factor levels may take several days, depending upon the vitamin K content of the patient's diet. To rapidly raise coagulant factor concentrations in patients with life-threatening hemorrhage, clotting factor concentrates are given.[15] The older concentrates were plasma-derived and consisted mainly of prothrombin complex factors. They had the disadvantages of thrombogenicity and potential for transmission of infectious agents. More recently, recombinant factor VIIa (NovoSeven) has been used with excellent control of bleeding, although thrombosis risk remains a concern. Fresh frozen plasma is an alternative therapy but usually does not completely correct the prothrombin time. Doses of at least 20 mL/kg are needed to raise clotting factor levels >20% of normal; such doses carry a substantial risk of producing circulatory overload. After an initial bolus of 200 mL, plasma may be given as a continuous infusion of 100 mL/hr with monitoring of venous pressure and administration of diuretics. Recently, plasma treated to inactivate infectious agents has become available.

Patients with warfarin-induced bleeding should also receive vitamin K, but the doses should be adjusted according to the intensity of bleeding. If bleeding is major, 5 mg to 10 mg of vitamin K is given subcutaneously. However, in most patients who do not have serious bleeding episodes and have an INR of <10, an oral dose of 2.5 mg vitamin K decreases the INR to between 2 and 4 by 48 hours.[16] And in nonbleeding patients, doses as low as 1 mg given by mouth reliably reduce the INR to the therapeutic range within 24 hours.[17]

■ Adverse Reactions Other Than Bleeding

Skin and muscle necrosis is a dreaded complication of warfarin therapy. The pathogenesis is related to the effect of warfarin on the levels of proteins C and S. Because these anticoagulant proteins disappear at a faster rate than prothrombin, an imbalance between procoagulant and anticoagulant proteins transiently develops. A recent investigation showed that prothrombin protects activated factor V (aFV) from degradation by activated protein C.[18] Low levels of protein C in the face of normal prothrombin concentrations are predictive of less inactivation of aFV with resultant hypercoagulability. The clinical manifestations of this disorder are necrosis of skin and fat, especially in such areas as the breast and abdominal wall. In addition, the veins of the lower extremities may become thrombosed, leading to venous gangrene.

This devastating syndrome is prevented by avoiding the use of warfarin in patients with low baseline levels of protein C and S; such patients are those with inherited deficiencies of these factors (detected by a positive personal or family history of thrombosis), patients suffering from poor nutrition (including those who are unable to eat because of gastrointestinal disease, recent surgery, or neurologic disease), and patients with heparin-induced thrombocytopenia (HIT) (see below). In patients with hereditary deficiencies of protein C or S, warfarin is introduced when therapeutic levels of heparin or low molecular weight heparin (LMWH) have been achieved. In other patients, warfarin therapy is delayed until the patient's nutri-

18

tion improves or the HIT has resolved; the starting dose should not exceed 5 mg daily. In patients who are receiving warfarin, the syndrome may be recognized by the development of skin discoloration and pain in a very localized body area and strongly suspected if the prothrombin time becomes greatly elevated with a single dose of warfarin, indicating extreme sensitivity of the vitamin K–dependent proteins to the vitamin K antagonist. The warfarin should be stopped immediately and the patient treated with vitamin K; in severe cases it is recommended that activated protein C, if available, or fresh frozen plasma be infused as a source of proteins C and S. A parenteral anticoagulant, such as heparin, LMWH, or recombinant hirudin, should also be given.

Another unusual complication of warfarin treatment is the "purple toes" syndrome. Patients with this syndrome usually have severe aortoiliac atheromatous disease; warfarin administration appears to promote plaque destabilization with distal embolization of cholesterol crystals, especially to the toes. Cessation of warfarin therapy generally resolves the problem, but vascular surgery may be necessary if there is extensive disease.[19]

Alopecia is an infrequent occurrence in patients on warfarin therapy. In two patients, hair loss was decreased with ubidecarenone (Coenzyme Q10), 30 mg daily.[20] Another potential but as yet undocumented complication of warfarin usage is osteoporosis. Warfarin effects osteocalcin, a vitamin K–dependent protein required for maintenance of bone matrix. Reassuringly, a recent study of 149 elderly women taking warfarin found no differences in bone mineral density as compared with control subjects matched according to age, weight, and estrogen use.[21]

The teratogenicity of warfarin is well recognized. The greatest risk is from week 6 to week 12 of gestation, but CNS malformations may occur later. During the third trimester, there is a risk of intracranial bleeding in the fetus. Therefore, warfarin should be discontinued when pregnancy is recognized in women who are taking the drug and alternative anticoagulation with heparin or LMWH substituted.[22] Warfarin may be resumed in the immediate postpartum period, even in women who nurse. Although some warfarin may appear in breast milk, the amounts are small and are counteracted by the vitamin K which is routinely given newborns at birth.

Heparin and Low Molecular Weight Heparin

The use of unfractionated heparin (UFH) and LMWH is associated with a variety of complications; as with warfarin, the most frequent problem is bleeding. However, other serious adverse effects also occur; these include HIT, osteoporosis, and less commonly, eosinophilia, alopecia, and transaminitis.

■ Bleeding

At the Sixth Consensus Conference on Antithrombotic Therapy, it was estimated that major bleeding occurs in from 0% to 7% of patients receiving intravenous (IV) UFH, and the rate of fatal bleeding is up to 2%.[23] For LMWH, the rates are 0% to 3.0% and up to 0.8%, respectively. Thus LMWH appears to be associated with a lesser risk of serious hemorrhage. One reason for this relates to the greater complexity of giving UFH. While LMWH is injected subcutaneously, UFH is usually given IV, requiring solution preparation, infusion pumps, and frequent laboratory monitoring. Errors have been discovered with infusion-pump precision, in making up solutions, in infusion and charting techniques, and with interruptions of infusions,[24] as well as with variations in the sensitivity to heparin of the partial thromboplastin time reagents in current use. Other pharmacologic problems with UFH, such as dose-dependent absorption and half-life, may likewise lead to under- or over-anticoagulation. LMWH is well absorbed at any dose and the anticoagulant effect is highly predictable.

Kitchens reviewed the sites of bleeding related to UFH or LMWH therapy in 474 patients.[25] Most common is wound and soft tissue hemorrhage (31%), followed by gastrointestinal (27%) and genitourinary (19%) bleeding. Less frequent (about 2%), but of great importance, is bleeding into the CNS, retroperitoneum, and adrenal glands. The clinical manifestations of adrenal hemorrhage may be very subtle, with only generalized weakness, hypotension, and hyperkalemia pointing to bleeding in these organs. A ma-

18

357

jor predisposing factor to bleeding appears to be the overall health of the patient, with those in good physical condition having a 2% frequency, whereas those who are severely ill having a 25% incidence.[26,27] Frail, elderly women in particular seem to be susceptible to heparin-associated hemorrhages, and such bleeding appears to occur with equal frequency with either UFH or LMWH.

Another important bleeding complication is spinal subarachnoid hematoma. This subject was reviewed in 1986; 33 patients were reported to have bleeding after attempted lumbar puncture.[28] Six had received heparin alone, and another six both heparin and warfarin. With intensive anticoagulant prophylaxis for orthopedic surgery and the widespread use of epidural anesthesia, many more cases of spinal epidural hematoma are now recognized.[29] As a consequence of this experience, guidelines for the use of anesthetic and anticoagulant agents have been established (**Table 18.4**).[30] As noted for other types of bleeding, most epidural hematomas have been in elderly women who should be given anticoagulants with considerable caution and close monitoring.

■ Management of Bleeding Due to Heparins

Bleeding in patients receiving heparin is managed by discontinuing the agent. Often this is all that is necessary, because the short half-life of the drug (90 minutes) ensures that the anticoagulant effect will disappear rapidly. However, if serious bleeding begins immediately after a dose is given or the patient has delayed heparin clearance (because of renal or hepatic disease), it may be necessary to neutralize the heparin with protamine. The dose is 1 mg for each 100 U of heparin suspected to be in the circulation; in practice, giving half this dose is usually safe and effective and can be repeated if necessary. Overdosing protamine may cause hypotension and even bleeding; allergic reactions to the drug have also been reported.

Reversal of LMWH is more challenging, since LMWH has a longer half-life and is less susceptible to inactivation by protamine. In a study of the neutralizing effects of protamine on UFH and LMWH, Wolzt and associates found that a dose of 1 mg/100 anti-Xa U of LMWH almost completely reversed the prolongation of the activated partial thrombo-

TABLE 18.4 — GUIDELINES FOR THE USE OF ANESTHETICS AND ANTICOAGULANTS IN PATIENTS UNDERGOING SURGERY

- Anti-Xa levels are not predictive of bleeding risk; therefore, monitoring is not recommended
- Antiplatelet or oral anticoagulant medications given in combination with low molecular weight heparin (LMWH) increase the risk of bleeding. The patient-care team should be educated regarding the dangers of this combination
- Traumatic needle or catheter placement may increase the risk of bleeding with LMWH
- In patients who have had preoperative LMWH, a single-dose spinal anesthetic may be safest and should be given no earlier than 10 to 12 hours after a prophylactic dose, and 24 hours after a therapeutic dose of LMWH
- Postoperative LMWH:
  - *Twice-daily dosing*: remove indwelling catheter and give first dose of LMWH 2 hours later and not earlier than 24 hours postoperatively
  - *Single-daily dosing*: catheter may remain in place. First dose of LMWH is given 6 to 8 hours postoperatively and repeated 24 hours later. Catheter should be removed 10 to 12 hours after the last dose of LMWH, and subsequent doses should be given a minimum of 2 hours after catheter removal

Horlocker TT, Wedel DJ. *Reg Anesth Pain Med*. 1998;23(suppl 2):164-177. Update, 2002.

plastin time (aPTT) and thrombin time, but had only a weak effect on anti-Xa activity.[31] However, since the subjects they studied were healthy volunteers, it is not known whether correction of the anti-Xa activity would be needed to control bleeding or whether normalization of the aPTT and thrombin time is sufficient.

■ Heparin-Induced Thrombocytopenia

18

Heparin-induced thrombocytopenia is a devastating complication that occurs in about 1% to 3% of patients who receive IV UFH, but in no more than 0.1% of patients treated with LMWH.[32] HIT is due to the formation of antibodies against a complex of heparin and platelet factor 4.[33] When these complexes attach to the membranes of platelets or endothelial cells, they provoke platelet activation, release of vasoconstrictors, formation of platelet microparticles, and exposure of tissue factor. The consequence of these effects is vascular occlusion due to platelet masses and fibrin (the white-clot syndrome). MI, ischemic stroke, peripheral artery occlusion, pulmonary embolism, and venous gangrene have all been reported. The diagnosis is based on the clinical history of prolonged or repeated exposure to heparin, a rapid decline in platelet count (which may still be in the normal range), and either a new thrombotic episode or worsening of existing thrombosis. Confirmation of the diagnosis requires laboratory testing using either a platelet-aggregation assay, the serotonin-release test, or an enzyme-linked immunoabsorbent assay.

Treatment includes immediate cessation of all forms of heparin, including LMWH; the latter invariably cross-reacts with the antibodies. Effective anticoagulation must be given, otherwise thrombosis is progressive. Warfarin is contraindicated because levels of protein C in these patients are low, increasing their susceptibility to warfarin-tissue necrosis (venous limb gangrene).[34] Two agents that do not cross-react with the HIT antibodies are available in the United States; they include lepirudin (Refludan) and argatroban. Dosing guidelines are presented in **Table 18.5**. Warfarin may be initiated when the platelet count is rising and it is clear that the patient is out of danger. Doses not exceeding 5 mg daily are suggested. Since both lepirudin and argatroban inhibit thrombin, they prolong the prothrombin time as well as the thrombin time. This complicates using the INR to monitor warfarin therapy. The INR can be estimated using the mathematical expression available in the argatroban dosing guidelines, or one can gradually decrease the dose of the thrombin inhibitor beginning 3 days after the initiation of warfarin therapy in anticipation of progressive lengthening of the prothrombin time by warfarin.

In a large, prospective study of patients with HIT, 418 individuals were treated with argatroban (2 µg/kg/min) adjusted to an aPTT of 1.5 to 3.0 baseline for a mean dura-

TABLE 18.5 — ANTICOAGULANT THERAPY IN PATIENTS WITH HEPARIN-INDUCED THROMBOCYTOPENIA	
Agent	**Dose and Monitoring**
Lepirudin	• IV bolus of 0.4 mg/kg • Continuous infusion of 0.15 mg/kg/h • Monitor with aPTT; do baseline and repeat 4 hours after initiation: ratio to normal should be 1.5-to-2.5 • Check aPTT at least twice daily during therapy • Reduce dose by ≥50% if renal failure present
Argatroban	• Continuous IV infusion of 2 mg/kg/min • Check aPTT 2 hours after initiation and adjust dose until target aPTT of 1.5 to 3.0 times control is attained (not to exceed 100 sec) • Reduce dose to 0.5 µg/kg/min if hepatic impairment
Abbreviations: aPTT, activated partial thromboplastin time; IV, intravenous.	

tion of 5 to 7 days. Compared with historical controls, the composite outcome of cardiovascular death, all-cause amputation, or new thrombosis (at 37 days) was reduced in argatroban-treated patients (38.8% vs 28.0%; $P = 0.04$). Among those with thrombotic events prior to treatment initiation, the comparative rates were 56.5% and 41.5%, respectively. In addition, argatroban reduced new thrombotic events and death due to thrombosis. Bleeding rates were similar between groups.[35]

A localized form of HIT, presenting as skin necrosis at the sites of injection of either UFH or LMWH, is also recognized and responds to cessation of heparin therapy. A vivid photograph of heparin-induced skin necrosis was published in the *New England Journal of Medicine* (1996;335: 715). Last, it should be noted that heparin-induced platelet antibodies are transient; in the study of Warkentin and Kelton, antibodies fell to undetectable levels at a median

18

of 50 to 85 days after the initial event.[36] Brief re-exposure to heparin after this time, in both their study and in that of Potzsch and associates[37] appeared to be safe. However, such re-exposure should only be done if there is a compelling indication such as cardiac surgery and the exposure time limited to just the time of operation. Testing for heparin antibodies should be performed using sensitive assays both prior to and following heparin administration. Early recognition and prompt treatment of HIT maybe lifesaving and limb-sparing.

■ Osteoporosis

Unfractionated heparin has been found to impair bone deposition and accelerate bone resorption, whereas LMWH only impedes bone deposition.[38] Furthermore, concentrations of LMWH 6- to 8-fold higher than those of UFH were required to inhibit osteoblast function *in vitro*.[39] The overall frequency of osteoporosis is somewhat <5% with UFH and lower with LMWH. It appears to occur more frequently with higher doses given for prolonged periods. Walenga and Bick recommend that if the duration of therapy is >12 months and the dose is ≤20,000 U daily, or if the duration is ≤3 months but the dose is >20,000 U daily, then baseline bone densitometry should be obtained and calcium supplements considered.[40]

■ Other Reactions

Eosinophilia occurs fairly commonly (estimates range from 10% to 50% in those exposed for long periods of time) and may be associated with eczematous plaques at injection sites.[41] More severe reactions, such as hypotension, chest pain, and shortness of breath, are probably manifestations of HIT. Alopecia occurs in <1% of patients. Patients will often show evidence of suppression of aldosterone secretion, manifested by hyperkalemia. A patient taking heparin subcutaneously for 4 years had hypoaldosteronism and at autopsy was found to have thinning of the adrenal cortex.[42] Hyperkalemia also occurs during therapy with LMWH.[43] During heparin treatment, serum transaminase levels may double, but there is no histologic evidence of liver damage, and other tests of liver function remain within the normal range.

■ Heparin During Pregnancy

Unfractionated heparin and LMWH may be safely given during pregnancy; they do not cross the placenta or appear in the maternal milk. However, pregnant patients taking heparin are at risk for all of the complications listed earlier. Prolongation of the aPTT may persist despite cessation of heparin 12 hours prior to predicted delivery, and serious bleeding has been reported.[44] Heparin should be discontinued at least 24 to 36 hours prior to labor induction, and the aPTT checked to ascertain whether it has returned to the normal range. In patients receiving heparin because of thromboembolic events during previous pregnancies, stopping heparin for 1 to 2 days prior to delivery is unlikely to result in recurrent thrombosis. However, it is important to resume anticoagulation soon after delivery because the risk of new thrombosis is greatest during the first 6 weeks postpartum.[45,46]

The choice of anticoagulant in pregnant women with prosthetic heart valves has been controversial. Anecdotal reports of fatal thromboembolism in women receiving enoxaparin led to a warning about the use of this LMWH in pregnancy. However, many women have received this and other LMWHs without adverse effects; these data are summarized in a Clinical Cardiology Consensus Report.[47] The panel felt that concerns about safety and efficacy are justified not only for enoxaparin, but for UFH, warfarin, and other LMWHs. When using LMWHs, monitoring weekly anti-Xa levels is appropriate and doses should be adjusted to maintain anti-Xa activity within the 0.5- to 1.2-U range.

Pregnancy is associated with bone loss, and this is aggravated by heparin exposure. Otherwise unexplained back pain may be the earliest sign of impending vertebral fracture. Douketis and associates performed a prospective, matched cohort study in pregnant women, and found that long-term heparin treatment was associated with a significant reduction in bone density that did not correlate with the dose or duration of heparin exposure.[48] Other studies have shown that LMWH causes less bone loss than UFH. Nevertheless, all pregnant women receiving heparin should be informed about the risks of bone loss and the possibility of fractures. Whether calcium supplementation and the use of calcitonin or other agents will be safe and effective in such women needs to be investigated.

Fibrinolytic Agents

Loscalzo[49] lists three principal shortcomings of fibrinolytic therapy:
- Bleeding
- Delayed lysis
- Reocclusion.

Serious bleeding occurs in about 1% of patients but may be intracranial and lead to considerable disability and even death. In 71,000 patients with MI treated with tissue plasminogen activator (tPA), the frequency of intracranial bleeding was 0.95%; 53% died during hospitalization and another 25% had residual neurologic deficit.[50] The major risk factors for bleeding were older age, female gender, black ethnicity, systolic blood pressure of ≥ 140 mm Hg, history of stroke, tPA dose >1.5 mg/kg, and lower body weight. In another study of 20,768 patients receiving either tPA or streptokinase (SK), the frequency of strokes was 1.14%; 0.36% were hemorrhagic, 0.48% were ischemic, and 0.3% were not further defined.[51] Patients treated with tPA had a small but significant excess of stroke as compared with those who received SK (1.33% vs 0.94%).

Any interruption of vascular integrity in a patient receiving fibrinolytic agents may lead to hemorrhage; for example, concurrent invasive procedures, such as coronary angioplasty and pulmonary artery catheter insertion, may result in hematoma formation at access sites. Gastrointestinal and retroperitoneal hemorrhage are also reported. Bleeding is due to the fibrinolytic activity of plasmin and also to the effects of fibrin degradation products, which interfere with platelet aggregation and fibrinogen polymerization.

Delayed lysis may be due to the depletion of plasminogen, which is the zymogen for plasmin. This may be due to consumption coagulopathy or prolonged administration of lytic agents and is corrected by plasma infusions. Several studies have shown that thrombolysis induces paradoxical activation of coagulation.[52] Plasmin can activate platelets and promote factor X activation. Furthermore, thrombin bound to fibrin may be exposed in the crevices of fissured plaques, where it may stimulate continued fibrin deposition. The consequences of this thrombin exposure are re-occlusion of vessels in patients who initially had successful thrombolysis. Heparin is unable to neutralize clot-bound thrombin; inactivation requires direct thrombin inhibitors such as hirudin.

Complications unique to SK therapy include fever, allergic reactions, and hypotension. A trial of anisolated human plasminogen streptokinase activator complex (anistreplase) was discontinued because several patients had severe hypotension, possibly related to dose and infusion rate.[53] In some patients, preformed antibodies to SK may dampen the response, although the doses of SK usually employed are sufficiently high to overcome most antibodies.

REFERENCES

1. Beyth RJ, Quinn LM, Landefeld CS. Prospective evaluation of an index for predicting the risk of major bleeding in outpatients treated with warfarin. *Am J Med.* 1998;105:91-99.

2. Gitter MJ, Jaeger TM, Petterson TM, Gersh BJ, Silverstein MD. Bleeding and thromboembolism during anticoagulant therapy: a population-based study in Rochester, Minnesota. *Mayo Clin Proc.* 1995;70:725-733.

3. Poller L, Shiach CR, MacCallum PK, et al. Multicentre randomised study of computerised anticoagulant dosage. European Concerted Action on Anticoagulation. *Lancet.* 1998;352:1505-1509.

4. Aithal GP, Day CP, Kesteven PJ, Daly AK. Association of polymorphisms in the cytochrome P450 CYP2C9 with warfarin dose requirement and risk of bleeding complications. *Lancet.* 1999;353:717-719.

5. Harrison L, Johnston M, Massicotte MP, Crowther M, Moffat K, Hirsh J. Comparison of 5-mg and 10-mg loading doses in initiation of warfarin therapy. *Ann Intern Med.* 1997;126:133-136.

6. Blickstein D, Shaklai M, Inbal A. Warfarin antagonism by avocado. *Lancet.* 1991;337:914-915. Letter.

7. Marongiu F, Sorano GG, Conti M, et al. Known vitamin K intake and management of poorly controlled oral anticoagulant therapy. *Lancet.* 1992;340:545-546. Letter.

8. Wells PS, Holbrook AM, Crowther NR, Hirsh J. Interactions of warfarin with drugs and food. *Ann Intern Med.* 1994;121:676-683.

18

9. Hylek EM, Heiman H, Skates SJ, Sheehan MA, Singer DE. Acetaminophen and other risk factors for excessive warfarin anticoagulation. *JAMA*. 1998;279:657-662.

10. Huber KC, Gersh BJ, Bailey KR, et al. Variability in anticoagulation control predicts thromboembolism after mechanical cardiac valve replacement: a 23-year population-based study. *Mayo Clin Proc*. 1997;72:1103-1110.

11. Palareti G, Manotti C, D'Angelo A, et al. Thrombotic events during oral anticoagulant treatment: results of the inception-cohort, prospective, collaborative ISCOAT study: ISCOAT Study Group (Italian Study on complications of Oral Anticoagulant Therapy). *Thromb Haemost*. 1997;78:1438-1443.

12. White RH, McKittrick T, Hutchinson R, Twitchell J. Temporary discontinuation of warfarin therapy: changes in the international normalized ratio. *Ann Intern Med*. 1995;122:40-42.

13. Kearon C, Hirsh J. Management of anticoagulation before and after elective surgery. *N Engl J Med*. 1997;336:1506-1511.

14. Beyth RJ, Quinn LM, Landefeld CS. Prospective evaluation of an index for predicting risk of major bleeding in outpatients treated with warfarin. *Am J Med*. 1998;105:91-99.

15. Makris M, Greaves M, Phillips WS, Kitchen S, Rosendaal FR, Preston FE. Emergency oral anticoagulant reversal: the relative efficacy of infusions of fresh frozen plasma and clotting factor concentrate on correction of the coagulopathy. *Thromb Haemost*. 1997;77:477-480.

16. Weibert RT, Le DT, Kayser SR, Rapaport SI. Correction of excessive anticoagulation with low-dose oral vitamin K_1. *Ann Intern Med*. 1997;125:959-962.

17. Crowther MA, Donovan D, Harrison L, McGinnis J, Ginsberg J. Low-dose oral vitamin K reliably reverses over-anticoagulation due to warfarin. *Thromb Haemost*. 1998;79:1116-1118.

18. Smirnov MD. Inhibition of activated protein C anticoagulant activity by prothrombin. *Blood*. 1999;94:3839-3846.

19. Abdelmalek MF, Spittell PC. 79-year-old woman with blue toes. *Mayo Clin Proc*. 1995;70:292-295.

20. Nagao T, Ibayashi S, Fujii K, Suimori H, Sadoshima S, Fujishima M. Treatment of warfarin-induced hair loss with ubidecarenone. *Lancet*. 1995;346:1104-1105. Letter.

21. Jamal SA, Browner WS, Bauer DC, Cummings SR. Warfarin use and risk for osteoporosis in elderly women. Study of Osteoporotic Fractures Research Group. *Ann Intern Med*. 1998;128:829-832.

22. Ginsburg JS, Hirsch J. Use of antithrombotic agents during pregnancy. *Chest.* 1998;114:524S-530S.

23. Levine MN, Raskob G, Landefeld S, Kearon C. Hemorrhagic complications of anticoagulant treatment. *Chest.* 2001;119(suppl 1):108S-121S.

24. Hattersley PG, Mitsuoka JC, King JH. Sources of error in heparin therapy of thromboembolic disease. *Arch Intern Med.* 1980;140:1173-1175.

25. Kitchens CS. Evaluation and treatment of bleeding associated with heparin and low-molecular-weight heparin administration. In: Alving BM, ed. *Blood Components and Pharmacologic Agents in the Treatment of Congenital and Acquired Bleeding Disorders.* Bethesda Md: AABB Press; 2000:167-184.

26. Landefeld CS, Beyth RJ. Anticoagulant-related bleeding: clinical epidemiology, prediction, and prevention. *Am J Med.* 1993;95:315-328.

27. Nieuwenhuis HK, Albada J, Banga JD, Sixma JJ. Identification of risk factors for bleeding during treatment of acute venous thromboembolism with heparin or low molecular weight heparin. *Blood.* 1991;78:2337-2343.

28. Owens EL, Kasten GW, Hessel EA. Spinal subarachnoid hematoma after lumbar puncture and heparinization: a case report, review of the literature, and discussion of anesthetic implications. *Anesth Analg.* 1986;65:1201-1207.

29. Wysowski DK, Talarico L, Bacsanyi J, Botstein P. Spinal and epidural hematoma and low-molecular-weight heparin. *N Engl J Med.* 1998;338:1774-1775. Letter.

30. Horlocker TT, Heit JA. Low molecular weight heparin: biochemistry, pharmacology, perioperative prophylaxis regimens, and guidelines for regional anesthetic management. *Anesth Analg.* 1997;85:874-885.

31. Wolzt M, Weltermann A, Nieszpaur-Los M, et al. Studies on the neutralizing effects of protamine on unfractionated and low molecular weight heparin (Fragmin) at the site of activation of the coagulation system in man. *Thromb Haemost.* 1995;73:439-443.

32. Warkentin TE, Chong BH, Greinacher A. Heparin-induced thrombocytopenia: towards consensus. *Thromb Haemost.* 1998;79:1-7.

33. Greinacher A, Potzsch B, Amiral J, Dummel V, Eichner A, Mueller-Eckhardt C. Heparin-associated thrombocytopenia: isolation of the antibody and characterization of a multimolecular PF4-heparin complex as the major antigen. *Thromb Haemost.* 1994;71:247-251.

34. Warkentin TE, Elavathil LJ, Hayward CP, Johnston MA, Russett JI, Kelton JG. The pathogenesis of venous limb gangrene associated with heparin-induced thrombocytopenia. *Ann Intern Med.* 1997;127:804-812.

18

35. Lewis BE, Wallis DE, Leya F, Hursting MJ, Kelton JG, for The Argatroban-915 Investigators. Argatroban anticoagulation in patients with heparin-induced thrombocytopenia. *Arch Intern Med*. 2003; 163:1849-1856.

36. Warkentin TE, Kelton JG. Temporal aspects of heparin-induced thrombocytopenia. *N Engl J Med*. 2001;344:1286-1292.

37. Potzsch B, Klovekorn WP, Madlener K. Use of heparin during cardiopulmonary bypass in patients with a history of heparin-induced thrombocytopenia. *N Engl J Med*. 2000;343:515. Letter.

38. Muir JM, Hirsh J, Weitz JI, Andrew M, Young E, Shaughnessy SG. A histomorphometric comparison of the effects of heparin and low-molecular-weight heparin on cancellous bone in rats. *Blood*. 1997;89: 3236-3242.

39. Bhandari M, Hirsh J, Weitz JI, Young E, Venner TJ, Shaughnessy SG. The effects of standard and low molecular weight heparin on bone nodule formation in vitro. *Thromb Haemost*. 1998;80:413-417.

40. Walenga JM, Bick RL. Heparin-induced thrombocytopenia, paradoxical thromboembolism, and other side effects of heparin therapy. *Med Clin North Am*. 1998;82:635-658.

41. Bircher AJ, Itin PH, Buchner SA. Skin lesions, hypereosinophilia, and subcutaneous heparin. *Lancet*. 1994;343:861. Letter.

42. Majoor CL. Aldosterone suppression by heparin. *N Engl J Med*. 1968; 279:1172-1173.

43. Canova CR, Fischler MP, Reinhart WH. Effect of low-molecular-weight heparin on serum potassium. *Lancet*. 1997;349:1447-1448. Letter.

44. Anderson DR, Ginsberg JS, Burrows R, Brill-Edwards P. Subcutaneous heparin therapy during pregnancy: a need for concern at the time of delivery. *Thromb Haemost*. 1991;65:248-250.

45. Brill-Edwards P, Ginsberg JS, Gent M, et al, for the Recurrence of Clot in This Pregnancy Study Group. Safety of withholding heparin in pregnant women with a history of thromboembolism. Recurrence of Clot in This Pregnancy Study Group. *N Engl J Med*. 2000;343:1439-1444.

46. Bates SM, Ginsberg JS. How we manage venous thromboembolism during pregnancy. *Blood*. 2002;100:3470-3478.

47. Topol EJ. Anticoagulation and enoxaparin use in patients with prosthetic heart valves and/or pregnancy. *American Health Consultants*. 2002;3:1-20.

48. Douketis JD, Ginsberg JS, Burrows RF, Duku EK, Webber CE, Brill-Edwards P. The effects of long-term heparin therapy during pregnancy on bone density. A prospective matched cohort study. *Thromb Haemost*. 1996;75:254-257.

49. Loscalzo J. Fibrinolytic therapy. In: Beutler E, Lichtman MA, Coller BS, eds. *Williams Hematology*. 5th ed. New York, NY: McGraw-Hill, Inc; 1994:1585-1591.

50. Gurwitz JH, Gore JM, Goldberg RJ, et al. Risk for intracranial hemorrhage after tissue plasminogen activator treatment for acute myocardial infarction. Participants in the National Register of Myocardial Infarction 2. *Ann Intern Med*. 1998;129:597-604.

51. Maggioni AP, Franzosi MG, Santoro E, White H, Van de Werf F, Tognoni G. The risk of stroke in patients with acute myocardial infarction after thrombolytic and antithrombotic treatment. Gruppo Italiano per lo Studio della Sopravvivenza nell 'Infarto Micardico II (GISSI-2), and the International Study Group. *New Engl J Med*. 1992;327:1-6.

52. Merlini PA, Ardissino D, Bauer KA, et al. Activation of the hemostatic mechanism during thrombolysis in patients with unstable angina pectoris. *Blood*. 1995;86:3327-3332.

53. Brenot F, Pacouret G, Meyer G, Sors H, Charbonnier B, Simonneau G. Adverse reactions with anistreplase. *Lancet*. 1991;338:114-115. Letter.

18

INDEX

Abciximab (ReoPro). See also *Glycoprotein IIb/IIIa receptor antagonists.*
  for acute coronary syndromes, 214t
  adverse effects of, 149, 173t, 251, 350t
  clinical experience and trials of, 69, *70,* 130, 132t-133t, 134-135, *136,* 146, *148,*
    220t-221t, 224, 248-249, *250*
  dosage of, 130, *131,* 214t
  duration of platelet effects after cessation of, 130, *131,* 144, 146, *146, 175*
  effectiveness of, 152t, 248, 250
  in elderly patients, 71
  heparin with, 71
  indications for, 152t, 214t, *227,* 231t
  mortality rate and, 135, *136*
  myocardial infarction and, 130, 133t, 134
  pharmacokinetics of, 129-130, *131,* 145t
  platelet defects from, 173t
  PTCA with, *136*
  reteplase with, 69, *70,* 71, 135, 248, 250, *252*
  revascularization and, 130, 133t, 134-135, *136*
  reversibility of, *147*
  source of, 129
  stenting and, 106, *136*
  streptokinase with, 248, 250
  tenecteplase with, 69, 71
  for thrombolytic resistance, 248-251, *250*
  tissue plasminogen activator with, 250, *250*
Abciximab before Directed Angioplasty and Stenting in Myocardial Infarction Regarding
  ©Acute and Long-term Follow-up (ADMIRAL) trial, 134, *136*
Abdominal surgery, 39t
ACE (angiotensin-converting enzyme) inhibitors
  for acute coronary syndromes, 213t
  aspirin and, 81
  for myocardial infarction, 246t
  preventive, *227*
Acenocoumarol, 49
Acetaminophen, 50, 352, 353t
Activated partial thromboplastin time
  heparin and, 35-36, 45t, 160, 363
  hirudin and, 45t, 46
  LMWH and, 36
  monitoring of, 164, 216, 217t
ACUTE trial, 220t
Adenosine diphosphate
  abciximab and, 130
  aspirin and, 79, 84, *86,* 92, *93*
  clopidogrel and, 111, *112*
  in dense bodies, 27
  platelet aggregation and, *112,* 168, 287, *288,* 323
  thrombus formation and, *172*
  ticlopidine and, 99, 108, *112*
ADMIRAL trial, 134, *136*
Adrenal glands, bleeding into, 358
AFASAK trial, 309
AFFIRM, 302, 304
Aggrastat. See *Tirofiban.*
Aggrenox (dipyridamole/aspirin), 107, 269, 282t
Alcohol, 51t, 307, 349, 352
Aldosterone, heparin and, 36, 362
Allergic reaction, 66
Alopecia, 350t, 356, 362
α₂-antiplasmin, 0, *20,* 59, *60,* 64, 71, 164
Alteplase. See also *Tissue plasminogen activator.*
  action mechanism of, *60*

Alteplase *(continued)*
  aspirin before, 61
  bleeding induced by, 43, 61
  chemical structure of, *61*
  clinical features of, 63t
  in clinical trials, 43, 67, 69, 71, 243t
  cost of, 63t
  dosage of, 60, 63t
  effectiveness of, 61, 63t
  half-life of, 60-61, 63t
  patency after, 60
Amiodarone, 51t, 353t
Amputation, 114t
Analgesics, 211
Androgens, 353t
Anesthetic
  anticoagulants and, in surgical patients, 353, 358, 359t
  in limb ischemia, 273t
Angina
  abciximab and, 134
  aspirin and, 83t, 94t
  Braunwald Classification System in, 210
  heparin and, 141t
  pathophysiology of, *202,* 216
  percutaneous coronary interventions in, 46
  ticlopidine and, 101, 103t
  TIMI risk score for, 210-211, 211t, *212*
  tirofiban and, 141t
Angiography, coronary, 203
Angiomax. See *Bivalirudin.*
Angioplasty. See also *Percutaneous coronary interventions; Percutaneous transluminal coronary angioplasty.*
  timing of, 72-73
Angiotensin-converting enzyme (ACE) inhibitors
  for acute coronary syndromes, 213t
  aspirin and, 81
  for myocardial infarction, 246t
  preventive, 227
Anisoylated plasminogen-streptokinase activator complex (APSAC). See *Anistreplase.*
Anistreplase
  action mechanism of, 66, *67*
  adverse effects of, 365
  aspirin with, 66
  clinical features of, 63t
  in clinical trials, 242t, 365
  contraindications for, 74t
  cost of, 63t
  dosage of, 63t, 66
  effectiveness of, 63t, 66
  half-life of, 63t, 66
  heparin with, 251, 253
  in ISIS-2 trial, 66
  patency after, 66
  pharmacokinetics of, 65-66
Annexins
  in antiphospholipid syndrome, 191-192
  thrombin generation and, 22
Antacids, 51t
Antibiotics, 51t, 334, 352, 353t
Anticoagulant factors, half-lives of, 16t
Anticoagulant proteins. See also *Protein* entries.
  in hemostatic balance, 15
Anticoagulants. See also *Factor* entries; specific agent, eg, *Heparin.*
  for acute coronary syndromes, 215t, 216, 217t, 217-218, *218-219,* 232t
  anesthetics and, in surgical patients, 359t
  aspirin with, 106
  contraindications for, 74t
  after coronary stenting, *106*
  under development, 52

19

371

Anticoagulants *(continued)*
  in hemostasis, 15
  lupus, 158, 160, 191, 193t
  monitoring of, 157-164, 293, 317t
    outpatient, 314-315, 317t
  oral, 225
  in patients with prosthetic heart valves, 159t
  speed of, 49
  thrombus formation and, 15, 332
  during vascular surgery, 281t
Anticoagulation in the Secondary Prevention of Events in Coronary Thrombosis
    (ASPECT) trial, 256t, 258t
Anti-factor Xa assay, 162
Anti-inflammatory drugs, 21. See also *Nonsteroidal anti-inflammatory drugs;* specific drug.
  statins as, 21
  warfarin interaction with, 51t, 352, 353t
Antiphospholipid antibody syndrome
  activated protein C resistance from, 189
  conditions associated with, 191
  diagnosis of, 191
  phospholipid-binding proteins recognized by, 192
  in pregnancy, 194
  protein C and protein S deficiency from, 190t
  thromboembolism risk in, 292t
  thrombophilia from, 183t
  warfarin for, 194
Antiplatelet agents. See also specific agent, eg, *Tenecteplase.*
  for acute coronary syndromes, 214t-215t, 230t-231t
  adverse effects of, 350t
  before alteplase infusion, 61
  aspirin as, 80, 84
  in atrial fibrillation patients, 309t, 309-311
  bleeding induced by, 84, 350t
  cerebrovascular disease and, 84, *85, 269*
  in clinical trials, 83-84, 87, 134
  myocardial infarction and, 84, *85,* 237-239
  percutaneous coronary interventions and, 91
  stenting and, 105-107, *106*
  stepwise approach to, *276-277*
  for surgical patients, anesthetics and, 359t
  thrombocytopenia induced by, 350t
  in thrombolytic resistance, 248, *249*
  vascular events and, 84, *85-86,* 87, *88-89,* 269
Antiplatelet Trialists' Collaboration, 83, *85,* 90, 268, 274
Antipyretics, 353t
Antithrombin, *18,* 22
  in acquired thrombophilia, 189, 190t, 193t
  in deep vein thrombosis, 333
  direct, 73, 253-254
  genetic mutations in, 182-183, 183t, *184,* 186
  half-life of, 16t
  heparin binding of, 35-36, 251
  idraparinux and, 52
  in inherited thrombophilia, 338
  LMWH and, 36, 253
  obesity and, 37
  in venous thromboembolism, in pregnancy, 339
Antithrombotics
  for atrial fibrillation, 302, 304-305
    dosage of, 312t, 313-314, *313-314*
    future challenges in, 316, *317*
    initiating and monitoring of, 311, 313-314
    risk vs benefits of, 313-314, *313-314*
  indications and dosages for, 280t-281t
  outpatient monitoring of, 314-315, 317t
  for peripheral vascular disease, 280t-281t
  statins as, 21
Antithrombotics in the Prevention of Reocclusion in Coronary Thrombolysis (APRICOT)
    trial, 256t

Aortic dissection, STEMI in, fibrinolytics and, 74t
Aortic valve. See also *Valvular heart disease.*
  blood flow across, 287, *288*
  disease of, 295t
Aortoiliac interventions, antithrombotics during, 281t
APRICOT trial, 256t
APSAC. See *Anistreplase.*
Argatroban
  action mechanism of, 46
  bleeding caused by, 361
  dosage of, 46-47, 360-361, 361t
  effectiveness of, 361
  for heparin-induced thrombocytopenia, 360-361, 361t
  indications for, 47
  monitoring of, 162
  pharmacokinetics of, 46
  prothrombin time and, 47, 160, 360-361
Arixtra. See *Fondaparinux.*
Arterial insufficiency, acute, 272, 274-275
Arterial occlusion/ischemia, acute, antithrombotics for, 280t
Arterial thrombosis. See *Thrombosis.*
Arteriosclerotic malformation, STEMI in, fibrinolytics and, 74t
L-Asparaginase, 190t
ASPECT trial, 256t, 258t
Aspirin
  ACE inhibitors and, 81
  action mechanism of, 79
  for acute coronary syndrome, 227
  adenosine diphosphate and, 79, 84, *86*, 92
  adverse effects of
    bleeding as, 80-81
    combined with other antithrombotics, 80
    neutropenia as, 271t
    platelet defects as, 173t
  allergy to, 61, 91, *260*
  before alteplase infusion, 43, 61
  anestreplase with, 66
  angina and, 94t
  for antiphospholipid antibody syndrome, 194
  benefits of, 239
  bivalirudin with, 46
  bypass grafting and, 87, 90
  cardiac events and, 82-83
  clinical efficacy of, 81-82, *82*, *86*, 92, 94t
  clopidogrel vs, Kaplan-Meier curves for, *117*
  clopidogrel with, 87, 111, 126, 216
  in combination therapy, 84, 87, *88-89*, 107
  contraindications to, 108, 216, 239
  coronary stenting and, *106*, 117-119
  development and history of, 79
  dipyridamole (Aggrenox) with, 91, 107
  dosage of, 80-81, 83t, 86-87, *88-89*, 214t, 238-239, 270t-271t, 280t-281t
    to avoid bleeding, 80
    erythrocytes and, 92
    in gastric erosions/ulcer patient, 81
    with streptokinase, 65
  effectiveness of, 216
  failure of, 84, *86*, 92-93
  Helicobacter pylori infection and, 81
  with and without heparin, 66, 191
  at hospital discharge, *260-261*
  indications for, 83t, 108, 213t, 216, 270t-271t, *276-277*, 280t
  intolerance of, 91
  in ISIS trial, 237-238
  limitations of, 93, 94t
  myocardial infarction and, 83t, 84, 94t, 113, 114t-115t, 138, *238*, 238-239
  percutaneous coronary interventions and, 214t-215t
  for peripheral vascular disease, 280t-281t

19

373

Aspirin *(continued)*
  pharmacokinetics of, 80
  platelet aggregation and, 79, 99
  in pregnancy, 194
  in primary prevention, 82-83, 83t, 94
  resistance to, 91-92, *93*
  revascularization and, 138
  in secondary prevention, 84, *85,* 94t
  streptokinase with, 65
  stroke and, 83t, *86,* 90-91, 113, 114t-115t
  thrombus formation and, *172*
  TIAs and, 90-91
  vascular events and, *82,* 94t, 268
  warfarin vs, after STEMI, 256t-258t
  warfarin with, 254-255
ASSENT trials, 69, *70,* 241, 250, *252,* 253
Assessment of the Safety and Efficacy of a New Thrombolytic (ASSENT) trials, 69, *70,*
  241, 250, *252,* 253
Atenolol, 51t
Atrial fibrillation
  antiplatelet agents for, 309t, 309-311
  antithrombotics for, 302, 304-305
    dosage of, 312t, 313-314, *313-314*
    future challenges in, 316, *317*
    initiating and monitoring of, 311, 313-314
    outpatient monitoring of, 314-315, 317t
    risk vs benefits of, 313-314, *313-314*
  management of, 312t
  prevalence and classification of, 301
  rheumatic valvular disease with, 257
  stroke risk in, 301-302, *303-304,* 304-305
    antiplatelet agents and, 309-311, *310*
    concept of number needed to treat in, 307
    echocardiographic findings in, 306t
    stratification of, 306t, 307, 308t
  thromboembolic risk and, 292t
  warfarin for, 306t, 307, 308t
    dosage of, 311, 312t, *313-314*
    initiating and monitoring of, 311, 312t, 313-314, *313-314*
    risks vs benefits in, 307, 309, 309t, *310*
    therapeutic window for, 313-314, *316*
Atrial Fibrillation Follow-up Investigation of Rhythm Management (AFFIRM), 302, 304

Baker's cyst, ruptured, 324
Balloon angioplasty, aspirin in, 91
Barbiturates, 51t, 353t
Bedside assays of hemostatic potential, 169, 172-174
Bernard-Soulier disease, 167, 170t
β-blockers
  for acute coronary syndromes, 213t, *227*
  for angina, 101
  for ischemia, 211
Biochemical markers for angina and myocardial ischemia, 225
Bivalirudin (Angiomax)
  for acute coronary syndromes, 215t
  aspirin with, 46
  bleeding caused by, 46
  in clinical trials, 224
  dosage of, 215t
  indications for, 46, 229
  monitoring of, 162, 163t
  pharmacokinetics of, 44, 45t, 46
  revascularization and, 46
  safety of, 46
Björk-Shiley mechanical heart valve, thromboembolic risk and, 292t
Bleeding. See also specific drug, eg, *Heparin, bleeding induced by.*
  from fibrinolytic therapy, 241, 244
  hemostatic potential assessment and, 167

Bleeding time, 167-168
Blood flow. See also *Valvular heart disease.*
  across aortic valve, 287, *288*
  across mitral valve, 287, *289*
  bypass grafting and, 275
  hemostatic balance and, 15
Bone marrow suppression, 108
Bradykinin, 66
Braunwald Classification System of unstable angina, 210
Bumetanide, 51t
Bypass grafting
  antiplatelets before, 230t
  aspirin and, 87
  blood flow and, 275
  indications for, 229t
  ticlopidine and, 103t-104t, 105

c7E3 antibody, 129
c7E3 Fab Antiplatelet Therapy in Unstable Refractory Angina (CAPTURE) trial, 134
CADILLAC, *136*
Caged-ball mechanical heart valve, thromboembolic risk and, 292t
Calcium channel blockers, 211, 213t
Canadian-American Ticlopidine Study (CATS), 102t, 107, 271t
Cancer. See *Malignancy.*
CAPRIE trial, 90, 113, 114t-115t, 116, *116,* 239, 270t
CAPTURE trial, 134
Carbamazepine, 51t, 353t
Cardiac drugs, 51t, 353t
Cardiomyopathy, dilated, thromboembolic risk and, 292t
Carotid endarterectomy, 280t
CARS, 254, 257t-258t
CAST, 270t
Catheterization, anticoagulants and, 359t
CATS, 102t, 107, 271t
Cellulitis, 325
Central nervous system, bleeding into, 48-49, 358
Central nervous system drugs, 51t, 353t
Cerebrovascular disease, 268-269, 270t-271t
Cerebrovascular lesion, STEMI in, fibrinolytics and, 74t
CHAMP trial, 256t, 258t
Chest pain. See also *Coronary syndromes, acute.*
  incidence of, 201
Children, LMWH in, 37
Chinese Acute Stroke Trial (CAST), 270t
Chlordiazepoxide, 51t, 353t
Cholestyramine, 51t, 352t, 353t
Cilostazol, *172,* 173t, 272, 280t, 282t
Cimetidine, 51t, 353t
Ciprofloxacin, 353t
CLASSICS, 117-118
Claudication, 280t
Clinical trials
  ACUTE, 220t
  ADMIRAL, 134, *136*
  AFASAK, 309
  AFFIRM, 302, 304
  Antiplatelet Trialists' Collaboration, aspirin in, 83, *85,* 90, 268, 274
  APRICOT, 256t
  ASPECT, 256t, 258t
  ASSENT, 69, *70,* 71, 241, 250, *252,* 253
  CAPRIE, 113, 114t-115t, 116, *116,* 239, 270t
  CAPTURE, 134
  CARS, 254, 257t-258t
  CAST, 270t
  CATS, 102t, 107, 271t
  CHAMP, 256t, 258t
  CLASSICS, 117-118
  COBALT, 243t

Clinical trials *(continued)*
  CREDO, 120-121, 124, *125-126*
  CURE, 87, 119-120, *121-123,* 124, 216, 239
  DREAM, 221t
  EAFT, 309-310
  EMATAP, 102t
  EPHESUS, *42*
  EPIC, 132t-133t
  EPILOG, 134
  EPISTENT, 100-101, 106
  ESPRIT, 142-143
  ESPS, 270t
  ESSENCE, 217, 220t
  ESTEEM, 254
  EXCITE, *150*
  EXTRACT, 62, 253
  FANTASTIC, 105-106
  Fibrinolytic Therapy Trialists, 244-245
  GISSI, 65, 240, 242t
  GUSTO, 65, 67, 69, *70,* 71, 134-135, 240-241, 243t, *244,* 250, *252*
  IMPACT, 139
  IMPACT-AMI, 142
  INJECT, 67, 242t
  INTERACT, 223
  InTIME-2, 71
  INTRO-AMI, 248
  ISAR, *136*
  ISIS
    anistreplase in, 66
    aspirin in, 237-238
    mortality outcomes in, *238,* 242t
    streptokinase in, 65-66, *238,* 240
  IST, 90, 270t
  MAST, 270t
  MATCH, 90-91
  MATISSE, 43
  MATTIS, 106
  NICE, 218-219, 220t, 253
  OPUS, *150*
  PCI-CURE, 118
  PENTALYSE, 43
  PENTAMAKS, *42*
  PENTATHLON, *42*
  PENTHIFRA, *42*
  PERSIST, 52
  POLONIA, 220t
  PREVENT, 332, 338
  PRISM, 138, 140t-141t
  PRISM-PLUS, 138, 140t-141t
  PURSUIT, 142, *143*
  RACE, 302, 304
  RAPPORT, *136*
  REDUCE, 221t
  REMBRANDT, 41, 43
  REPLACE, 224
  RESTORE, 137, 146
  SALT, 271t
  SPAF, 158, 309-310
  SPEED, 249-250
  SPORTIF, 47-48, 306
  Swedish Ticlopidine Multicentre, 102t, 107
  SYMPHONY, *150*
  SYNERGY, 223-224
  TACTICS, 138-139
  TACTICSTIMI, 138
  TARGET, 118, 146, *148*
  TASS, 102t, 107, 271t
  THRIVE, 48-49

Clinical trials *(continued)*
  TIMI. See *Thrombolysis in Myocardial Infarction trials.*
  TISS, 102t
  TMD, 103t
  UK-TIA, 271t
  WARIS, 253-254, 256t-257t
  Women's Health Initiative, 82
Clofibrate, 51t, 353t
Clopidogrel (Plavix)
  absorption and metabolism of, 111-112, 239
  action mechanism of, 111-112
  for acute coronary syndromes, 119, 214t, *227,* 230t, 232t
  adenosine diphosphate and, 111
  before alteplase, 61
  amputation and, 114t
  in aspirin failure, 84, *86*
  aspirin vs, Kaplan-Meier curves for, *117*
  aspirin with, 84, 111, 126, 216
  bypass grafting and, 90, 124, 126
  cardiovascular event prevention with, 83, *125-126*
  cardiovascular-related death and, *120-121*
  cerebrovascular disease and, 269
  coronary artery disease and, 275
  coronary stenting and, 117-119, 255
  dosage of, 111-112, 270t, 280t-281t
  drug combinations with, 224
  duration of therapy with in thrombosis prevention, 119
  effect on platelets, 111, 173t
  hemorrhagic risk with, 124, 126
  after hospital discharge, *260-261*
  at hospital discharge, *260-261*
  indications for, 81, 91, 213t, 239, 270t, *276-277,* 311
  for ischemic stroke, 90-91
  myocardial infarction and, 114t-115t
  percutaneous coronary interventions and, 91, 230t
  peripheral occlusive disease and, 269, 275, *276-277,* 280t-282t
  peripheral vascular reconstructive surgery and, 275
  placebo vs, Kaplan-Meier curves for, *119*
  platelet defects caused by, 173t
  potency of, 111, *112*
  for recurrent embolism, 294t
  renal impairment and, 112
  safety of, 108, 112-113
  stroke and, 90-91, 107, 114t-115t
  thrombus formation and, *172*
  for TIA, 90-91
  TIA and, 90-91, 295t
  vascular disease and, 113, 114t-115t, *116*
  warfarin vs, *261*
Clopidogrel for the Reduction of Events During Observation (CREDO) trial, 120-121, 124, *125-126*
Clopidogrel in Unstable Angina to Prevent Recurrent Events (CURE) trial, 87, 119-120, *121-123,* 124, 216, 239
Clopidogrel Plus ASA vs Ticlopidine Plus ASA in Stent Patients Study (CLASSICS), 117-118
Clopidogrel vs Aspirin in Patients at Risk for Ischemic Events (CAPRIE) trial, 113, 114t-115t, *116,* 239, 270t
Clot retraction assay, 172-173
Coagulation. See also *Thrombosis.*
  activation of, 15, *17*
  cell-based model of, 28, *29-32*
  disseminated intravascular, 190t
  negatively charged surface and, 21-22
  platelet-binding proteins in, *32*
Coagulation factors. See *Factor* entries.
Coagulation protease assembly, 26
COBALT trial, 2243t
Combination Hemotherapy and Mortality Prevention (CHAMP) trial, 256t, 258t
Compression stockings, 332, 340-341

19

377

Contact activation system, 16
Continuous Infusion vs Double-Bolus Administration of Alteplase (COBALT) trial, 243t
Controlled Abciximab and Device Investigation to Lower Late Angioplasty Complications
    (CADILLAC), *136*
Coronary angiography, 203
Coronary artery, occluded infarct-related, reperfusion of, 72-73
Coronary artery bypass grafting. See *Bypass grafting.*
Coronary artery disease. See also *Coronary syndromes, acute; Myocardial* entries.
    atheromatous plaque characteristics in, 201
    pathophysiology of, 201, *202,* 203
    peripheral vascular disease with, 267, 274-275
    risk factors for, 203
    ticlopidine and, 101, 102t-103t
Coronary heart disease, 217t
Coronary interventions, percutaneous. See *Percutaneous coronary interventions.*
Coronary stenting, 106, 117-119
    abciximab and, 106, *136*
    clopidogrel and, 117-118, 255
    management at hospital discharge, *260-261*
    ticlopidine and, 105-106, *106,* 117-118
    tirofiban and, 137-138
    warfarin and, 105
Coronary syndromes, acute. See also *Angina; Coronary artery disease; Myocardial* entries.
    ACE inhibitors for, 213t
    anticoagulants for, 215t, 216, 217t, 217-218, *218-219,* 232t
        oral, 225
    anti-ischemic therapy for, 211-212, 213t, 224
    antiplatelets for, 214t-215t, *227,* 230t-231t
    β-blockers for, 213t
    biochemical markers of, 225
    calcium channel blockers for, 213t
    direct thrombin inhibitors in, 224
    electrocardiogram in, 203-204, 204t-205t, *206-209*
    fibrinolysis for, 225
    in hospitalized patients, 211, 213t
    incidence of, 201
    lipid-lowering agents for, 213t
    LMWH for, 217-219, *227*
    LMWH with glycoprotein IIb/IIIa antagonists for, 223
    management algorithm for, *226-227*
    management strategies in, 225
    monitoring in, 211
    nitroglycerin for, 213t
    pathobiology of, 201, *202,* 203
    patient characteristics in, 203, 204t
    percutaneous interventions for. See *Percutaneous coronary interventions.*
    platelet aggregation in, 27-28
    platelet antagonists for, 216
    revascularization in, 229t
    risk factors for, 203, 210t
Co-trimoxazole, 43t, 51t, 309t, 353t
Coumadin. See *Warfarin.*
Coumadin Aspirin Reinfarction Study (CARS), 254, 257t-258t
Coumarins. See also *Warfarin.*
    oral, 225
    vitamin K epoxide and, 49
CREDO trial, 120-121, 124, *125-126*
CURE trial, 87, 119-120, *121-123,* 124, 216, 239
Cyclooxygenase
    in aspirin action mechanism, 79-81
    in aspirin resistance, 92, *93*
    clopidogrel and, 112
    thrombus formation and, *172*
CYP2C9 enzyme, genetic polymorphisms of, 50

D-dimers, *19,* 326, 328
Dalteparin (Fragmin)
    for acute coronary syndromes, 215t

Dalteparin (Fragmin) *(continued)*
  clinical trials of, 47-48, 221t, 332
  for deep vein thrombosis, 334t
  dosage of, 38, 39t-40t, 221t, 332, 334t
  efficacy of, 41, 47-48
  indications for, 39t
  for percutaneous coronary interventions, 221t
Danish Atrial Fibrillation Aspirin Coagulation (AFASAK) trial, 309
Deep vein thrombosis
  anatomy and pathophysiology of, 321-3324, *322*
  D-dimer in, *19*
  diagnosis of, 324, 328
    algorithm for, *327*
  incidence of, 3321
  laboratory testing for, 326-328
  management of
    complications of, 340-343
    compression stockings in, 340-341
    dalteparin in, 334t
    duration of, 336-338
    heparin in, 333
    LMWH in, 334t, 334-335
    as outpatient, 335-336
    ximelagatran in, 48-49
  postphlebitic syndrome and, 181, 340-341
  signs and symptoms of, 324-325
  stages of, 323
  thrombophilia and, 181-182, 187
Dense bodies, 27
Dermatan sulfate, 21
Diabetes Reduction Approaches with Ramipril and Rosiglitazone Medications (DREAM) trial, 221t
Diabetic retinopathy, 103t
Diflunisal, 51t
Dipyridamole, *88,* 91, 270t
Dipyridamole/aspirin combination (Aggrenox), *89,* 107, 269, 282t
Direct thrombin inhibitors. See also specific drug, eg, *Lepirudin.*
  clinical trials of, 47-49, 224
  for clot-bound thrombin, 365
  monitoring of, 162, 163t, 164
  for percutaneous coronary interventions, 229
  prothrombin time and, 160
  for pulmonary embolism, 329
  sources of, 43-44
Disseminated intravascular coagulation, 190t
Do Tirofiban and ReoPro Give Similarly Efficacy Trial (TARGET), 118, 146, *148*
DREAM trial, 221t
Dual vascular bed disease, 274-275, *276-277*

EAFT, 309-310
Efficacy and Safety of Subcutaneous Enoxaparin in Non-Q-Wave Coronary Events (ESSENCE) trial, 217, 220t
Electrocardiogram, diagnostic, 203-204, 204t-205t, *206-209*
EMATAP, 102t
Embolic arterial occlusion, 272, 274
Embolism. See *Pulmonary embolism; Thromboembolism.*
Embolization, distal, 201
Endarterectomy, carotid, 21, 280t
Endothelium, in thrombus formation, 21
Endotoxemia, 183t, 190t
Enhanced Suspension of Platelet Receptor GPIIb/IIIa Using Integrilin Therapy (ESPRIT) trial, 142-143
Enoxacin, 51t
Enoxaparin (Lovenox)
  for acute coronary syndromes, 215t, 217, 223, *227,* 232t
  bleeding induced by, 223
  in bridging therapy, 296
  clinical trials of, 221t, 223-224, *252*

19

Enoxaparin (Lovenox) *(continued)*
  for deep vein thrombosis, 334, 334t
  dosage of, 38, 39t-40t, 41, 219, 222t, 334t
  indications for, 39t-40t, 41, 43
  mechanical heart valves and, 296
  for percutaneous coronary interventions, 162, 218-219, 222t-223t, 224
  in pregnancy, 363
  safety of, 47, 224
  tenecteplase with, 69, 250, *252*, 253
  for thromboprophylaxis, 332
  tissue plasminogen activator with, 62, 69, 71, 250, 253
  venous thromboembolism and, *42*, 48, 334, 334t
Eosinophilia, 306t
EPHESUS, *42*
EPIC, 132t-133t
Epidural bleeding, 38
EPILOG, 134
EPISTENT, 100-101, 106
Eptifibatide (Integrilin). See also *Glycoprotein IIb/IIIa receptor antagonists.*
  for acute coronary syndrome, 230t-231t
  for acute coronary syndromes, 214t
  clinical trials and experience with, 139, 142-143, *143*, 152t, 223-224
  dosage of, 143
  duration of platelet effects after cessation of, 143-144, 145t
  FDA approval of, 129
  myocardial infarction incidence with, *143*
  pharmacodynamics of, 139
  pharmacokinetics of, 139, 143-144, 145t
  platelet defects from, 173t
  reversibility of, *146-147*
  source of, 139
  thrombolytic resistance and, 248
  tissue plasminogen activator with, 248
Erythrocytes, 22, 92, 100
Erythroleukemia, 100
Erythromycin, 51t, 353t
ESPRIT trial, 142-143
ESPS, 270t
ESSENCE trial, 217, 220t
ESTEEM trial, 254
Estrogen replacement, 183t, 189, 190t, 356
Estudio Multicentrico Argentino de la Ticlopidine en las Arteriopatias Perifericas
      (EMATAP), 102t
European Atrial Fibrillation Trial (EAFT), 309-310
European Stroke Prevention Study (ESPS), 270t
Evaluation in PTCA to Improve Long-term Outcome with Abciximab GPIIb/IIIa
      Blockade (EPILOG), 134
Evaluation of Oral Xemilofiban in Controlling Thrombotic Events (EXCITE), *150*
Evaluation of Platelet GPIIb/IIa Inhibitor for Stenting (EPISTENT), 100-101, 106
Evaluation of Platelet IIb/IIIa Inhibition for Prevention of Ischemic Complications (EPIC),
      132t-133t
EXCITE, *150*
EXTRACT, 62, 253

Factor(s), heparin effect on, 35-35
Factor II, prothrombin time and, 49
Factor V
  half-life of, 16t
  HR2 haplotype of, 184-185
  Leiden mutation of, 183t
    incidence of, 182, *184*
    thrombophilia and, 182, 183t
    thrombophlebitis and, 321, 323
    thrombosis management in, 192-194
  prothrombin time errors and, 158, 160
  secretion of, 27
Factor Va
  inactivation of, 19
  in thrombin activity regulation, *18*

Factor VII
half-life of, 16t, 49
prothrombin complex concentrate dosage and, 52
prothrombin time and, 49
warfarin effect on, 49
Factor VIIa, in coagulation process, *17*
Factor VIII
activation of, *17*
elevated levels of, 182, *184*
genetic mutations in, 183t, 187
half-life of, 16t
von Willebrand factor and, 21, 183t
Factor VIIIa, in thrombin activity regulation, *18*
Factor IX
activation of, *17*
half-life of, 16t
warfarin effect on, 49
Factor IXa, formation of, *17*
Factor X
half-life of, 16t
prothrombin time and, 49
warfarin effect on, 49
Factor Xa. See also specific drug, eg, *Fondaparinux*.
LMWH and, 36
monitoring of, 37
selective inhibitors of, 40-41, *42, 43*
Factor XI
binding to activated platelets, 16
glycoprotein Ib as receptor for, 18
Factor XII, in contact activation system, 16
Factor XIII, half-life of, 16t
Famotidine, 51t
FANTASTIC trial, 105-106
Felodipine, 51t
Femorofemoral graft patency, 104t
Femoropopliteal graft patency, 104t
Fetal embryopathy, 50, 351t, 356
Fibrin
generation of, 19, *19*
lysis of, in hemostatic balance, 15
Fibrinogen
genetic mutations in, 183t, 183-184
half-life of, 16t
platelet aggregation and, 28
secretion of, 27
in thrombolysis pathway, *60*
Fibrinolysis, *19*, 19-20, 225
Fibrinolytic agents, 63t, 65, 239. See also specific agent, eg, *Tissue plasminogen activator*.
action mechanisms of, 59, 239
angioplasty after, 73, 247-248
benefits of, 350t
bleeding induced by, 350t, 364
clinical features of, 63t
comparative trials of, 240-241, 242t-243t, *244*
complications of, 241, 244-245, 364-365
contraindications to, 342-343
future developments of, goals for, 73, 75
glycoprotein IIb/IIIa receptor antagonists with, 135, *137*, 248
indications for, 245, 246t, 247
monitoring of, 164
for peripheral vascular disease, 280t-281t
for postphlebitic syndrome, 340-341
resistance to, 248, *249,* 250
third generation, 66-67, 68t, 69, *70,* 71-72
Fibrinolytic system, 59, *60*
Fibrinolytic Therapy Trialists, 244-245
Fibronectin, 28
Flow cytometry, 169

Fluconazole, 51t, 353t
Fluoxetine, 51t, 353t
Folate deficiency, 181
Fondaparinux (Arixtra)
  action mechanisms of, 40
  clinical trials of, 41, *42,* 43
  current investigations of, 41
  dosage of, 39t, 41, 43
  hemorrhage and, 43
  indications for, 41
  long-acting, 52
  pharmacokinetics of, 40-41
  reocclusion and, *44*
  safety of, 41, 43
  for thromboprophylaxis, 41, *42,* 43, 332
Fragmin. See *Dalteparin.*
Full Anticoagulation vs Aspirin and Ticlopidine (FANTASTIC) trial, 105-106
FURY algorithm, in thrombophilia diagnosis, 192, 193t

Gangrene, 50, 360
Gastrointestinal bleeding, 357
Gastrointestinal drugs, 51t
Gastrointestinal erosion, aspirin dose in, 81
Genetic disorders, platelet function and, 169, 170t-171t. See also *Thrombophilia.*
Genitourinary bleeding, 357
Ginkgo, 50
Ginseng, 50
GISSI, 240, 242t, 665
Glanzmann's thromboasthenia, 170t
Global Use of Strategies to Open Occluded Arteries (GUSTO) trials, 65, 67, 69, *70,* 71,
  134-135, 240-241, 243t, *244,* 250, *252*
Glycoprotein(s)
  antithrombotic activity of, 22-23
  platelet activation and, 27
Glycoprotein Ia, genetic mutations in, 183t
Glycoprotein Ib
  as factor XI receptor, 18
  von Willebrand factor adhesion to, 22
Glycoprotein Ib/IX, platelet adhesion and, 25
Glycoprotein Ib/IX receptor deficiency, 167
Glycoprotein IIb/IIIa
  before alteplase infusion, 61
  fibrinogen binding of, 28
  platelet activation and, 27
  platelet aggregation and, *26,* 28
  as prothrombin receptor, 18
  thrombus formation and, *172*
  von Willebrand factor adhesion to, 22
Glycoprotein IIb/IIIa receptor
  deficiency of, 167
  as therapeutic target, 129
Glycoprotein IIb/IIIa receptor antagonists. See also specific drug, eg, *Abciximab.*
  for acute coronary syndrome, *227,* 230t
  angioplasty after, 73, 247-248
  evolution of, 129
  fibrinolytic agents with, 135, *137,* 248
  intravenous, 129-143
    advantages of, 216
    clinical trials of, 118, 132t-133t, 137-139, 140t-141t, 142-143
    dosage of, 213t
    duration of platelet effects after cessation of, *131,* 143-144, 145t, *175,* 177-178
    indications for, 213t
    individual characteristics of, 145t
    major clinical end points of, 144, 146
    nonfatal myocardial infarction and, *143*
    platelet defects induced by, 173t
    safety and efficacy of, 118, 144, 146
    similarities and differences among, 143-144, 145t

382

Glycoprotein IIb/IIIa receptor antagonists (continued)
  LMWH with, for acute coronary syndromes, 223
  mortality rates and, 147
  oral, 149
    clinical trials of, 149, 150
    clinician's approach to, 149, 151
  platelet inhibition by, percutaneous coronary intervention outcome and, 87, 176-177
  thrombocytopenia and, 149
Griseofulvin, 51t, 353t
Gruppo Italiano per lo Studio della Streptochinasi nell'Infarcto Miocardio (GISSI) trial,
  65, 240, 242t
GUSTO trials, 65, 67, 69, 70, 71, 134-135, 240-241, 243t, 244, 250, 252

Head trauma, STEMI in, fibrinolytics and, 74t
Heart valves. See also Coronary entries; Valvular heart disease.
  prosthetic, anticoagulant dosage and, 159t
Hematoma, spinal, 38, 358
Hematoma wound, 357
Hemostatic balance, 15
  statins and, 21, 22
Hemostatic potential assessment, 167
  acquired platelet defects and, 169
  bedside assays and instruments in, 169, 172-173
  bleeding time in, 167-168
  clot retraction assay in, 172-173
  congenital platelet abnormalities and, 169, 170t-171t
  dermatan sulfate and, 21
  flow cytometry in, 169
  platelet adhesion tests in, 25, 27, 168
  platelet aggregometry in, 168
  platelet function analysis in, 172-174
Heparin. See also Low molecular weight heparin.
  acquired thrombophilia and, 190t
  action mechanism of, 35-36, 251
  activated partial thromboplastin time and, 35-36, 45t, 160, 363
  for acute coronary syndromes, 215t, 230t-232t
  aldosterone and, 36
  alopecia from, 350t, 362
  angina and, 141t
  for antiphospholipid antibody syndrome, 194
  aspirin with and without, 66, 216
  bleeding induced by, 61, 350t, 357-358, 359t
    frequency of, 61
    management of, 358-359
    risk of, 38
    sites of, 357
  clinical trials of, 70
  coronary stenting, 105
  dosage of, 61, 217t
    difficulties in, 35
    after streptokinase, 65
    for thromboembolism, 161t
  drug interactions with, 38
  effect on myocardial infarction mortality and reinfarction, 250-251
  eosinophilia caused by, 350t
  fibrinolytics with, 71, 251, 253
  immunogenicity of, 45t
  indications for, 251, 333
  LMWH advantages over, 38-39, 217-218, 253
  molecular characteristics of, 35
  monitoring of, 162, 216-217, 217t
  myocardial infarction and, 139, 140t-141t, 142-143
  osteoporosis caused by, 36, 350t, 362
  in percutaneous coronary intervention, therapeutic index in, 217, 218-219
  for peripheral vascular disease, 280t-282t
  pharmacokinetics of, 35-36, 45t
  platelet factor 4 and, 35-36, 218
  in pregnancy, 37, 194, 339, 363

19

Heparin *(continued)*
  properties of, 45t
  protamine reversal of, 38, 45t
  prothrombin time and, 35-36, 45t
  revascularization and, *44*, 46, 137-138, 140t-141t
  skin/muscle necrosis caused by, 37, 350t, 355-356
  thrombin and, 35-36, 45t
    rebound generation of, 216
  thrombocytopenia caused by, 37, 45t, 350t, 359-362, 361t
    argatroban for, 360, 361t
    danaparoid for, 360
    lepirudin for, 46, 360, 361t
    thrombophilia and, 183t
Heparin cofactor II mutation, 187
Heparinoids, 39t
Herbal remedies, 50
High molecular weight kininogen (HMWK), 16
Hip surgery, 39t
Hirudin
  action mechanism of, 44, 46
  in acute coronary syndromes, 224
  adverse effects of, 356
  immunogenicity of, 45t, 46
  indications for, 365
  lack of antidotes for, 45t
  pharmacokinetics of, 44, 45t
  platelet factor 4 and, 46
  prophylactic, 224
  prothrombin time and, 45t, 46, 160
  renal toxicity of, 46
  source of, 43
Histamine blockers, 352, 353t
Homans' sign, 324
Hospitalized patients
  coronary syndromes in, 211, 213t
  monitoring of, 211
  STEMI management at discharge, *260-261*
HR2 haplotype, of factor V, 184-185
Human immunodeficiency virus infection, 190t
3-Hydroxy-3-methylglutaryl coenzyme A reductase inhibitors, hemostatic effects of, 21, *22*
Hyperhomocysteinemia, 181, 183t, 185, 186t
Hyperkalemia, 362
Hyperlipidemia, 183t
Hypertension, STEMI in, fibrinolytics and, 74t
Hypoaldosteronism, 350t
Hypotension, 66

Ibuprofen, in acquired aspirin resistance, 92, *93*
Idraparinux, 52
Immobilization, 183t
IMPACT trial, 139
IMPACT-AMI trial, 142
Inflammatory bowel disease, 190t
Inflammatory response modulating agents, 73
Infrainguinal prosthetic bypass, antithrombotics during, 281t
Infrainguinal vein bypass, antithrombotics during, 281t
INJECT trial, 67, 242t
Innohep (tinzaparin)
  for deep vein thrombosis, 40t, 333-334, 334t
  dosage of, 38, 39t-40t, 333, 334t
  for thromboprophylaxis, 39t, 333
INR. See *International normalized ratio.*
Integrilin. See *Eptifibatide.*
Integrilin and Enoxaparin Randomized Assessment of Acute Coronary Syndrome
  Treatment (INTERACT) trial, 223
Integrilin and Reduced Dose of Thrombolytics in Acute Myocardial Infarction
  (INTRO-AMI) trial, 248
Integrilin to Minimize Platelet Aggregation and Coronary Thrombosis (IMPACT) trial, 139

Integrilin to Minimize Platelet Aggregation and Coronary Thrombosis-After Myocardial Infarction (IMPACT-AMI) trial, 142
INTERACT trial, 223
International Joint Efficacy Comparison of Thrombolysis (INJECT) trial, 67, 242t
International normalized ratio (INR). See also specific drug.
    in patients with prosthetic heart valves, 159t
    prothrombin time in, 49-50
    in thrombotic disorders, 158
    vitamin K dosage and, 50, 52
International sensitivity index (ISI), 49
International Stroke Trial (IST), 90, 270t
International Study of Infarct Survival (ISIS) trials
    anistreplase in, 66
    aspirin in, 237-238
    mortality outcomes in, 238, 242t
    streptokinase in, 65-66, 238, 240
InTIME-2 trial, 71
Intracoronary radiation therapy, 118-119
Intracoronary Stenting and Antithrombotic Regimen (ISAR) trial, 136
Intracranial bleeding, 65, 251
Intracranial hemorrhage, before STEMI, fibrinolytics and, 74t
Intravenous nPA Treatment of Infarcting Myocardium Early II (InTIME-2) trial, 71
INTRO-AMI trial, 248
ISAR trial, 136
Ischemia. See Myocardial ischemia; Transient ischemic attack.
ISI, 49
ISIS. See International Study of Infarct Survival trials.
Isoniazid, 51t, 353t
IST, 90, 270t

Ketorolac, 51t
Knee surgery, 39t

Lanoteplase, 66-67, 68t, 71
Laser angioplasty, 91
L-asparaginase, 190t
Leiden mutation of factor V, 183t
    incidence of, 182, 184
    thrombophilia and, 182, 183t
    thrombophlebitis and, 321, 323
    thrombosis management in, 192-194, 323
Lepirudin (Refludan), 43
    for acute coronary syndrome, 215t
    for heparin-induced thrombocytopenia, 360, 361t
    indications for, 46
    monitoring of, 162, 163t
Leukocytes, platelet interactions with, 27
Limb ischemia
    classification of, 273t
    critical, 269, 274
    pathogenesis of, 272t
Lipid-lowering agents, 213t
Liver disease
    acquired thrombophilia and, 189, 190t
    vitamin K absorption and, 50
    warfarin and, 51t
Liver enzymes, ximelagatran and, 47, 306
LMWH. See Low molecular weight heparin.
Lovastatin, 353t
Lovenox. See Enoxaparin.
Low molecular weight heparin (LMWH). See also specific drug, eg, Enoxaparin.
    action mechanism of, 36
    for acute coronary syndrome, 230t-232t
    advantages over unfractionated heparin, 38-39, 217-218, 253
    alopecia caused by, 350t
    anti-factor Xa assay of, 162
    for antiphospholipid antibody syndrome, 194
    antithrombin and, 36

19

Low molecular weight heparin (LMWH) *(continued)*
  bleeding induced by, 350t
    frequency of, 38, 357
    management of, 358-359
    risk of, 38
    sites of, 38, 357
  in children, 37
  dosage of, 38
  drug interactions with, 38
  effectiveness of, 216-217
  eosinophilia caused by, 350t
  FDA approval pending, 38-39, 39t
  glycoprotein IIb/IIIa receptor antagonists with, for acute coronary syndromes, 223
  hyperkalemia from, 362
  indications for, 251, 334t, 334-335
  molecular structure of, 36
  monitoring of, 37, 162
  obesity and, 37
  osteoporosis caused by, 37, 350t, 362
  in percutaneous coronary interventions, 218-219, 220t-221t
  pharmacokinetics of, 36
  platelet factor 4 and, 37
  in pregnancy, 37, 162, 194, 363-364
  protamine neutralization of, 38, 45t
  for pulmonary embolism, 341-343
  self-administered, 255
  skin/muscle necrosis from, 350t
  thrombin and, 36-37
  thrombocytopenia from, 37, 45t, 350t, 360, 361t
  for thromboembolism, 334t
Low-density lipoprotein cholesterol oxidation, aspirin and, 79
Lower extremities
  chronic ischemia in, antithrombotics for, 280t
  venous anatomy of, 321, *322*
Lupus anticoagulant, 158, 160, 191, 193t
Lysosomes, 27

Macrophages, 15, 22
Malignancy
  STEMI in, fibrinolytics and, 74t
  thrombophilia and, 183t
  vitamin K absorption and, 50
Management of Atherothrombosis with Clopidogrel in High-Risk Patients with Recent
  Transient Ischemic Attach or Ischemic Stroke (MATCH) trial, 90-91
MAST, 270t
MATCH trial, 90-91
MATISSE, 43
MATTIS, 106
Melagatran, pharmacokinetics of, 47
Metoprolol, 51t
Metronidazole, 51t, 353t
Miconazole, 353t
Mitral valve. See also *Valvular heart disease.*
  blood flow across, 287, *289*
  diseases of, 294t-295t
Monitoring. See specific drug, eg, *Warfarin (Coumadin), monitoring of.*
  in acute coronary syndromes, 211
  of anticoagulant therapy, 157-164, 293, 317t
  of antithrombotics for atrial fibrillation, 311, 313-314, 317t
  of direct thrombin inhibitors, 162, 163t
  of factor Xa and LMWH, 37
  of fibrinolytic agents, 164
  of heart valve implant patient, 293
  of heparin therapy, 162, 216-217, 217t
  of hospitalized patients, 211
  of LMWH therapy, 37, 162
  of oral anticoagulant therapy, 293
  of platelets, 174, 178t
  of warfarin, 49, 157-158, 311, 313-314, *313-314,* 317t

Monocytes, 15, *17*
MTHFR 677 mutations, 183t, 185, 187
Multicenter Acute Stroke Trial (MAST), 270t
Multicenter Aspirin and Ticlopidine Trial After Coronary Stenting (MATTIS), 106
Muscle necrosis, 350t, 355-356
Myeloproliferative disorders, 183t
Myocardial infarction. See also *Chest pain; Coronary artery disease; Coronary syndromes, acute; ST-segment elevation myocardial infarction.*
  abciximab and, 130, 133t, 134
  antiplatelet agents and, 237-239
  aspirin and, 83t, 84, 94t, 113, 114t-115t, 138, *238,* 238-239
  clopidogrel and, 114t-115t
  heparin and, 139, 140t-141t, 142-143
  management of
    goals in, 237
    thrombolytic agents in. See *Fibrinolytic agents;* specific drug, eg, *Streptokinase.*
  nonfatal, incidence of, *143*
  non-ST-segment elevation, antithrombotic therapy after, 256t-258t, *260-261*
  outcome of, antiplatelet therapy and, 84, *85-86*
  platelet antagonists for, 270t-271t
  primary angioplasty for, 247
  as risk factor for coronary artery disease, 203
  secondary prevention of, 84
  streptokinase and, 237-238, *244*
  systemic embolization after, 251, 253t
  ticlopidine and, 104t, 105
  TIMI risk score for, 210-211, 211t, *212*
  tirofiban and, 135, 140t-141t
  warfarin plus aspirin after, 255
Myocardial ischemia. See also *Chest pain.*
  early evaluation steps in, 205t
  electrocardiographic features in, 204t, *206-207*
  management of, 205t
    pharmacologic, 216
  revascularization for, *212*

Nafcillin, 51t, 353t
Naproxen, 51t
National Investigators Collaborating on Enoxaparin (NICE), 218-219, 220t, 253
Necrosis of skin and muscle, 37, 350t, 355-356
Nephrotic syndrome, 183t, 190t
Neurosurgery, 39
Neutropenia
  aspirin-induced, 271t
  ticlopidine-induced, 100
Neutrophils, 15
NICE, 218-219, 220t, 253
Nitrates, for myocardial infarction, 101, 134, 211-212
Nitrazepam, 51t
Nitric oxide, 21-22, 79, 185
Nitroglycerin, 213t, *227,* 246t
Nonsteroidal anti-inflammatory drugs
  acquired aspirin resistance and, 92, *93*
  heparin/LMWH interaction with, 38
  warfarin interaction with, 51t

Obesity, anti-Xa level in, 37
Omeprazole, 51t, 353t
OPUS trial, *150*
Oral contraceptives, 183t, 190t
Orbofiban in Patients with Unstable Coronary Syndromes (OPUS) trial, *150*
Orthopedic surgery, thromboprophylaxis in, 41, 358
Osteoporosis, 36-37, 350t, 362

Patency rate, 60. See also specific drug, eg, *Anistreplase, patency after.*
  alteplase and, 60-61
  fibrinolytic agents and, 63t, 68t
PCI-CURE trial, 118
PENTALYSE trial, 43

19

PENTAMAKS, *42*
Pentasaccharide. See also *Factor Xa, inhibitors of; Fondaparinux.*
  binding site for thrombin, on LMWH chain, 36
  as heparin sequence, 35
  in ischemia/thrombosis prevention, 224
  thrombocytopenia induced by, 318
Pentasaccharide as an Adjunct to Fibrinolysis in ST-Elevation Acute Myocardial
    Infarction (PENTALYSE) trial, 43
PENTATHLON, *42*
PENTHIFRA, *42*
Pentoxifylline, 282t
Peptic ulcer, STEMI in, fibrinolytics for, 74t
Percutaneous coronary interventions, 91
  abciximab with, *136*
  antithrombotics during, 281t
  aspirin during, 87, 91, 214t-215t
  bleeding after, 124
  clinical trials of, 118, 120-121, 124, *125-126, 136,* 247
  clopidogrel after, 120-121, 124, *125-126*
  fibrinolysis or platelet glycoprotein before, 247-248
  heparin in, therapeutic index in, 217, *218-219*
  indications for, 253t
  LMWH in, 218-219, 220t-221t
  outcome of
    cumulative hazard rates for, 118, *119-120*
    platelet inhibition and, *176-177*
  study by CURE investigators (PCI-CURE), 87, 118, *121*
  timing of, 72-73, 247
  in unstable angina, 46
Percutaneous transluminal coronary angioplasty (PTCA)
  abciximab with, *136*
  in clinical trials, 110, 114, 199t
Peripheral vascular disease. See also *Myocardial infarction; Stroke;*
    Transient ischemic attack.
  Aggrenox for, 282t
  antiplatelet therapy for, *276-277*
  antithrombotic therapy for, 280t-281t
  aspirin for, 280t-282t
  causes of, 267
  cilostazol for, 282t
  classification of, 273t
  clopidogrel for, 280t-282t
  coronary artery disease with, 267, 274-275
  heparin for, 282t
  occlusive, 269, 272t, 275
  pathogenesis of, 272t
  pentoxifylline for, 282t
  platelet antagonists for, 270t-271t
  sites of, by frequency, 267
  ticlopidine and, 102t, 104t, 107
  warfarin for, 281t
Peripheral vascular reconstructive surgery, 275, 281t
Persantine, 280t
PERSIST, 52
Phenylbutazone, 51t, 353t
Phospholipid-binding proteins, 192
Picotamide, *89*
Piroxicam, 51t, 353t
Plaque, atheromatous, 201
Plasmin, in fibrinolysis, *19,* 19-20
Plasminogen, 22-23
  functions of, 59, *60*
  genetic mutations in, 183t
  streptokinase interaction with, 62, 64, *64*
Plasminogen activators. See also *Tissue plasminogen activator.*
  third generation, 66-67, 68t, 69, *70,* 71-72
Platelet(s)
  acquired defects of, 169, 173t. See also *Thrombophilia.*

Platelet(s) (continued)
  activation of, 27
    biochemical and physical changes from, 27
    erythrocytes in, 92
    thrombolytic resistance and, 249
  coagulation supported by, 28, 29-32
  congenital disorders and, 169, 170t-171t
  factor XI binding to, 16
  functions of, 25
    analyses of, 172-174
  leukocyte interactions with, 27
  monitoring of, 174, 178t
  in secretion from storage granules, 27
  sticky, 188
  in thrombin generation, 16-18, 21, 176-177, 179
Platelet adhesion
  in arterial thrombosis, 26
  tests of, 25, 27, 168
  von Willebrand factor and, 21, 25, 26
Platelet aggregation, 27-28
  abciximab and, 129-130, 131, 134
  aspirin and, 79, 99
  clopidogrel and, 111-112, 112
  glycoprotein IIb/IIIa complex and, 26, 28
  interval to, after cessation of glycoprotein receptor antagonists, 131, 144, 145t, 175
  sticky platelet syndrome and, 188
  thrombus formation and, 21, 26, 29
  ticlopidine and, 99, 111, 112
  von Willebrand factor and, 21
Platelet aggregometry, 168
Platelet α-granules
  aggregation and, 28
  secretion of, platelets and, 27
Platelet antagonists
  for acute coronary syndromes, 216
  for peripheral vascular disease, 270t-271t
Platelet antibodies, heparin-induced, 361
Platelet factor 4
  detection of, 37
  heparin and, 35-36, 218
  heparin-induced thrombocytopenia and, 360
  hirudin and, 46
  LMWH and, 37
Platelet Function Analyzer-100, 172
Platelet glycoprotein(s). See Glycoprotein entries.
Platelet Glycoprotein IIb/IIIa in Unstable Angina Receptor Suppression Using Integrilin
    Therapy (PURSUIT) trial, 142, 143
Platelet plug formation, 27-28, 167
Platelet Receptor Inhibition in Ischemic Syndrome Management (PRISM) trials, 138,
    140t-141t
Platelet-binding proteins, in coagulation, 32
Platelet-derived growth factor, secretion of, 27
Plavix. See Clopidogrel.
Polish-American Local Lovenox NIR Assessment (POLONIA) study, 220t
POLONIA, 220t
Postphlebitic syndrome, 181, 340-341
Pregnancy
  antiphospholipid antibody syndrome in, 194
  aspirin in, 194
  heparin, 37, 194, 339, 363
  LMWH in, 37, 162, 194, 339, 363-364
  mechanical heart valves in, anticoagulants for, 296
  STEMI in, fibrinolytics for, 74t
  thrombophilia and, 190t
  venous thromboembolism in, management of, 339-340
  warfarin in, 50, 194, 339-340, 356-357, 363
Prekallikrein (PK)
  in contact activation system, 16
  in fibrinolysis, 19-20

PREVENT, 332, 338
PRISM in Patients Limited by Unstable Signs and Symptoms (PRISM-PLUS) trial, 138, 140t-141t
PRISM trial, 138, 140t-141t
Procoagulant factors, 16t
Propafenone, 51t
Propranolol, 51t, 353t
Prostacyclin, 21-22, 79
Prostaglandin metabolism, 79
Prosthetic heart valves
  anticoagulant therapy in
    in bioprosthetic valves, 296t
    dosage of, 159t
    hemorrhage risk in, 293t
    in mechanical valves, 297t
  bridging therapy in, 296-297
  frequency of, 285
  ideal, 285
  in pregnancy, 296
  thrombogenic surface of, 287, *288-289,* 290
  thrombosis conditions in, 287, 290
  tissue vs mechanical
    durability of, 290
    thromboembolism risk in, 290-291, 292t
Protamine, 38, 45t
Protein C
  activated, 18
    acquired resistance to, 189
    thrombus formation and, 20
  in antiphospholipid antibody syndrome, 190t
  genetic mutations in, 182, 183t, *184,* 186
  half-life of, 16t, 49
  thrombophilia and, 189, 190t
  tissue necrosis and, 50
  warfarin effect on, 49
Protein S
  in antiphospholipid antibody syndrome, 190t
  enhancing anticoagulant effect of, 18-19
  genetic mutations in, 182, 183t, *184,* 186
  half-life of, 16t
  structure of, 18
  thrombophilia and, 189, 190t
  tissue necrosis and, 50
Prothrombin
  glycoprotein IIb/IIIa as receptor for, 18
  half-life of, 16t
Prothrombin 20210A mutation, 183t, 185
  smoking and, 187
Prothrombin complex concentrate, 52
Prothrombin time
  argatroban and, 47, 160
  heparin and, 35-36, 45t
  hirudin and, 45t, 46, 160
  INR and ISI in, 49-50
  sample storage and, 158, 160
  warfarin and, 49-50, 52, 157-158, 160
  warfarin effect on, 49
Prothrombinase complex, 16
PTCA. See *Percutaneous transluminal coronary angioplasty.*
Pulmonary embolism
  D-dimer in, *19*
  diagnosis of, 324
    algorithm for, *330-331*
  incidence of, 321
  laboratory testing for, 328-329
  management of, 329, 332-338, 334t, 341-343, 342t
  signs and symptoms of, 325-326
Purple toes, 50, 350t-351t, 356
PURSUIT trial, 142, *143*

RACE trial, 302, 304
Radiation therapy, intracoronary, 118-119
Ramipril, 221t
Randomized Efficacy Study of Tirofiban Outcomes and Restenosis (RESTORE), 137, 146
Randomized Evaluation in PCI Linking Angiomax to Reduced Clinical Events
    (REPLACE), 224
Rapid Platelet Function Assay, 173-174, *176-177*
RAPPORT, *136*
Rate Control vs Electrical Cardioversion for Persistent Atrial Fibrillation (RACE) trial,
    302, 304
REDUCE, 221t
Reduction of Restenosis after PTCA, Early Administration of Reviparin in a Double-blind
    Unfractionated Heparin and Placebo-controlled Evaluation (REDUCE), 221t
Refludan. See *Lepirudin.*
REMBRANDT study, 41, 43
Renal impairment, 37
    clopidogrel in, 112
Renal percutaneous coronary intervention, antithrombotics during, 281t
ReoPro. See *Abciximab.*
ReoPro and Primary PTCA Organization and Randomized Trial (RAPPORT), *136*
Reperfusion, selecting optimal strategy for, 72-73
REPLACE, 224
RESTORE, 137, 146
Reteplase
    abciximab with, 69, *70*, 71, 135, 248, 250, *252*
    clinical features of, 63t
    clinical trials of, 67, *70*, 135
    cost of, 63t
    dosage of, 63t, 69
    effectiveness of, 49t, 241, 243t
    in elderly patients, 71
    heparin with, 71
    mortality outcome with, 243t, *252*
    pharmacokinetics of, 67
    reocclusion and, 67, 69
Retinopathy, diabetic, 103t
Retroperitoneum, bleeding into, 358
Revascularization
    abciximab and, 130, 133t, 134-135
    in acute coronary syndromes, *227*, 229t
    aspirin and, 138
    heparin and, 137-138, 140t-141t
    rates of, *212*
    reteplase and, 67, 69
    thrombolytic therapy and, 245
    tirofiban and, 137-138, 140t-141t
Reviparin, 221t
Rifampin, 51t, 353t
Rosiglitazone, 221t
Rotational atherectomy, 91

SALT, 271t
Saphenous vein graft patency
    aspirin and, 87, 90
    flow and, 275
    ticlopidine and, 103t-104t, 105
Saruplase, 66-67, 68t, 71-72
Selectin, in cell-based coagulation model, *30-31*
Shock, cardiogenic, 248
Sibrafiban vs Aspirin to Yield Maximum Protection from Heart Events Post Acute
    Coronary Syndromes (SYMPHONY), *150*
Sickle cell disease, 190t
Skin necrosis, induced by antithrombotic agents, 37, 350t, 355-356
Smoking, 187
Soft tissue hemorrhage, 357
SPAF trials, 158, 309-310
SPEED trial, 249-250
Spinal hematoma, 38, 358

SPORTIF trials, 47-48, 306
St. Jude mechanical heart valve, thromboembolic risk and, 292t
Staphylokinase, 66-67, 68t, 72
Statins
  for acute coronary syndrome, *227*
  hemostatic effects of, 21, *22*
STEMI. See *ST-segment elevation myocardial infarction.*
Stents, coronary
  abciximab and, 106, *136*
  clopidogrel and aspirin in, 117-119, 255
  management at hospital discharge, *260-261*
  ticlopidine and, 105-106, *106,* 117-118
  tirofiban and, 137-138
  warfarin and, 105
Sticky platelet syndrome, 188
Stockings, compression, 332, 340-341
Storage pool disease, 170t
Strategies for Patency Enhancement in the Emergency Department (SPEED) trial, 249-250
Streptokinase
  abciximab with, 248, 250
  action mechanism of, 62, 64
  administration route of, 63t, 64-65
  adverse effects of
    allergic, 65, 365
    hemorrhage as, 65, 364
    hypotension as, 365
  aspirin with, 65
  clinical features of, 63t
  contraindications for, 74t
  cost of, 63t
  dosage of, 63t, 64, 237, 342t
  effectiveness of, 63t, 65, 237, 240-241
  half-life of, 62, 63t
  heparin after, dosage of, 65
  mortality rate with, *244*
  myocardial infarction and, 237-238, *244*
  patency after, 63t, 64-65
  for postphlebitic syndrome prevention, 340
  for pulmonary embolism, 342t
  readministration of, 65
  stroke/TIA and, 270t, 364
  studies of, 65, *238,* 240
Streptokinase-plasminogen activator complex, *64.* See also *Anistreplase.*
Stroke
  anticoagulants after, 269
  antiplatelet prevention of, 84, *85,* 87, *88-89,* 268-269, 270t-271t
  aspirin and, 83t, *86,* 90-961, 113, 114t-115t
  aspirin with and without clopidogrel for, 90-91
  in atrial fibrillation patients, 301-302, *303-304,* 304-605
    antiplatelet agents for, 309-311, *310*
    concept of number needed to treat in, 307
    echocardiographic findings in, 306t
    initiating and monitoring antithrombotic therapy in, 311, 312t, *313,* 313-314
    risk stratification in, 306, 307, 308t
    warfarin and, 304, 306t, 307, 309
  clopidogrel and, 107, 114t-115t
  ischemic, STEMI in, fibrinolytics and, 74t
  outcome of, antiplatelet therapy and, 84, *85-86*
  outpatient coagulation for, monitoring of, 314-315, 317t
  platelet antagonists for, 270t-271t
  thromboprophylactic LMWHs in, 38-39
  ticlopidine and, 102t, 104t, 107-108
Stroke Prevention in Atrial Fibrillation (SPAF) trials, 158, 309-310
Stroke Prevention Using Oral Thrombin Inhibition in Atrial Fibrillation (SPORTIF) trials, 47-48, 306
ST-segment elevation myocardial infarction (STEMI)
  aspirin vs warfarin after, 256t-258t
  fibrinolytics in, contraindications for, 74t-75t

ST-segment elevation myocardial infarction (STEMI) *(continued)*
  management at hospital discharge, *260-261*
  on PENTALYSE, 43
  on TIMI, 253, 256t-258t
  TIMI risk score for, 210-211, 211t, *212*
  ximelagatran and, 48
ST-segment shifts, *206, 211*
Sucralfate, 51t, 353t
Sulfinpyrazone, 51t, *88-89*, 353t
Suloctidil, *88*
Sulotroban, *89*
Superior Yield of the New Strategy of Enoxaparin, Revascularization and Glycoprotein
  IIb/IIIa Inhibitors (SYNERGY) trial, 223-224
Swedish Aspirin Low-Dose Trial (SALT), 271t
Swedish Ticlopidine Multicentre Study, 102t, 107
SYMPHONY trial, *150*
SYNERGY trial, 223-224

TACTICS trial, 138-139
TACTICSTIMI, 138
Tamoxifen, 353t
TARGET, 118, 146, *148*
TASS, 102t, 107, 271t
Tenase complex, 16
Tenecteplase
  for acute coronary syndromes, 246t
  clinical trials of, 69, *70,* 71, *252*
  combined with other drugs, 69, *70,* 71, 250, *252,* 253
  in elderly patients, 71
  heparin with, 71
  structure of, 66
THRIVE trials, 48-49
Thrombin
  activation of, thrombolytic resistance and, 248, *249,* 250-251
  arterial sclerosis and, 216
  in arterial thrombosis, *26*
  aspirin and, 79, 92, *93*
  bivalirudin and, 45t
  in blood flow across heart valves, *288-289*
  in cell-based coagulation model, 28, *29, 32*
  in clot retraction assay, 173
  in coagulation, *17,* 28, 46
  direct inhibitors of. See *Direct thrombin inhibitors.*
  endothelium and, 21
  factor activation by, 16
  generation of
    in hemostatic balance, 15
    platelets in, 16-18, 21, 176-177, *179*
    rebound, 216
    regulation of, *18,* 18-19
    tests of, 164
    Xa and prothrombin in, 16, *19*
  heparin and, 35-36, 45t, 216, 251
  hirudin and, 44, 45t
  LMWH and, 36-37
  melagatran and, 47
  in Rapid Platelet Function Assay, 173
  selective factor Xa inhibitors and, 40
  statins and, 21, *22*
  in thrombolytic resistance, 248
  warfarin and, 49
Thrombin activatable fibrinolysis inhibitor, 20
Thrombin Inhibitor in Venous Thromboembolism (THRIVE) trials, 48-49
Thrombocytopenia
  abciximab-induced, 149
  antiplatelet-induced, 350t
  glycoprotein IIb/IIIa receptor antagonists and, 149

Thrombocytopenia *(continued)*
  heparin-induced, 37, 45t, 350t, 359-362, 361t
    argatroban for, 360, 361t
    danaparoid for, 360
    lepirudin for, 46, 360, 361t
    thrombophilia and, 183t
  hirudin and, 45t
  LMWH-induced, 37, 45t, 350t, 360, 361t
  ticlopidine-induced, 100, 350t
Thromboembolic disease, INR in, 158
Thromboembolism. See also *Deep vein thrombosis; Pulmonary embolism; Venous thromboembolism.*
  in antiphospholipid antibody syndrome, 292t
  in heart valve, risk of, 290-291, 292t
  LMWH for, 41, *42,* 48, 332, 334, 334t
  repeated, 181
  vena caval filters for, 343
Thrombolysis in Myocardial Infarction (TIMI) trials
  alteplase on, 60
  anistreplase on, 66
  fibrinolytic combinations on, 62
  fibrinolytics compared on, 63t, 68t, 241
  flow grades on, 43
  infarct artery patency on, 250, *250*
  lanoteplase on, 71
  LMWH on, 217, 253
  myocardial infarction risk score on, 210-211, 211t, *212,* 229
  percutaneous coronary interventions on, 245, 247-248
  reocclusion rates on, *44*
  reperfusion on, 73, 142
  risk score for angina and STEMI on, 210-211, 211t, *212, 226*
  STEMI on, 256t-258t
  streptokinase on, 64
  tenecteplase on, 69
  thrombolytic resistance on, 248-249
  tPA dosage on, 245
Thrombolytic agents. See *Fibrinolytic agents.*
Thrombomodulin
  effect on thrombin generation, 18
  genetic mutations in, 183t
Thrombophilia
  acquired
    antiphospholipid antibody syndrome and, 183t
    antithrombin, protein C, and protein S deficiencies in, 189, 190t
    management of, 193-194
  causes of, 183t, 189-192
  deep vein thrombosis and, 181-182
  definition of, 181
  diagnosis of, 192-193, 193t
    FURY algorithm in, 192, 193t
  incidence of, 182, *184*
  indications of, 181
  inherited, 182-187, 183t
  platelet abnormalities in, 188
  in pregnancy, 339
  thrombi location in, 187-188
  thrombosis risk in, 182
Thromboplastins. See also *Activated partial thromboplastin time.*
  lupus anticoagulant and, 158, 160, 191, 193t
Thromboprophylaxis, LMWHs for, 39
Thrombosis. See also *Pulmonary embolism; Thromboembolic disease; Thrombophilia.*
  arterial, *26,* 182
  atherosclerosis progression and, 267, *280*
  deep vein. See *Deep vein thrombosis.*
  initiation of, 15-18, *17*
  INR in, 158
  regulation of, 18-19
  vessel wall injury and, 15
  warfarin and, 49-50

Thrombotic arterial occlusion, 274-275
Thrombotic microangiopathy, 183t
Thrombotic thrombocytopenic purpura, 100-101
Thromboxane A$_2$
  aspirin and, 79
  in aspirin resistance, *93*
  in platelet activation, 27
  statins and, 21
  suppression of, 92, *93*
  synthesis of, 92
Thrombus formation
  adenosine diphosphate and, *172*
  pharmacological control of, *172*
  vascular factors in, 20-21
TIA. See *Transient ischemic attack.*
Ticlopidine (Ticlid)
  action mechanism of, 99-100
  for acute coronary syndromes, 214t
  adenosine diphosphate and, 99, 108
  adverse effects of, 100-101, 108, 112-113, 173t, 350t
  angina and, 101, 103t
  bypass grafting and, 103t-104t, 105
  cerebrovascular disease and, 269
  coronary artery disease and, 101, 102t-103t
  coronary stents and, 105-106, *106*, 117-118
  diabetic retinopathy and, 103t
  dosage of, *88*, 102t-103t, 217t
  indications for, 271t, *276-277*
  myocardial infarction and, 104t, 105
  nonplatelet effects of, 100
  peripheral vascular disease and, 102t, 104t, 107
  pharmacokinetics of, 100, 108
  platelet function and, 99, 101, *112*, 173t
  stroke and, 102t, 104t, 107-108, 269, 311
  thrombocytopenia induced by, 100, 350t
  thrombus formation and, 172
  TIAs and, 102t, 104t
  trials of, 102t-103t
  vascular events and, *88*
  in vitro effects of, 99
Ticlopidine Aspirin Stroke Study (TASS), 102t, 107, 271t
Ticlopidine Ibuprofen Stroke Study (TISS), 102t
Ticlopidine Microangiopathy of Diabetes (TMD) trial, 103t
TIMI. See *Thrombolysis in Myocardial Infarction study.*
Tinzaparin (Innohep)
  for deep vein thrombosis, 40t, 333-334, 334t
  dosage of, 38, 39t-40t, 333, 334t
  obesity and, 37
  for thromboprophylaxis, 39t, 334t
Tirofiban (Aggrastat). See also *Glycoprotein IIb/IIIa receptor antagonists.*
  for acute coronary syndromes, 215t, 230t-231t
  angina and, 141t
  clinical experience and trials of, 137-139, 140t-141t, 146, *148*, 152t, 220t
  in coronary stenting, 137-138
  dosage of, 136-137
  duration of platelet effects after cessation of, 144, 145t, *146-147*
  myocardial infarction and, 135, 140t-141t
  for percutaneous coronary interventions, 230t-231t
  pharmacodynamics of, 136-137
  pharmacokinetics of, 135, 145t
  platelet defects and, 173t
  revascularization and, 137-138, 140t-141t
  source of, 135
TISS, 102t
Tissue factor activation, 15
Tissue factor pathway inhibitor
  in coagulation process, 15, *17*, 22-23
  genetic mutations in, 183t

Tissue factor pathway inhibitor *(continued)*
  half-life of, 16t
  LMWH and, 36, 218
Tissue necrosis, 37, 350t, 355-356
Tissue plasminogen activator (tPA), 20. See also *Alteplase.*
  abciximab with, 248, 250, *250*
  action mechanism of, 60, *62*
  for acute coronary syndromes, 246t
  adverse effects of, 245, 343, 364
  alteplase and, 60-61
  clinical features of, 63t
  dosage of, 251, 281r, 342t, 364
  effectiveness of, 240-241, 242t-243t
  endothelial release of, *20,* 21
  enoxaparin with, 62, 69, 71, 250, 253
  eptifibatide with, 248
  fibrin with, 60
  in fibrinolysis, 19, 23, 59, *137*
  heparin with, 61
  infarct artery patency and, *250*
  myocardial infarction mortality and, 142, *244*
  for postphlebitic syndrome prevention, 340-341
  for pulmonary embolism, 342t
  structure of, 59-60, *61, 72*
  in thrombolytic resistance, 248
TMD trial, 103t
Toes, purple, 50, 350t-351t, 356
Transaminase elevation, induced by antithrombotic agents, 350t
Transient ischemic attack (TIA)
  antiplatelet therapy and, 87
  antithrombotic therapy after, 280t
  aspirin and, 90-91
  aspirin with and without clopidogrel for, 90-91
  recurrent, 295t
Trauma, thrombophilia and, 183t
Treat Angina with Aggrastat and Determine Cost of Therapy with an Invasive or
  Conservative Strategy (TACTICS) trial, 138-139
Treat Angina with Aggrastat and Determine Cost of Therapy with an Invasive or
  Conservative Strategy-Thrombolysis in Myocardial Infarction (TACTICSTIMI), 138
Trials. See *Clinical trials.*
Triflusal, *89*
Troponin I, 134, 203, 210t, 216, 225, 230t

UK-TIA trial, 271t
Ulcer, aspirin dose in, 81
United Kingdom Transient Ischemic Attack (UK-TIA) trial, 271t
Urokinase, 20
  dosage of, 342t
  in fibrinolytic system, 59, 66, 71
  for postphlebitic syndrome prevention, 340-341
  for pulmonary embolism, 342t

Valvular heart disease
  anticoagulant therapy in
    with bioprosthetic valves, 296t
    early postoperative, 291, 293
    hemorrhage risk in, 291, 293t
    with mechanical valves, 297t
    monitoring of, 293
    with native valves, 294t-295t
    threshold level of, 290
  aortic, 295t
  atrial fibrillation with, 301
  blood flow in
    across aortic valve, 287, *288*
    across mitral valve, 287, *289*
  incidence of, 285
  mechanisms of, 285-286

Valvular heart disease *(continued)*
  mitral
    annular calcification, 294t
    prolapse of, 295t
    rheumatic, 294t, 305t
  natural history of thrombi in, 286
  prosthetic. See *Prosthetic heart valves.*
  thromboembolic risk in, 290-291, 292t
Vascular disease. See also *Peripheral vascular disease.*
  antiplatelet therapy and, 87, *88-89*
  aspirin and, *85,* 94t, 268
  clopidogrel and, 113, 114t-115t, *116*
  primary prevention of, 82-83
  secondary prevention of, 83-84, *85-86*
Vascular puncture, STEMI in, fibrinolytics and, 74t
Vascular surgery, anticoagulation during, 281t
Vasculature, in thrombus formation, 20-21
Vasospasm, 267
Vena caval filters, 343
Venous thromboembolism
  in pregnancy, 339-340
  prevention of, 332
  recurrent, 337-338
  risk factors for, 329, 332
Venous thrombosis
  deep. See *Deep vein thrombosis.*
  thrombophilia in, 181, 187
  treatment of, *42,* 48, 193-194, 334, 334t
  vena caval filters for, 343
Vitamin K
  dosage of, 50, 52
  malignancy and, 50
  as warfarin antidote, 50, 51t, 351-352, 354-355
Vitronectin, platelet aggregation and, 28
von Willebrand disease, 167, 170t-171t
von Willebrand factor
  in cell-based coagulation model, *29-32*
  in coagulation process, *17,* 22
  glycoprotein binding by, 22
  platelet adhesion and, 21, 25, *26*
  platelet aggregation and, 21

Warfarin (Coumadin)
  acetaminophen and, 50, 353t
  acquired thrombophilia and, 189, 190t
  action mechanism of, 49
  adverse effects of
    alopecia as, 350t, 356
    bleeding as. See *Warfarin (Coumadin), bleeding caused by.*
    embryopathic, 50, 356-357
    gangrene as, 50, 360
    purple toes as, 50, 350t-351t, 356
    skin/muscle necrosis as, 37, 50, 350t, 355-356
  aspirin vs, 310-311
    after STEMI, 256t-258t
  aspirin with, 254-255
  for atrial fibrillation
    dosage of, 311, 312t, *313-314*
    initiating and monitoring of, 311, 312t, 313-314, *313-314*
    risk vs benefits of, 307, 309, 309t, *310, 315*
    therapeutic window for, 313-314, *316*
  bleeding caused by, 43, 350t
    diet and, 351-352
    drug interactions and, 46-47, 50, 51t, 352
    genetics and, 351
    incidence of, 309t
    management of, 354-355
    risk factors for, *315,* 349, 351t, 351-352

Warfarin (Coumadin) *(continued)*
  spinal hematoma from, 358
  treatment dosage and duration and, 352-354
 coagulation factors and, 49
 contraindications for, 360
 in coronary stenting, 105
 diet and, 50, 351-352
 direct thrombin inhibitors with, 47-48
 dosage of
  bleeding and, 352-354
  initial, 311, 313, *313*
  lowest possible, *314*
  maintenance, 335
  to prevent stroke, 310
  to prevent thrombosis, 49, 52, 158, 193-194, 253-254, 254, 338
 drug interactions with, 50, 51t, 239, 352, 353t
 duration of, 194, 239, 251, 255, 336, 352-354
 effectiveness of, 253-254
 herbal remedy interactions with, 50
 hirudin and, 46
 at hospital discharge, *260-261*
 increased use of, 316, *317*
 indications for, 65
 initiating therapy with, 311, 313, *313*
 metabolism of, 50
 monitoring of, 49, 157-158, 311, 313-314, *313-314*, 317t, 360
 in native and prosthetic heart disease, 291, 293
 for peripheral vascular disease, 281t
 in peripheral vascular reconstructive surgery, 275, 281t
 pharmacokinetics of, 49-50
 in pregnancy, 50, 194, 339-340, 356-357, 363
 protein C and S mutations in, 50
 prothrombin time and, 49-50, 52, 157-158, 160
 reinfarction and, 254
 after STEMI, 256t-258t, *260-261*
 after stroke, 269
 in stroke prevention, 269, 304-307, 306t, 308t, 309, 318
  concept of number needed to treat in, 307
  risks vs benefits of, 307, 309, 309t, *310*
 therapeutic window for, 313-314, *316*
 for venous thrombosis, 193, 255, 332-333, 338
 vitamin K and, 50, 51t, 351-352, 354-355
Warfarin-Aspirin Reinfarction Study (WARIS), 253-254, 256t-257t
WARIS, 253-254, 256t-257t
White-clot syndrome, 360
Women's Health Initiative, 82
Wound hematoma, 162
Wound hemorrhage, 357

Xemilofiban, *150*
Ximelagatran
 aspirin with, 254
 bleeding caused by, 47-48, 306, 318
 in clinical trials, 47-48, 254, 306
 for deep vein thrombosis, 48
 dosage of, 47-48, 254
 effectiveness of, 47, 306, 318
 FDA approval of, 47, 305-306
 liver enzymes and, 47, 306
 in myocardial infarction, 48
 pharmacokinetics of, 306
 recurrent thromboembolism and, 48-49
 safety of, 47